53	54	55	56	57	58	59	60	61	62	63	64	65	66	67	68	69	70
✓	✓	✓	✓	✓	✓	✓	✓	✓	✓	✓	✓	✓	✓	✓	✓	✓	✓
✓	✓	✓	✓	✓	✓	✓	✓	✓	✓	✓	✓	✓	✓	✓	✓	✓	✓
✓	✓	✓	✓	✓	✓	✓	✓	✓	✓	✓	✓	✓	✓	✓	✓	✓	✓
✓	✓	✓	✓	✓	✓	✓	✓	✓	✓	✓	✓	✓	✓	✓	✓	✓	✓
✓	✓	✓	✓	✓	✓	✓	✓	✓	✓	✓	✓	✓	✓	✓	✓	✓	✓
							✓	✓	✓	✓	✓	✓	✓	✓	✓	✓	✓
							✓	✓	✓	✓	✓	✓	✓	✓	✓	✓	✓
							✓										✓
												✓	✓	✓	✓	✓	✓
												✓					
		✓					✓					✓					
							✓										✓
							✓		✓		✓		✓		✓		✓
✓		✓				✓			✓			✓			✓		
✓	✓	✓	✓	✓	✓	✓	✓	✓	✓	✓	✓	✓		✓		✓	

sexual practices, dental health, injury prevention.

A
Clinical Guide
for the Care of
Older Women

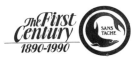

A Clinical Guide for the Care of Older Women

Richard L. Byyny, M.D.

Professor of Medicine
University of Colorado School of Medicine
Denver, Colorado

Leon Speroff, M.D.

Professor of Obstetrics and Gynecology
Oregon Health Sciences University
Portland, Oregon

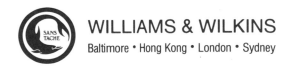

WILLIAMS & WILKINS
Baltimore • Hong Kong • London • Sydney

Editor: Carol-Lynn Brown
Associate Editor: Victoria M. Vaughn
Copy Editor: Thomas Lehr
Designer: Wilma Rosenberger
Illustration Planner: Lorraine Wrzosek
Production Coordinator: Barbara J. Felton
Illustrator: Nancy A. Burgard

Copyright © 1990
Williams & Wilkins
428 East Preston Street
Baltimore, Maryland 21202, USA

Accurate indications, adverse reactions, and dosage schedules for drugs are provided in this book, but it is possible that they may change. The reader is urged to review the package information data of the manufacturers of the medications mentioned.

Printed in the United States of America

Library of Congress Cataloging-in-Publication Data

Byyny, Richard L.
   A clinical guide for the care of older woman / Richard L. Byyny, Leon Speroff.
      p.   cm.
   Includes bibliographical references.
   ISBN 0-683-01150-2
   1. Aged women—Diseases   I. Speroff, Leon, 1935–   II. Title.
   [DNLM: 1. Geriatrics.   2. Women.   WT 100 B998c]
RC952.5.B98   1990
618.97′8—dc20
DNLM/DLC
for Library of Congress   90-12146
                                                              CIP

                                        90   91   92   93   94
                        1   2   3   4   5   6   7   8   9   10

Preface

In 1968, an internist and an obstetrician-gynecologist met during their tour of duty at Vandenberg Air Force Base in California. Over the next year and a half, they presented to each other, every Wednesday at lunchtime, reviews of endocrine topics and problems. Eventually they became the elected officers and sole members of the Vandenberg Endocrine Society. From that beginning came an intellectual relationship and a close friendship which now, years later, are manifested in this book.

We are fast attaining a society which contains 40 million women beyond the age of menopause. The health care of older women has become a major public health concern. Society, and the medical profession in particular, cannot expect older people to be totally cared for by geriatric specialists. All clinicians who interact with women will have to share in this care. The purpose of this book is to help all health care providers improve the health of older women.

This book is a guide, an easy to use quick resource, for day-to-day clinical practice. It deliberately was designed and constructed not to be encyclopedic. We offer a specific method for the screening, diagnosis, and management of frequently encountered health problems in older women. The focus is on common problems, leaving the esoteric and complicated for thicker texts and specialized consultations.

At all times our aim has been to project an attitude of preventive health care. We wish to encourage clinicians, and ultimately patients, to think of the postmenopausal years as a special, positive time of life in which good health plays a vital role in making these years productive and enjoyable. As we ourselves enter these older years, this philosophy looks more and more attractive, and we dedicate this book to the achievement of a vital, happy, long life.

We don't regret that we are not women, but we do miss the added insight of the feminine point of view. With that limitation in mind, we have done our best and hope that the results will benefit women and their families.

Richard L. Byyny, M.D.
Denver, Colorado

Leon Speroff, M.D.
Portland, Oregon

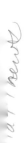

Contents

1 The Rectangularization of Life

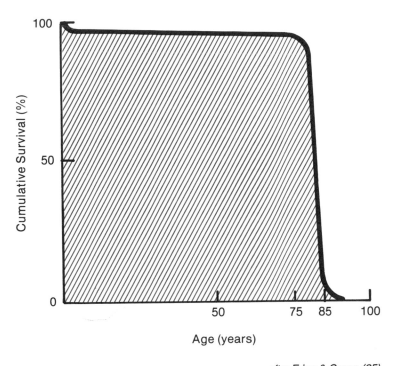

after Fries & Crapo (25)

We are experiencing a relatively new phenomenon: we can expect to become old. We are on the verge of becoming a rectangular society; this is a society in which nearly all individuals survive to advanced age and then succumb rather abruptly over a narrow age range centering about the age of 85. When George Washington was president, half the people in the country were under age 16, and only a tiny handful were over 65. In 1000 B.C., life expectancy was only 18 years. By 100 B.C., the time of Caesar, it had reached 25 years. In 1900, in the United States, life expectancy still had reached only 49 years. But by 1987, the average life expectancy had reached 75 years. Today, once you reach 65, if you are a man you can expect to reach 80, if a woman, age 84.

A good general definition of elderly is 65 and older, although it is not until age 75 that a significant proportion of older people show the characteristic decline and problems. Today the elderly population is the largest contributor to illness and human need in the United States. At a time (1980s) when those over the age 65 constituted 12% of the population, they accounted for the following: (1,2)

25% of all medications.

33% of physicians' time.

69% of health care expenditures.

1

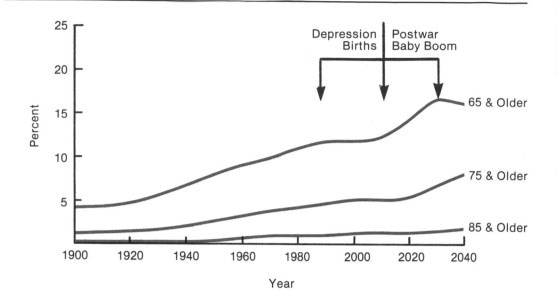

after Lowenstein & Schrier (2)

In the 1980s, only 6% of older people lived in institutions; 64% lived in a family setting, and 30% lived alone. Importantly, elderly blacks, Chicanos, and other ethnic elderly (such as Native Americans) experience no greater loss of psychological well-being beyond what might be expected on the basis of low socioeconomic status. (3)

There are more old people (with their greater needs) than ever before. (4) In 1900, there were approximately 3 million Americans 65 and older (about 4% of the total population). By 2030, the elderly population will reach about 57 million (17% of the total population).

Another way of looking at the change is the demographic shape of our society. In the year 1900, it was a true pyramid. In the 1900s, the shape is becoming more rectangular. By 2050, the shape will be nearly a perfect rectangle. But there are qualitative changes as well.

In viewing demographic data, don't lose sight of the remarkable heterogeneity among older people. There are wider physiological and psychological differences between two people at age 65 than between two 20 year olds. In addition, there is a remarkable turnover. At the present time, about 5000 new people reach age 65 every day, and 3300 die. (2) Thus every day, the mix changes, with a group of people with more health, more wealth, and more education. The result is a changing socioeconomic profile of older people, an increasingly less disadvantaged elderly cohort.

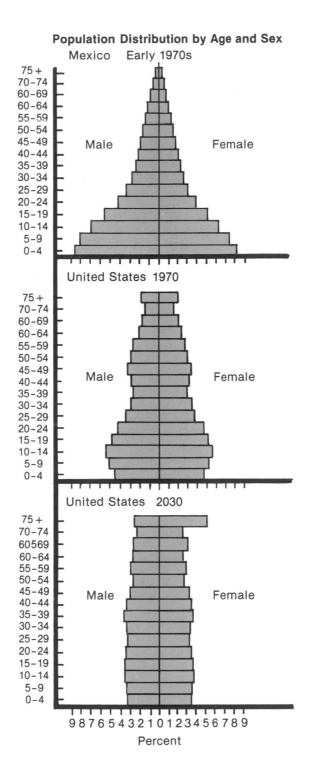

Population Distribution by Age and Sex

Mexico   Early 1970s

Male	Female

75+
70-74
60-69
60-64
55-59
50-54
45-49
40-44
35-39
30-34
25-29
20-24
15-19
10-14
5-9
0-4

United States 1970

Male	Female

75+
70-74
60-69
60-64
55-59
50-54
45-49
40-44
35-39
30-34
25-29
20-24
15-19
10-14
5-9
0-4

United States   2030

Male	Female

75+
70-74
60569
60-64
55-59
50-54
45-49
40-44
35-39
30-34
25-29
20-24
15-19
10-14
5-9
0-4

9 8 7 6 5 4 3 2 1 0 1 2 3 4 5 6 7 8 9

Percent

This is a growing resource for our society. Older people are better citizens. They vote and volunteer more often; they commit fewer crimes; and they carry our history and culture. And the older we get, the more we are convinced that older people bring wisdom and experience into our lives.

A World-Wide Change

This is a world-wide development, not limited to affluent societies. (5) The population of the earth will continue to grow until the year 2100 or 2150, when it is expected to stabilize at approximately 11 billion. 95% of this growth will occur in developing countries, and the number of women over age 45 will exceed 700 million by the year 2000. The poorest countries today (located in Africa and Asia) account for about half of the global population, and by 2000, 87% of the world's population will be living in what are now called developing countries. In 1950, only 40% of people 60 and older lived in developing countries. By 2025, more than 70% will live in those countries.

Projected Size of World Population Age 60 and Older (5)

Year	World	Developing Countries	
1950	200 million	80 million	(40%)
1975	350	178	(51%)
2000	590	355	(60%)
2025	1,100	792	(72%)

The Female Problem

It has been estimated that shortly after the year 2000, American internists will be spending about 75% of their time with patients who are older than 65. (2) The burden of physicians who care for women is even more significant, and only beginning to be appreciated. In 1900, older men outnumbered women 102 to 100. In the 1980s, there were only 68 men for every 100 women over age 65. By age 85, only 45 men are alive for every 100 women. In 1985, 40% of American white women reached age 85, compared to only 20% of white men. Nearly 90% of white American women can expect to live to age 70.

The Older U.S. Female Population (6)

Age	1990		2000		2010		2020	
55–64	10.8 mill	(8.6%)	12.1 mill	(9.0%)	17.1 mill	(12.1%)	19.3 mill	(12.9%)
65–74	10.1	(8.1%)	9.8	(7.3%)	11.0	(7.8%)	15.6	(10.4%)
>75	7.8	(6.2%)	9.3	(7.0%)	9.8	(6.9%)	11.0	(7.3%)
TOTAL	28.7		31.2		37.9		45.9	

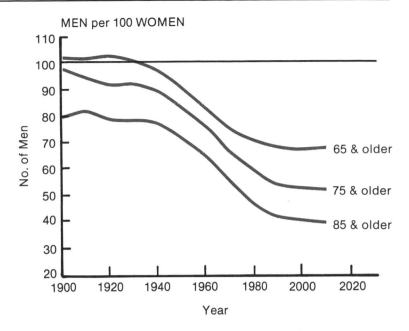

MEN per 100 WOMEN

No. of Men

65 & older

75 & older

85 & older

Year

after Lowenstein & Schrier (2)

The sex differential in cigarette smoking has been considered to be a major factor in the sex differential in mortality, and because of the growing equivalence in cigarette smoking between the sexes, a narrowing of the sex differential in mortality may occur in the future. Nevertheless, men and women reach old age with different prospects for older age, a sex differential which (it can be argued) is due to the sex hormone-induced differences in the cholesterol-lipoprotein profile, and thus the greater incidence of atherosclerosis and earlier death in men. (7) Therefore, the use of postmenopausal estrogen replacement therapy, with its protective effect on atherosclerosis, may in fact exaggerate the sex differential in mortality. From a public health point of view, the greatest impact on the sex differential in mortality would be gained by concentrating on lifestyle changes designed to diminish atherosclerosis in men: low cholesterol diet, no smoking, optimal body weight, and active exercise.

Because improvements in medical care are not the only explanation for the growing elderly population, a similar situation (the male-female difference) is facing the developing countries. (8) Here the major contribution is the numbers of births combined with the high death rates in younger ages (changes in the initial size of a cohort).

Men Per 100 Women (8)

	Population 65 and Older			
	1975	**1980**	**1990**	**2000**
World	74	74	74	77
Developing	88	87	85	85
Developed	64	63	63	68

5

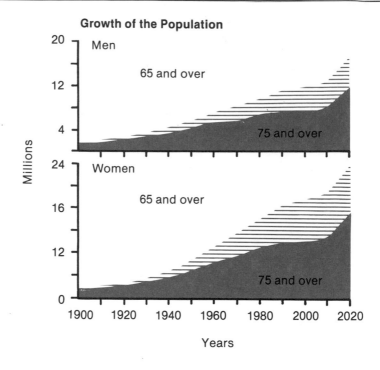

Growth of the Population

Data from U.S. Bureau of the Census (6)

The determinants of a population's age structure include the following:

1. Fertility.

2. Mortality.

3. Migration.

It is incorrectly and widely believed that decreases in mortality in older people represent the only reason for population aging. (9) The decline in mortality has been greatest in the young. The reproduction of this increased younger population (fertility) ultimately yields more old people. Another contribution to aging of a national population is control of fertility; a decrease in fertility results in a decrease in the proportion of the younger population. Thus control of fertility has an impact, but paradoxically, undeveloped countries with high fertility rates also develop a growing elderly population.

In developed countries, mortality rates in the young are near nadir levels, thus the main contribution to population aging in America in recent years has come from reduction in mortality in older ages (38% overall). The countries of northwestern Europe have reached a point of nearly stationary population; a population in which mortality and fertility rates are constant and there is no population growth. At this point about 18% of the total population is 65 or older.

6

In addition to the growing numbers of elderly people, the older population itself is getting older. (10) For example, in 1984, the 65–74 age group was over 7 times larger than in 1900, but the 75–84 group was 11 times larger and the 85 and older group was 21 times larger. The most rapid increase is expected between 2010 and 2030 when the baby boom generation hits 65. In the next century, the only age groups in the U.S. expected to experience significant growth will be those past age 55.

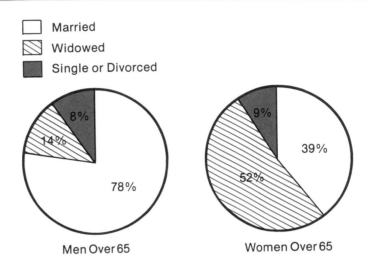

Married
Widowed
Single or Divorced

8%
14%
78%

Men Over 65

9%
39%
52%

Women Over 65

after Lowenstein & Schrier (2)

The unmarried will be an increasing proportion of the elderly. By 1983, 50% of American women ages 65–74 were unmarried (partly divorced, but largely widowed), and after age 75, 77%! (11) Because the unmarried tend to be more disadvantaged, there will be a need for more services for this segment of the elderly population. Older unmarried people are more vulnerable, demonstrating higher mortality rates and lower life satisfaction.

The death rate is higher for men at all ages. Coronary heart disease accounts for 40% of the mortality difference between men and women. (2) Another one-third is from lung cancer, emphysema, cirrhosis, accidents, and suicides. It is interesting to note that in our society the mortality difference between men and women is largely a difference in lifestyle. Smoking, drinking, coronary prone behavior, and accidents account for most of the higher male mortality rate over age 65. It has been estimated that perhaps two-thirds of the difference has been due to cigarettes alone. (2)

7

Health Conditions in Women Age 65 and Older, 1984 (12)

Arthritis	52.2%
Hypertension	30.2%
Hearing impairment	25.9%
Visual impairment	23.1%
Heart conditions	19.0%
Chronic sinusitis	13.4%
Varicose veins	9.7%
Diabetes mellitus	9.4%
Back or spine impairment	8.5%
Constipation	7.5%
Urinary system diseases	7.1%
Hip, extremity impairment	7.1%
Upper GI disorders	4.9%
Thyroid conditions	4.2%
Anemia	3.5%
Cerebrovascular disease	3.5%
Gall bladder condition	3.0%
Migraine	1.8%

Women lag behind men in the incidence of coronary heart disease by 10 years, and for myocardial infarction and sudden death, women have had a 20 year advantage. (13) After menopause, the risk of coronary heart disease doubles for women. In women all the atherogenic lipids rise to about age 60 and then decline. The ratio of total cholesterol to HDL-cholesterol rises with age, from 3.4 at ages 25–34 to 4.7 at ages 75–89. At all ages, HDL-cholesterol values in women are 10 mg/dl higher than in men. When the total cholesterol/HDL-cholesterol ratio exceeds 7.5, women have the same risk as men. For every 10 mg/dl change in HDL-cholesterol there is a corresponding 50% change in coronary heart disease risk.

Perhaps because more women are smoking, drinking, and working, the mortality sex difference has begun to lessen. The U.S. Census Bureau projects that the difference in life expectancy between men and women will increase until the year 2050, then level off. (12) In 2050, life expectancy for women will be 81 years and for men, 71.8 years. There will be 33.4 million women 65 and older, compared to 22.1 million men.

Year	Men per 100 U.S. Women (12)
1900	96.3 (75 and older)
1979	45.0 (85 and older)
2000	39.4 (85 and older)
2050	38.8 (85 and older)

8

The elderly woman represents a new challenge for us. Indifference to the elderly is to some extent an iatrogenic problem. Considerable disease and symptoms among elderly people pass by untreated or unnoticed because we haven't learned to deal with these problems. For example, up to 30% of older people diagnosed as having senility have been found to have a reversible problem such as malnutrition or a drug dosage problem. (2) The frequency and amount of drugs taken per person increase progressively with age. Yet our understanding of the pharmacology is based on studies in young people.

Here is an example of the kind of new learning required of physicians: The ability to continue living independently is a critical issue for all elderly people. Manual function has been demonstrated to correlate best with the probability that a patient will lose independence. (14) No traditional assessment in the usual history and physical examination is as sensitive as the assessment of manual function, measured simply, for example, by timing the writing of a sentence or the stacking of checkers.

The Quest for Long Life

The Fountain of Youth legend led Ponce de Leon to discover Florida in 1513, and before you discount the power of this theme, consider the market for megavitamins, mineral supplements, and even plastic surgery. The fountain theme is an important theme of aging: the idea that long life without the preservation of youth is unacceptable.

The most dramatic story is the Greek legend of Eos and Tithonus. The goddess Eos requested that Zeus give her mortal lover Tithonus eternal life. The request was granted, and Tithonus lived forever. But like the portrait in Oscar Wilde's *The Picture of Dorian Gray*, he became more and more decrepit because Eos had failed to request eternal youth as well. Eventually Eos shut Tithonus away in a room, where presumably he still is.

What is the greatest age ever reached? In 1973, a Russian died at the reputed age of 168, but there was no written documentation of his age. Charlie Smith in America was reputed to be 137 in 1979, but was found to be actually two months short of his 104th birthday. *Guinness Book of World Records* has accepted as documented only 5 people living beyond the age of 112. The oldest was a Japanese man of 117. Over and over again, reputed long life spans have turned out to be son, father, and grandfather all with the same name.

The new record holder is Arthur Reed who died in 1984, in Oakland, California, 2 months short of his 124th birthday. In an interview just before his death, he said: "They took time and they made me good. I don't drink or smoke, but I eat plenty of candy bars and lots of Coca-Cola." Born in Buffalo in the year Abraham Lincoln was elected president, his age was verified in 1944 when the Social Security Administration began paying him benefits.

There is a misconception that there are small secluded places in the world where the very old can live, that without our stresses and pollutants, long life is attained. Alexander Leaf studied the lifestyles of three different mountain people: (15,16)

The District of Abkhazia in the Caucasus Mountains of Russia.

The Province of Hunza in the Karakoram Mountains of Pakistan.

And the Village of Vilcabamba in the Andes Mountains of Ecuador.

Several common patterns were apparent in people at least 80 to 100 years old in these regions. Diets were low in calories and animal fats; physical activity and fitness levels were high; and moderation in alcohol and tobacco was common. One man alleged to be 117 said that his prescription for longevity was: "active physical work, and a moderate interest in alcohol and the ladies." Perhaps most importantly, there was no retirement in these communities. Elderly people remained active in social and economic life, giving them a sense of usefulness and purpose.

After Alexander Leaf's publications, hordes of sociologists descended on these villages. They found that just as age reduction is a common practice among the middle aged, age exaggeration is prevalent in the very old. Critical analysis of these societies discovered systematic age exaggeration after age 70, and there was no evidence of an increase in older people. (17) For example, in Ecuador, none of the 23 individuals claiming to be over 100 was actually that old. Indeed, not a single individual over 100 was found.

The Rectangularization of Life

The life span is the biological limit to life, the maximal obtainable age by a member of a species. The general impression is that human life span is increasing. Actually life span is fixed, and is a biological constant for each species. In fact, differences in species' life spans argue in favor of a species-specific genetic basis for longevity. If life span were not fixed, it would mean an unlimited increase of our elderly. But a correct analysis of survival reveals that death converges at the same maximal age; what has changed is life expectancy—the number of years of life expected from birth. Life expectancy cannot exceed the life span, but it can closely approximate it. Thus the number of old people will eventually hit a fixed limit, but the percentage of a typical life spent in the older years will increase.

Our society has almost eliminated premature death. Diseases of the heart and the circulation, and cancers, are now the leading causes of death. The reason for this is not an increase or an epidemic; it is a result of our success in virtually eliminating infectious diseases.

Now the major determinant is chronic disease, affected by genetics, lifestyle, the environment, and aging itself. The major achievement left is in cardiovascular diseases. With control of this health problem, approximately 12 years of additional life can be expected, compared to an additional 2 years if cancer is eliminated and only 0.2 years for diabetes mellitus. (18)

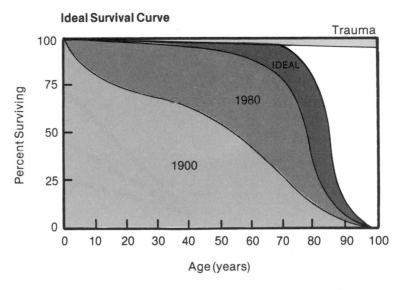

Ideal Survival Curve

after Fries & Crapo (25)

Disregarding violent death, progress in eliminating premature death since 1900 had, by 1980, removed about 80% of the area between the ideal curve and the 1900 curve. And notice that the greatest change occurred in the earlier years of life; most of the remaining premature death is now concentrated in the years over the age of 60 and is due to chronic illnesses. The change is dramatic: the white female in 1980 was only 7 years short of the theoretical limit. It is now time to concentrate on the later years. An appropriate goal is to have healthy and independent elders who maintain physical and cognitive functions as long as possible. Said in a different way, our goal is to maximize "active life expectancy," the duration of functional well-being, the maintenance of independence in the activities of daily living. (19)

Fries describes 3 eras in health and disease. (20) The first era existed until sometime in the early 1900s, and was characterized by acute infectious diseases. The second era, highlighted by cardiovascular diseases and cancer, is now beginning to fade into the third era, marked by problems of frailty (fading eyesight and hearing, impaired memory and cognitive function, decreased strength and reserve). Much of our medical approach is still based on the first era (find the disease and cure it), and now we have conditions that require a combination of medical, psychological, and social approaches.

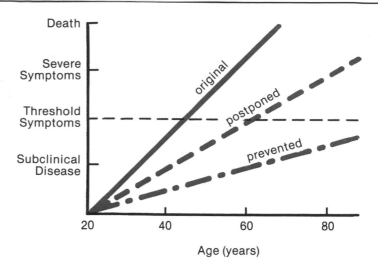

after Fries & Crapo (25)

**The Concept of
the Compression
of Morbidity**

Chronic illnesses are incremental in nature. The best health strategy is to change the slope, the rate at which illness develops, thus postponing the clinical illness, and if it is postponed long enough, effectively preventing it. The methods for postponing illness are obvious to us all: exercise, elimination of cigarette smoking, discipline over excessive alcohol consumption, elimination of obesity—and something newly appreciated in the elderly, a sense of personal choice in dealing with problems.

The relationship between individual health and one's sense of control is significantly affected by aging. (21) The very issue of control increases with aging due to stereotyping of old folks, loss of coping and feedback mechanisms (e.g. death of family and friends), loss of ability—all influenced by accumulated experience which gives control great importance. Furthermore, increased dependency with aging is a side effect of increasing interaction with medical care.

Studies among older people have emphasized the importance of self-determination. When older people are being relocated and given choices about when and where to move, and about aspects of the living arrangements, there is less decline in health and psychological status. In nursing homes, patients responsible for their own care do better and feel happier. Enhanced control even leads to improvements in memory. Most importantly, elders with a sense of control are more likely to seek answers and adhere to programs of preventive health care.

It is not surprising, therefore, that career involvement is accompanied by greater satisfaction in aging, and it also eases both economic and psychologic problems that accompany the loss of a spouse. (23)

Postponing illness is expressed by J.F. Fries as the *compression of morbidity*. (23–25) We would live relatively healthy lives and compress our illnesses into a short period of time just before death. Is this change really possible? The mean national body weight has decreased by 5 pounds despite a slight increase in the national average height. There has been a decrease in atherosclerosis in the U.S. (26) Reasons include changes in the use of saturated fat, more effective detection and treatment of hypertension, increased exercise, and decreased smoking. The number of American adults who smoke dropped from 37% in 1974 to 26.5% in 1987. Smoking initiation has decreased markedly in men, but unfortunately has remained essentially unchanged in women. (27) Physician smokers have declined from a high of 79% to a small minority of about 6%. It is interesting, and amusing, to note that the greatest decrease is among pulmonary surgeons, not surprising, while the least decrease is among proctologists. In repeated unscientific and personal surveys of our medical students, virtually all medical students by the time of graduation are nonsmokers! Projected to the year 2000, approximately 30% of people who have not obtained a high school diploma will be smokers, but less than 10% of those with higher education will be smoking.

Physicians and older patients may be skeptical that quitting smoking after decades of smoking could be beneficial. In a longitudinal study of 2674 people, aged 65–74, the mortality rates for exsmokers were no higher than for nonsmokers. (28) The effects are at least partly reversible within one to five years after quitting. Even older patients who already have coronary artery disease have improved survival if they quit smoking. (29) No matter how old you are, if you continue to smoke, you have an increased relative risk of death. But no matter how old you are, if you quit smoking, your risk of death decreases.

There has been a profound change in public consciousness towards disease. Disease is increasingly seen as something not necessarily best treated by medication or surgery, but by prevention, or more accurately, by postponement. How many runners are there in America today? The number of militant antismokers grows and grows.

This concept has been criticized. (30) The first criticism hinged on the interpretation that compression of morbidity means that natural death will occur without disease. But the concept does not deny the role of pathological insult as an instrument of death. Disease occurs, but later in life.

The second criticism contends that life span is increasing and eventually will reach into the ninth decade. The contention is based on the observation that the numbers of the very old are increasing, rather than falling off as they should after the peak mortality at age 85. However, the critics failed to take into consideration the increase in total population. The increase in numbers by itself is responsible for an increase in the numbers of old people. Furthermore, if better data indicate that life span is a little longer than 85, that still does not invalidate the compression of morbidity concept as a health strategy.

Criticism number three argues that no improvement in the health of old people is a statement against compression of morbidity. Instead, this fact argues in favor of the need to attack this problem. We have focused on disease in the younger population, and it is not surprising that the health of old people fails to show improvement.

A 5 year study of 263 initially healthy elderly men and women supported the concept of the compression of morbidity. (31) The mortality rate averaged 1.8% compared to the 5% rate for the general population, and the average duration of terminal illness in this population was 4.9 months, a relatively short time period. These individuals had successfully maximized their health potential and demonstrated that individuals who reach old age in good health tend to maintain good health until shortly before death.

Fries argues that the primary purpose of health promotion is to improve quality of life; this is in fact being achieved in that preventive health programs have a greater impact on morbidity than on mortality. (24) Because our greatest health problems are now concentrated in our senior population, it makes sense to direct health promotion to older people as well as the young.

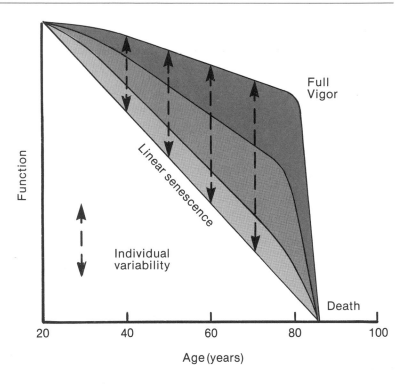

after Fries & Crapo (25)

The choice is between what Fries calls linear senescence or maximizing the vigor in life. Some linear decline is unavoidable, but the slope can be changed by effort and practice. The bad news is that life span is fixed. The good news is that most aspects of what we think of as aging can be modified. And most appealing, the issues of human aging depend upon individual personal choices which require personal effort—a very rewarding process.

And here is a revolutionary message for health care providers: it can be cheaper. Currently our society is seeing a shift from acute illnesses to lingering illnesses with a dramatic increase in costs and the number of years of impaired health per person. By postponing the onset of chronic illness, a dramatic reversal is possible.

Compressed into the remaining years before the fixed life span, illness can become less lingering. Logically there will be more attention to home care, more attention to a humane way of dying. The result could be a need for fewer medical services, less intensive care for the terminally ill, fewer hospitalizations. That adds up to decreased costs. The projected decline in health care costs has been estimated to be as much as 20%. (32)

The Menopause as an Opportunity

All physicians who interact with women at the time of the menopause have a wonderful opportunity and, therefore, a significant obligation. Medical intervention at this point of life offers women years of benefit from preventive health care. This represents an opportunity which should be seized.

What is needed for women today is preventive health care, and menopause gives us the opportunity to provide what is needed. The issues of preventive health care for women are familiar ones, and this book repeatedly addresses many of those issues. They include: family planning, cessation of smoking, prevention of heart disease and osteoporosis, maintenance of mental well-being including sexuality, cancer screening, and treatment of urologic problems.

There are four components of health care management:

1. Entry of the patient into a health care system.

2. Maintenance of continuity of care.

3. Appropriate referrals when needed.

4. Supervision of the cost-effectiveness of care.

A health care manager provides all of the above. In some circles, this is called being a gatekeeper, the contact point which allows the interaction between patient and the health care system. In other circles, it's called being a primary care provider. Let's expand the vision of health bureaucrats beyond the concept of a gatekeeper, a primary care provider, to that of a health care manager whose charge is to keep patients in a preventive health program, not necessarily to provide every bit of care.

The menopause (like pregnancy) serves a useful purpose in more ways than one. This physiologic event brings clinicians and patients together, providing the opportunity to enroll patients in health maintenance. The failure to respond appropriately (by either clinician or patient) easily leads to a loss of the patient from a practice, but equally, if not more, importantly is the probability that the loss of a patient from a practice means that another woman has lost her involvement in a preventive health care program. Contrary to popular opinion, the menopause is not a signal of impending decline, but rather a wonderful phenomenon that can signal the start of something positive, a good health program.

15

References

1. **Rowe JW, Grossman E, Bond E, et al,** Special report. Academic geriatrics for the year 2000, New Engl J Med 316:1425, 1987.

2. **Lowenstein SR, Schrier RW,** Social and political aspects of aging, in Schrier RW, editor, *Clinical Internal Medicine in the Aged*, W.B. Saunders Co., Philadelphia, 1982, pp 1–23.

3. **Markides KS,** Minority status, aging, and mental health, Intl J Aging Human Develop 23:285, 1986.

4. **Cutler NE, Harootyan RA,** Demography of the aged, in Woodruff DS, Birren JS, editors, *Aging: Scientific Perspectives and Social Issues*, D. Van Nostrand Co., New York, 1975.

5. **Diczfalusy E,** Menopause, developing countries and the 21st century, Acta Obstet Gynecol Suppl 134:45, 1986.

6. **U.S. Bureau of the Census,** Projections of the population of the United States: 1977 to 2050, Current Population Reports, Series P-25, No. 704.

7. **Hazzard WR,** Biological basis of the sex differential in longevity, J Am Geriatrics Soc 34:455, 1986.

8. **Siegel JS,** Demographic background for international gerontological studies, J Gerontol 36:93, 1981.

9. **Grundy E,** Demography and old age, J Am Geriatrics Soc 31:325, 1983.

10. **Manton KG, Soldo BJ,** Dynamics of health changes in the oldest old: New perspectives and evidence, Health and Soc 63:206, 1985.

11. **Keith PM,** The social context and resources of the unmarried in old age, Intl J Aging Human Develop 23:81, 1986.

12. **Lewis, M,** Older women and health: an overview, in Golub S, Freedman RJ, editors, *Health Needs of Women as They Age*, The Haworth Press, New York, 1985, pp 1–16.

13. **Kannel WB,** Metabolic risk factors for coronary heart disease in women: Perspective from the Framingham Study, Am Heart J 114:413, 1987.

14. **Williams ME, Hadler NM, Earp JAL,** Manual ability as a marker of dependency in geriatric women, J Chronic Dis 35:115, 1982.

15. **Leaf A, Lannois J,** Search for the oldest people, Natl Geographic 143:93, 1973.

16. **Leaf A,** Long-lived populations: extreme old age, J Am Geriatrics Soc 30:485, 1982.

17. **Mazess RB,** Health and longevity in Vilcabamba, Ecuador, JAMA 240:1781, 1978.

18. **Hayflick L,** The cell biology of human aging, Scientific American 242:58, 1980.

19. **Katz S, Branch LG, Branson MH, Papsidero JA, Beck JC, Greer DS,** Active life expectancy, New Engl J Med 309:1218, 1983.

20. **Fries JF,** The future of disease and treatment, J Prof Nursing, Jan–Feb, 1986.

21. **Rodin J,** Aging and health: effects of the sense of control, Science 233:1271, 1986.

22. **Holahan CK,** Lifetime achievement patterns, retirement and life satisfaction of gifted aged women, J Gerontol 36:741, 1981.

23. **Fries JF,** Aging, natural death and the compression of morbidity, New Engl J Med 303:130, 1980.

24. **Fries JF, Green LW, Levine S,** Health promotion and the compression of morbidity, Lancet i:481, 1989.

25. **Fries JF, Crapo LM,** *Vitality and Aging*, W.H. Freeman and Co., San Francisco, 1981.

26. **Cooper R,** Recent health gains for adults, New Engl J Med 307:631, 1982.

27. **Fiore MC, Novotny TE, Pierce JP, Hatziandreu EJ, Patel KM, Davis RM,** Trends in cigarette smoking in the United States, JAMA 261:49, 1989.

28. **Jajich CL, Ostfeld AM, Freeman DH Jr,** Smoking and coronary heart disease mortality in the elderly, JAMA 252:2831, 1984.

29. **Hermanson B, Omenn GS, Kronmal RA, Gersh BJ,** Beneficial six-year outcome of smoking cessation in older men and women with coronary artery disease. Results from the CASS registry, New Engl J Med 319:1365, 1988.

30. **Schneider EL, Brody JA,** Aging, natural death, and the compression of morbidity: another view, New Engl J Med 309:854, 1983.

31. **Thomas PD, Garry PJ, Goodwin JS,** Morbidity and mortality in an initially healthy elderly sample: findings after five years of follow-up, Age and Ageing 15:105, 1986.

32. **Gordon TJ, Gerjuoy H, Anderson M,** editors, *Life-extending Technologies: A Technology Assessment*, Pergamon Press, New York, 1979.

2   The Biology of Aging

Biologic aging is universal and inevitable. The rate of aging is determined by the interaction between genetic factors and environmental influences. Peak physiologic performance and maximal homeostatic capacity occur between 30 and 40 years of age. Subsequently, a progressive decline occurs in most organ functions. While baseline function is often maintained at levels similar to younger people, dynamic testing frequently reveals a ''limitation of reserve'' in older age.

Some organ systems escape the adverse effects of aging. Cognitive function, for example, as measured by intelligence tests, demonstrates the maintenance of intellect until late in life. Metabolic disorders, such as progeria, Werner's syndrome, and diabetes mellitus accelerate the aging process.

Environmental influences, including social pressures, alter physiologic functions, and the effects often are erroneously attributed to aging. In addition, many of the changes attributed to aging can be due to disease. Despite the evidence that aging is inevitable, the rate of change can be significantly modified by healthy lifestyles, regular use of organ systems, and avoidance of illnesses.

The Basis of Aging

The growth of organs proceeds until adolescence when adult proportions are achieved. Most tissues then maintain little replicative activity until injury or physiologic stress occurs. Organs can respond to injury or stress with increased cellular proliferation as well as hypertrophy of existing cells, with the latter becoming more important with increasing age. Some cells, such as those in the nervous system, never regenerate after fetal formation. On the other hand, the proliferative capacity of hematopoietic, gastrointestinal, epidermal, and endometrial cells is enormous. However, hematopoietic cells and stem cells decrease in number with advancing age, increasing the potential for anemia and leukopenia, especially when subjected to additional stresses. In addition, the germinal cell layer of the epidermis atrophies with age, resulting in delayed repair of skin wounds, and a decrease in hair follicles and sweat glands. The aging of the immune system leads to impairment of antigen processing. The growth potential of cells is progressively modified with increasing age, until eventually sufficient impairment results in the death of the organism.

Biologic and environmental differences lead to different rates of aging in women.(1) Currently most older women fall between "normal" aging and premature aging, and most men tend to follow the curve associated with premature aging.

The deterioration of functional capacity leads to more impairments for the elderly than the decrease in cellular replication. (2) The effects of aging in systems which do not regenerate, such as nerve and muscle, can be attributed to a decline in function due to a decrease in metabolic capacity. Vital cellular functions like oxidative phosphorylation decrease with aging. Critical molecules, including DNA, RNA, and other important proteins, are diminished in production.

Women can maintain good health and function by decreasing "unnecessary cell turnover," for example by avoiding excessive sunlight and cigarettes, and by eating a healthy diet to decrease the damaging effects of increased cholesterol and high blood pressure. Maintenance of the metabolic capacity of organ cells is encouraged by regular use, such as physical exercise and constant learning. Overuse and abuse diminish the maximal period of physiologic function and ultimately decrease the quality and quantity of life.

Organ Changes with Aging

Typically, elderly people have been classified as normal or diseased (clinically evident disease). Rowe and Kahn have recommended stratification of the "normal" group into a "successful aging" subgroup (with minimal organ system changes) and an "usual aging" subgroup (with complicating and confounding factors influencing the effects of aging). (3) These factors include poor diet, smoking, excessive alcohol use, use of drugs and medications, and low level of physical and mental activity.

Old Classification	New Classification
Normal	Normal: Successful Aging / Usual Aging
Diseased	Diseased

Obviously many of the factors which contribute to usual aging are preventable (or "postponed"—see Chapter 1) with appropriate attitudes, activities, lifestyles, and personal relationships. The challenge of aging deserves a plan by physician and patient to postpone the normal consequences of aging.

Organ/System	Morphologic Changes	Physiologic Effects	Clinical Effects
CNS	Declining neuron numbers Decrease in brain size	Decreases in neuro- transmitters	Decreased reaction time, speed of movement Slow shuffling gait, unsteadiness Decreased memory Slower learning and processing
Vessels	Atherosclerosis Calcification	Stiffness and decreased compliance	Systolic hypertension Increased cardiac work
Heart	Atherosclerosis Amyloid deposition Collagen accumulation Left ventricular hypertrophy	Stiff ventricle Decreased compliance Decreased cardiac output Decreased receptor activity	Decreased exercise tolerance Limited cardiac reserve Arrhythmias Diastolic dysfunction
Immune	Thymic atrophy	Decreased antibody response	Increase in infections
Endocrine	Decreased weight and size of organs Fibrosis and adenomas Vascular changes	Decreased hormone secretion and clearance Decreased receptors	Diabetes mellitus Menopause Hypothyroidism Vitamin D deficiency
Bones/joints	Loss of bone Degeneration of cartilage	Decreased height Stooped posture Arthritis	Falls and fractures Pain Immobility
Renal	Loss of nephrons Arterial sclerosis	Decreased GFR	Drug toxicity Dehydration, volume overload
Pulmonary	Coalescence of alveoli Loss of compliance	Decreased vital capacity Decreased reserve Decreased cough reflex	Decreased response to hypoxia and hypercapnia Pneumonia
Skin	Decreased fat Deterioration of collagen	Wrinkles Decreased padding and insulation	Pressure sores Hypothermia

Endocrine Systems. Part of the aging process has been described as the incapacity to regulate the internal environment in response to changes in the internal or external milieu. (3) Endocrine changes lead to a decrease in physical reserve and influence the expression of disease and the response to treatment. The most common endocrine change with aging, the menopause, is discussed in Chapter 5. Thyroid and parathyroid function is discussed in Chapter 15.

Most endocrine organs decrease in weight with aging and often develop vascular changes leading to atrophy and fibrosis. Most endocrine organs tend to form adenomas with increasing age, most notably the pituitary and adrenal glands. Secretion rates of most hormones decline with increasing age, but there is a decrease in clearance rate, resulting in little or no change in blood concentrations. Some cell surface receptors are decreased, but the majority are unchanged. Post-receptor response to hormones often decreases with advancing age, including insulin, catecholamines, steroid hormones, and somatomedins. The clinical results include diabetes mellitus, hypothyroidism, and decreased absorption of calcium.

Catecholamines. Catecholamines serve as hormones and as neurotransmitters. The adrenal medulla has little role in aging, but the adrenergic nervous system is important in homeostatic control, regulating body temperature, energy metabolism, and blood pressure. In general, adrenergic responsiveness diminishes with increasing age, influencing many biologic functions in the elderly.

Plasma norepinephrine concentration increases with increasing age. The normal circadian rhythm in plasma norepinephrine continues in the elderly, but the difference between young and older subjects is very dramatic at night. (4) The increase represents increased sympathetic nervous system activity. Why this occurs is not clear, but some hypothesize that it is due to altered baroreceptor reflexes resulting in higher sympathetic tone with alterations in adrenergic receptor responsiveness.

Altered Receptors and Catecholamine Responsiveness. Beta-adrenergic mediated responses, including forearm blood flow, heart rate response, and renin release, diminish with increasing age. (5) The evidence implicates post-receptor response in the presence of normal numbers of cell surface adrenergic receptors. Alpha-adrenergic receptors appear to maintain normal responsiveness, including vasoconstriction, with aging.

Decreased beta-adrenergic mediated vasodilatation and unaltered alpha-adrenergic mediated vasoconstriction with high catecholamine release can play a role in the development of hypertension in older people. The decrease in myocardial beta-adrenergic inotropic and chronotropic response is also associated with decreased myocardial functional reserve.

The cause of the altered catecholamine response has been attributed to down regulation of adrenergic receptors due to the high levels of circulating norepinephrine. (6) However, other factors including a decrease in exercise and physical conditioning and increased fat may account for the adrenergic changes with aging. The high plasma norepinephrine levels can by modified by changes in lifestyle, for example, exercise has been demonstrated to decrease plasma norepinephrine.

Central and Peripheral Nervous System. The nervous system reaches its maximal number of neurons in fetal life with no subsequent replication to replace lost cells. Neural tissue maintains function in the presence of declining numbers of neurons in the following ways: having a significant reserve supply of neurons, increased production and release of neurotransmitters, the extension of axons from neurons to other neurons that have lost innervation, modulation of the number, affinity, and effects of receptors to increase sensitivity to neurotransmitters at times of declining input from presynaptic pathways, and end organ increases in functional capacity to cope with declining neural stimulation. Essentially, the remaining cells increase their workload to compensate for lost cells. However, this increased work may accelerate the aging in the remaining structures. (7)

Aging of the Brain.   The brain decreases in size as atrophy develops over the surface of the cerebral hemispheres. The loss of brain tissue leads to ventricular dilatation after age 60. However, there is no consistent relationship between intellectual performance and the degree of cerebral atrophy.

Growth of dendritic trees probably increases in aging brains. Neurofibrillary tangles (argyrophilic, tortuous masses of fibrils in the neuronal cytoplasm) appear in increasing numbers in some gray matter. However, in nondemented elderly, they occur predominantly in the hippocampus and rarely in the cortex. Senile plaques of amyloid appear in neurons of most people over age 70. Characteristically, the dopamine content decreases in the striatum, accelerating between ages 60–90. Norepinephrine content decreases in the brain stem, while serotonin levels do not appear to change. Basal ganglia catecholamine synthetic enzymes decrease rapidly early in life, and later in life, decrease more gradually. Glutamic acid decarboxylase which is associated with gammabutyric acid (GABA) synthesis falls early in the aging process. Acetylcholine synthesis declines moderately in normal individuals, and markedly in those with Alzheimer's disease. Dopamine receptors decrease in selected anatomic areas, but cholinergic receptors appear to be maintained. (8)

What are the functional changes related to these changes? Neuropsychologic tests indicate a decline in the ability to perform tasks. On the other hand, verbal performance remains relatively stable. Short-term memory decreases, but immediate recall is unchanged. Older people have a reduced ability to retrieve stored information and have a diminished ability to use strategies for effective memory processing. They manipulate knowledge normally, but learn at a slower rate. Older people tend to perseverate and have trouble with tasks requiring selective attention since they have difficulty screening out irrelevant stimuli.(9) Older people have decreased motor function with a reduction in the speed of movement and an increase in reaction time. The gait tends to slow and becomes shuffling. Starting, turning, walking, and running become more difficult. Unsteadiness with standing increases after age 60. And finally, the elderly demonstrate difficulty in voluntary muscle relaxation leading to elderly tremors.

The Peripheral Nervous System.   Sensory and motor nerve conduction velocity declines 10–15% with aging. This results in a loss of the sense of vibration distally and sometimes the impairment of light touch, pain, and joint position sense in the toes and feet. Tendon and abdominal reflexes decrease with aging, and ankle jerks may be lost. Muscle size decreases in the elderly with a reduction in muscle fiber size and number, with fast twitch (anaerobic) fibers affected more than slow twitch (aerobic) fibers. Mitochondrial enzymes and the ability to increase oxidative metabolism in muscle with exercise decline in the elderly. Muscle strength decreases about 25% after age 60, and the maximal muscular work rate decreases even more. These changes vary considerably in "healthy" older people and are very dependent upon physical activity and conditioning.

The Auditory System. Presbycusis, a bilateral, predominantly high tone hearing loss, becomes more frequent with increasing age. The loss is due to a degeneration of the organ of Corti and the loss of elasticity in the basilar membrane of the inner ear. Auditory evoked response slows with a decrease in central processing of sensory information.

The Vestibular System. From age 40 to 70, provocative stimuli demonstrate hyperresponsiveness of the vestibular system, probably because of decreased central inhibitory control. The result is an increase in vertigo. After age 70, there is a progressive decline in vestibular response, attributed to a deterioration of end-organ function. This probably contributes to the postural instability seen in the elderly.

The Visual System. Visual acuity and contrast sensitivity decrease rapidly after age 60. Central factors seem more important than optical factors in these changes. Aging of the eye is characterized by decreasing pupil size, progressive yellowing of the lens, and a decrease in visual fields. Photoreceptor function declines with aging. Corneal sensitivity declines, and the corneal reflex may be lost. There is a reduction in the ability to converge, gaze upward, and smoothly track objects. Cataracts tend to form, and vision declines.

The Immune System. The major changes in the immune system result in decreased cell-mediated immunity, diminished primary and secondary antibody responses, and aberrant immunoglobulin and antibody production. This results in the increased prevalence and severity of some bacterial infections, especially urinary tract infection and pneumonia. In addition, there is an increased susceptibility to viral infections, including herpes zoster and influenza. The immune system is important in protecting against the development of cancer, and the increased incidence of many cancers relates to some degree to this decreased immune responsiveness. The elderly develop high monoclonal immunoglobulin protein levels and high autoantibody levels, but do not have a significantly higher risk of autoimmune disease. Most of these changes are thought to be a consequence of aging rather than the cause of aging. (10)

The Heart. Differentiating "normal" aging from the effects of cardiac disease has been difficult. (11) Subclinical coronary heart disease is very frequent in older women. The level of physical fitness varies tremendously in elderly women, further confusing the influence of physical fitness on cardiovascular performance. Advanced age has no effect on cardiac output in the sitting position. However, cardiac output is lower in the supine position, indicating that the elderly do not increase cardiac output with increased preload. The basal heart rate declines. Left ventricular mass thickness increases with aging, but this is probably due to the increase in systolic blood pressure. Early diastolic filling of the left ventricle falls with advancing age secondary to prolongation of isometric relaxation time and a decrease in cardiac compliance due to collagen accumulation in the ventricle. The left ventricle stiffens and relaxation is impaired, with slow filling. If cardiac rate increases then diastolic filling time decreases, which may result in inadequate filling with a risk of pulmonary venous congestion and dyspnea. This is referred to as diastolic dysfunction. However, these changes in the absence of disease or hypertension are not necessarily inevitable. At low levels of exercise, cardiac output increases at the same rate as in younger people, but at maximal exercise, the elderly cannot achieve the same heart rate and must increase cardiac output by an increase in left ventricular end-diastolic volume and stroke volume. Cardiac function in the elderly is normal at rest, but with exercise there is a decrease in the maximal heart rate with a compensatory increase in stroke volume required to maintain cardiac output. The elderly may not compensate for sudden changes in heart rate, and heart failure can result.

The Renal System. Renal mass progressively decreases with increasing age, with a decrease in glomeruli proportional to the decrease in total mass. (12) The renal cortex is predominantly involved as there is relative sparing of the medulla. Renal arteries develop sclerotic changes resulting in abnormal tapering and tortuosity. The smallest vessels are usually spared. Renal plasma flow decreases about 50%, reaching about 300 ml/min at age 80. The renal blood flow does not increase normally in response to a sodium load or other provocative stimuli.

The glomerular filtration rate decreases about 8 ml/min/1.73 m^2 after age 30. However, about one-third of older people show no change or an increase in GFR. In the two-thirds with a decline in renal function, about half have some renal disease and the remainder have an identifiable risk factor for renal dysfunction. These effects can predispose an older person to drug toxicity from renally excreted compounds, and alter responses to sodium load or restriction. Despite the dramatic decrease in GFR in many older people, the serum creatinine does not usually increase proportionately because of the age-related decrease in muscle mass and the resultant decrease in creatinine production.

The Pulmonary System. Pulmonary reserve is substantially reduced with aging. (13) With aging, the chest wall and lungs become stiffer with a tendency to expand and a limited capacity for collapse. This results in an increase in functional residual capacity of the lungs and a decrease in vital capacity. Most studies demonstrate that the usual flow rate studies of pulmonary function, including forced vital capacity and forced expiratory volume in one second, decrease with aging. The changes in lung and chest wall compliance result in closure of airways in the lower portion of the lung during the respiratory cycle, resulting in a mismatch of ventilation and perfusion. There is also an increase in the physiologic dead space. These changes result in a progressive decline in arterial oxygen concentration with age. The normal arterial Po_2 can be estimated by the following formula:

$$Po_2 = 100 - (0.34 \times age)$$

There is no change in arterial CO_2 content or in pH. There is progressive blunting of respiratory drive as evidenced by a decreased ventilatory response to hypoxia and hypercapnia. Local changes in the cough reflex, laryngeal reflexes, and in mucus clearance in the trachea predispose to pneumonia.

The Gastrointestinal System. Gastric acid secretion decreases about 10 mEq/hr/decade with aging in women. The effect is to decrease gastric emptying, lower intrinsic factor levels, enhance propensity for bacterial overgrowth, and elevate proximal small intestine pH which can alter drug absorption. (14) Small intestine functions and absorption, however, are usually well preserved with increasing age. Calcium absorption decreases due to decreases in estrogen and circulating 1,25-dihydroxyvitamin D. Hepatic blood flow and oxidizing systems decrease with age, but hepatic function tests do not usually change, although the clearance of drugs can be altered. Despite a common problem with constipation, large bowel function is unaltered with aging, and the reflex responsible for defecation remains normal.

The Oral Cavity. Taste usually remains normal except for complex flavors. There is no effect of aging on either the composition or volume of saliva. Masticatory muscle function decreases with age with lengthening of the time required to chew food and create a bolus for swallowing. There is also a loss of tone in the circumoral muscles. This accounts for the tendency of some older people to drool because of inadequate closure of their mouths. Although there is an increased prevalence of tooth loss and edentulousness, the loss of teeth with aging is now decreasing due to better care and diets. However, dental and periodontal disease is so prevalent in the elderly that this problem deserves special attention by physicians.

Drugs and Drug Metabolism (15)

Drug absorption is usually normal in the elderly. However, the decrease in gastric acid secretion can affect absorption of some drugs. Aging decreases the metabolic capacity of the liver, and one would expect drugs with a high hepatic clearance to have reduced systemic bioavailability. However, hepatic clearance of drugs is so variable that this cannot be predicted. The administration of drugs such as propranolol and many calcium channel blockers has the potential to achieve higher dose-related blood concentrations with prolonged half lives, and more care is required than with younger patients.

Dosage Adjustments Required with Aging

Reduced Doses Due to Decreased Renal Clearance	Increased Doses Due to Decreased Hepatic Clearance
Aminoglycosides	Lidocaine
Atenolol	Levothyroxine
Cimetidine	Propranolol
Digoxin	Theophylline
Disopyramide	
Lithium	
Phenobarbital	
Procainamide	
Quinidine	
Ranitidine	
Salicylate	
Tocainide	

Drug distribution is altered in the elderly because of changes in body composition and plasma protein binding. Aging is associated with a 10–15% reduction in total body water and lean body mass and a marked increase in total body fat. The plasma concentration of albumin decreases, decreasing plasma protein binding of acidic drugs like phenytoin, phenylbutazone, warfarin, some oral hypoglycemic drugs. Because of the decrease in total body water, drugs which distribute predominantly in water would have a smaller volume of distribution in the elderly. Ethanol is an example, and it is more potent in the elderly. Some drugs, like diazepam, which are lipophilic have an increase in volume of distribution and are less effective. Because of a decline in muscle, drugs, like digoxin, with extensive tissue binding, have a large volume of distribution.

In general, the greater the volume of distribution, the longer the half-life, and the smaller the distribution, the shorter the half-life. With high volume of distribution for a drug, it may take a long time to achieve steady state blood concentrations, and with small volume of distribution, it should take less time.

Many drugs are excreted by the kidney. Because renal function declines with age, the metabolism of many drugs is affected, including digoxin, procainamide, aminoglycoside antibiotics, penicillin, thiazide diuretics, clonidine, and some beta blockers like atenolol and nadolol. With many drugs one can assess the clinical response to determine the appropriate dose in the elderly. However, with other drugs, one may have to estimate the creatinine clearance (see Chapter 13) and measure drug concentrations to safely achieve a therapeutic concentration. The clinician should be aware that end organ response to drugs can be exaggerated or attenuated with age.

References

1. **Hazzard WR,** Basis for geriatric content in the clinical curriculum, *Proceedings of the Regional Institutes on Geriatrics and Medical Education,* Association of American Medical Colleges, 1983, p 111.

2. **Scoggin CH,** The cellular, biochemical, and genetic basis of aging, in Schrier RW, editor, *Clinical Internal Medicine in the Aged,* W.B. Saunders Co., Philadelphia, 1982, pp 24–28.

3. **Rowe JW, Kahn RL,** Human aging: usual versus successful, Science 237:143, 1987.

4. **Prinz PN, Halter J, Benedetti T, Raskind M,** Circadian variation of plasma catecholamines in young and old men: relation to rapid eye movement and slow wave sleep, J Clin Endocrinol Metab 49:300, 1979.

5. **Scarpace PJ,** Decreased beta-adrenergic responsiveness during senescence, Fed Proc 45:51, 1986.

6. **Feldman RD, Limbird LE, Nadeau J, Robertson D, Wood AJJ,** Alterations in leukocyte B-receptor affinity with aging. A potential explanation for altered beta-adrenergic sensitivity in the elderly, New Engl J Med 310:815, 1984.

7. **Creasey H, Rapoport SI,** The aging human brain, Ann Neurol 31:225, 1985.

8. **McGeer E, McGeer PL,** Neurotransmitter metabolism in the aging brain, in Terry RD, Gershon S, editors, *Aging, Vol 3: Neurobiology of Aging,* Raven Press, New York, 1976, pp 389–397.

9. **Peppard RF, Callne DB,** Central and peripheral nervous system alterations (in the elderly), in Hazzard WR, editor, *Geriatrics,* J.B. Lippincott Co., Philadelphia, 1989, pp 2577–2581.

10. **Weksler M,** Biologic basis and clinical significance of immune senescence, in Rossman I, editor, *Clinical Geriatrics,* J.B. Lippincott, Philadelphia, 1986, p 57.

11. **Weisfeldt ML,** editor, *The Aging Heart. Its Function and Response to Stress,* Raven Press, New York, 1980, Vol. 12.

12. **Brown WW, Davis BB, Spry LH, et al,** Aging and the kidney, Arch Intern Med 146:1790, 1986.

13. **Muiesan G, Sorbini CA, Grassi V,** Respiratory function in the aged, Bull Physiopath Resp 7:973, 1971.

14. **Holt P,** Aging in the gut, Geriatric Med Today 4:44, 1985.

15. **Montamat SC, Cusack BJ, Vestal RE,** Management of drug therapy in the elderly, New Engl J Med 321:303, 1989.

3   Successful Aging: Health Maintenance and Preventive Care

A healthy 50 year old American woman can expect to live another 30.9 years to approximately age 81. When she reaches age 65, an American woman can expect another 18.6 years, but it is likely that she will live only two-thirds of that time independently.

Women in America live an average of 8 years longer than men, have higher rates of illness, experience more days of disability, and utilize more health services than men. (1) Some aspects of preventive care and health maintenance in older women are well-established and some remain controversial. Data continue to become available leading to an on-going evolution of recommendations. This chapter considers current principles and guidelines for preventive care and health maintenance, and proposes strategies and recommendations specific for older women. This information is intended to enable the practicing physician to incorporate appropriate prevention measures, health goals, and interventions into clinical practice.

General Considerations

The decline in mortality from infectious disease right after the turn of the century, and the recent decline in cardiovascular mortality in the U.S., provide strong evidence that we can have an impact on illness and mortality. At the turn of the century, infectious disease accounted for most of American mortality. Social and environmental changes, followed by immunizations and antibiotics, reduced premature mortality from these illnesses to a minimum. Chronic diseases which occur with an aging population have taken the place of infections.

In the last 30 years, stroke mortality has declined by 60% and mortality from coronary heart disease by 30% in the U.S. Improvements in medical and surgical care can account for some of this decline, but 60–70% of the improvement is due to preventive measures. (2) Excellent data from epidemiologic studies and clinical trials demonstrate a decline in morbidity and mortality from smoking cessation, blood pressure reduction, and lowering of cholesterol. We can now recognize that there is a strong and growing scientific basis for preventive medicine and health promotion efforts in clinical practice.

29

At the close of the 20th century, nearly 13% of the U.S. population will be over age 65 and 60% will be women. Personal, social, and environmental factors determine the health status of these women, their risk of disease or disability, and their premature mortality.

Personal Factors. Although characteristics of age, race, ethnicity, and heredity affect women's health, personal health behavior and lifestyle are also significant determinants of health risks. These include smoking, alcohol and drug abuse, nutrition, physical activity, response to stress, use of seat belts, adherence to preventive laws (e.g. speed limits), and personal hygiene.

Social Factors. Social factors which influence women's health include marital and household status, urban or rural living, education, occupation, and income. Physicians and other health care professionals should be aware that the 3 most important current social changes affecting women's health care are the increasing numbers of women living in poverty, the large number of women entering the labor force, and the continuing increase in the longevity of women.

The relationship between poverty and ill health needs to be emphasized. Currently, a disproportionate number of women live in poverty and are unable to meet their financial demands or deal with unanticipated events. The problem is complicated for single heads of households and those who provide the sole support for their families. (3) Poverty and ill health are related. Illness develops because of poor nutrition, poor living conditions, stress, and reduced access to health care. The "new" poor includes elderly women living on low fixed incomes. Among the elderly poor, 74% are women. (3) An additional problem is the fact that employed women earn 59% of what men earn.

Mortality rates are higher for minority women, unmarried women, and rural women. A common characteristic of these groups is a high prevalence of poverty. Women married for more than 20 years divorce at increasing rates, and their longevity results in women seeking employment with limited experience in finding employment. As most working women know, the average work week for a woman working and running a home is 80 hours compared to 50 hours for men. Because of lower employment rates and lower income, Social Security benefits for women are two-thirds those of men. Divorced older women have incomes 50% lower than married women and have higher rates of illness. Although health care providers cannot solve all these social problems, they need to consider them in dealing with older women and become advocates for changes to resolve them.

Environmental Factors. Environmental factors include the sociocultural factors mentioned above, plus the many different conditions and influences in which a person lives and develops. The environment contains the food we eat, the air and pollutants we breathe, the water we drink, the geographic regions and structures we live in, the climatic conditions, the communities we live in, and exposures to pathogens and toxins. It also embraces the health services available, exposure to preventive measures, and the potential adverse consequences of treatment and technology. We should never lose sight of the fact that we have control over a number of environmental factors and exposures which can influence health.

Goals for
Older Women

The overall objectives for preventive medicine and health promotion in older women are to prevent premature mortality and to maintain physical and mental function with independent living. Significant steps towards achieving these objectives include reducing heart attacks and strokes by prevention, early detection, and treatment of hypertension, elevated cholesterol, and diabetes; and changing unhealthy behaviors such as smoking, sedentary lifestyle, and a diet high in saturated fat content and alcohol. Prevention of mental illness and periodontal disease are also important priorities.

Because of changes with increasing age, the goals for individuals are age specific. Age-related recommendations can be incorporated into a strategy which applies to three major age groups: older middle age (40–59), the elderly (60–74), and the old (75 and older).

Older Middle Age
(40–59 Years)

Health Goals:

1. To prolong the period of maximal physical energy and optimal mental and social activity.

2. To detect as early as possible any of the major chronic diseases, including hypertension, heart disease, diabetes mellitus, and cancer, as well as impairments of vision, hearing, and teeth.

3. To smoothly traverse the menopausal period of life.

Professional Services:

1. Four professional visits, once very 5 years (at about 40, 45, 50, and 55) with complete physical examination and medical history, tests for specific chronic conditions, appropriate immunizations, and counseling regarding changing nutritional needs, physical activities, injury prevention, occupational, sexual, marital, and parental problems, and use of cigarettes, alcohol, and drugs. Annual visits should include a breast and pelvic examination with hemoccult testing and Pap smear.

2. For those over 50, annual tests for hypertension, obesity, and certain cancers.

3. Annual dental prophylaxis.

The Elderly
(60–74 Years)

Health Goals:

1. To prolong the period of optimal physical, mental, and social activity.

2. To minimize handicapping and discomfort from the onset of chronic conditions.

3. To prepare for retirement.

Professional Services:

1. Professional visits at 60 years, and every 1–2 years thereafter, including the same tests for chronic conditions as in older middle age, and professional counseling regarding changing lifestyle related to retirement, nutritional requirements, absence of children, possible

loss of spouse, and probable reduction in income as well as reduced physical capabilities. Annual visits should include a breast and pelvic examination with hemoccult testing and Pap smear.

2. Annual immunization against influenza.

3. Annual dental prophylaxis.

4. Periodic podiatry treatment as needed.

Old Age
(75 and Older)

Health Goals:

1. To prolong the period of effective activity and ability to live independently, and to avoid institutionalization so far as possible.

2. To minimize inactivity and discomfort from chronic conditions.

3. When illness is terminal, to assure as little physical and mental distress as possible and to provide emotional support for patient and family.

Professional Services:

1. Professional visit at least once a year, including complete physical examination, medical and behavioral history, and professional counseling regarding changing nutritional requirements, limitations on activity, mobility, and living arrangements.

2. Annual immunization against influenza.

3. Periodic dental and podiatry treatments as needed.

4. For low-income women and patients not sick enough to be institutionalized but not well enough to cope entirely alone, counseling regarding sheltered housing, health visitors, home help, day care and recreational centers, meals-on-wheels, and other measures designed to help patients remain in their own homes and as independent as possible.

5. Professional assistance with family relations and preparations for death if needed.

General Principles

Several prestigious groups have provided recommendations for an optimal preventive medicine program based upon the available scientific evidence. (4–11) We have utilized this material for the construction of the screening program displayed on the endpapers of this book.

These recommendations are based upon the following criteria:

1. The effectiveness of prevention or early treatment of the condition.

2. Potential severity of the condition.

3. Quality of screening tests, including sensitivity, specificity, predictive value, cost, safety, and acceptability to patients and physician.

Good evidence from epidemiologic studies and clinical triumphs demonstrate the efficacy of many interventions. However, some interventions are based on less solid data and require consideration of the potential benefits compared to cost. The proposals are for minimal, not maximal, standards. Individuals at specific risk based upon family and health habits will require more intensive screening and intervention.

Each physician should develop an individualized preventive health program for each asymptomatic patient. Evidence has accumulated that lifestyle is largely responsible for health and the acquisition of risk factors for chronic disease or premature mortality and disability. (12) This is not a complicated story. The lifestyle factors of diet, activity, use of alcohol, and smoking significantly determine health and how long one lives.

Preventive measures may involve the individual or groups of patients living in communities. Because lifestyle factors have such an important impact on health, there is increasing use of social psychology in attempts to change unhealthy behaviors. Preventive strategies can be divided into 3 levels based upon the point of intervention.

Primary Prevention. Primary prevention incorporates positive strategy to change unhealthy lifestyles and to prevent the acquisition of risk factors. This strategy includes the usual methods aimed at diet, activity, smoking, and alcohol. It includes safety habits such as wearing seat belts and driving carefully. It also includes preventive dental health care and immunization to prevent infectious disease.

Secondary Prevention. Many patients in older age already have identifiable risk factors for chronic disease or premature disability. Ideally, these risk factors should be detected early, followed by appropriate and specific interventions to decrease the risk. This includes disease in early undetected stages, where early diagnosis and treatment will influence mortality and prevent advancement to later stages of disease (e.g. cervical, breast, and colon cancers).

Tertiary Prevention. Many older women already have a chronic disease. The goal here is to maintain function as long as possible. This often involves prevention of another acute episode using drugs or lifestyle changes (e.g. the management of arthritis).

Screening

Proficient preventive medicine involves screening and assessment. Effective screening separates asymptomatic patients into groups at lower and higher risk for the disease or outcome of concern. Screening tests do not make definitive diagnoses, but identify individuals requiring more detailed evaluation. An excellent example of effective screening is the use of mammography to detect early breast cancer. The abnormal mammogram does not provide a diagnosis of breast cancer, but identifies women who require further evaluation or biopsy.

33

The clinician should understand the criteria for incorporating screening measures in the practice of medicine. These include the following:

1. The characteristics of the disability or disease.

2. The characteristics of the test for screening and assessment.

3. The characteristics of the treatment regimen.

4. The prevalence of the disease or condition in the population.

5. The impact on the individual and society.

6. The presence of a subclinical phase which allows for effective screening.

7. The false positive and false negative rates.

8. The risk of harm from the screening procedure.

9. The likelihood of compliance with the procedure by both patient and physician.

As one can appreciate from a review of these criteria, not all health problems will allow for screening. Lung cancer is common and devastating in women, but screening for lung cancer is not effective. There is neither a good method for early detection nor an efficacious treatment that would justify the effort and expense of screening.

Many of the recommendations for the oldest women have limits because they are derived from primary and secondary prevention strategies indicated for biomedical disorders in young people. Although preventive measures begun in early adulthood should be continued into old age, new strategies are needed with frail, old patients. Health maintenance for the elderly requires more personalized measures, an emphasis on the reduction of iatrogenic problems, attention to the needs of family care givers, maintenance of functional ability, and the strengthening of important social supports.

Special Considerations

Have the right attitude! Physicians usually have little problem relating to middle aged women, but often have personal biases about the elderly which interfere with patient care. It's important to ask yourself, "How do I feel about old people? How do I relate to older patients?" The right attitude is very important in order to be maximally effective in caring for older patients. Complaints from patients reveal the following: Many physicians shout at old people as if none can hear or understand. Many treat older women like children. Many picture older women as deteriorated, confused, agitated, querulous, apathetic, dependent, depressed, rigid, and unattractiave. A more positive physician views older women as senior to be sure, but experienced, proud, knowledgeable, independent, interesting, reliable, respectable, and active. It is important not to believe that we have little to offer older people, or that our skills will be wasted because death is near.

Old age does not justify diagnostic nihilism. Decisions regarding screening in the oldest women are complex. They cannot be based on age alone. The decision must consider the biologic age as well as the chronologic age, the short and long term prognoses for survival and function, the presence of other chronic diseases, institutionalization or independent living, and last but not least, patient preference.

A patient's preferences are important. We should minimize unnecessary changes in lifestyle in older women. Maintenance of quality of life is a predominant aim. Interventions such as restriction of diet, exercising, and sometimes even smoking cessation may have an adverse effect on the patient's perceived quality of life. Therefore the patient's right for self determination deserves respect. With the exception of the mentally incompetent older woman, the physician and family must involve the patient in decision making. At times the family may feel that the judgment of an older person is impaired, especially in making a decision to enter a nursing facility or stay at home. A physician can be helpful in bringing out the patient's desires and reasoning.

Target patients at high risk for losing functional independence. An older woman who is deteriorating and is at risk of losing her independence should become a special target for preventive efforts. One may be able to avoid a crisis during which rapid deterioration occurs and institutionalization is inevitable. Interventions should not foster dependency or cost the patient and family too much by over-utilizing scarce resources.

Individualize therapeutic decisions. The risks of treatment in older women must be weighed against the potential benefit. For many patients, a high risk procedure may be justified to prevent irreversible loss of functional independence. An old woman who has a bed to bathroom existence because of severe incapacitating angina may welcome the chance for coronary bypass surgery despite the very high risks, if there is a prospect that she can be returned to a functional, independent life.

Recognize that screening tests may perform differently in older women than younger women. Most of the screening recommendations are appropriate for women between the ages of 50 and 65. There are limited data, however, for women over 65, and almost no data for those over 75. Since there are many important changes in biologic characteristics in old age, these will have be considered on an individualized basis when one considers testing in old women.

Recognize that preventive interventions vary with age. A good example is the use of pneumococcoidal vaccine for older women. There is good evidence that this vaccine protects against pneumonia in younger people, but there is some doubt whether the elderly sustain the protection derived from immunizations.

Identify screening and intervention opportunities. Most older women present to physicians for recognizable illnesses. It is important at this time to seek out unreported problems. Approximately 90% of elderly patients contact a primary care provider each year. (13) This provides an excellent opportunity for screening, intervention, and early case finding.

35

Common Hidden Problems in Older Patients

Sexual dysfunction	Incontinence
Alcoholism	Depression
Musculoskeletal prolems	Hearing loss
Dementia	Falls

Multiple health professionals provide comprehensive preventive care. Teams of individuals, including physicians, nurses, psychiatrists, physical and occupational therapists, dentists, pharmacists, and social workers, are useful in performing together the collective tasks of assessment and prevention. Comprehensive assessment is especially useful in bringing order and guidance to the multiple problems of the very old.

Accept that death might be a legitimate end point. At some point, every patient has the right to die peacefully and with dignity. This is incontestable when a patient is suffering from an untreatable, fatal disease. Health maintenance in older women has as its principal goal *improvement in quality of life rather than prolongation of life*.

Recommendations for Older Women

"Health in older women includes the absence of disease, optimal functional status, and an adequate support system." (14) Recommendations for older women, therefore, include components in disease prevention, functional status, and support systems. These recommendations are proposed mainly for ambulatory women. For women who are severely ill or are institutionalized, one should refer to a textbook of geriatric medicine. Many of these subjects are discussed in greater detail in other chapters.

DISEASE PREVENTION

Cardiovascular Disease:
   Hypertension
   Hypercholesterolemia
   Smoking
   Sedentary lifestyle
   Obesity

Cancer:
   Lung cancer
   Breast cancer
   Uterine cancer
   Ovarian cancer
   Gastrointestinal cancer
   Skin cancer
   Melanoma

Infectious Disease:
   Influenza
   Pneumonia
   Hepatitis B
   AIDS
   Immunizations for travel

Chronic Obstructive Pulmonary Disease

Diabetes Mellitus:
 Proper weight maintenance

Accidents and Injuries:
 Seat belts
 Speed limits
 Drinking and driving

Periodontal Disease:
 Gum and teeth hygiene
 Regular exams

Osteoporosis:
 Hormone replacement therapy
 Calcium supplementation

Foot Care:
 Good footwear
 Trim nails

Iatrogenic Disease:
 Unnecessary medication
 Unnecessary support
 Unnecessary institutionalization

Hypothyroidism

Incontinence

Excessive Alcohol Use

MAINTENANCE OF FUNCTION

Immobility:
 Adapt home environment
 Avoid overprotection
 Guard against falls
 Orthostatic hypotension
 Walking aids

Poor Vision:
 Periodic exams
 Improve lighting
 Low vision aids

Hearing Loss:
 Periodic evaluation
 Hearing aids

Mental Health:
 Evaluate stresses
 Memory aids
 Depression and anxiety

MAINTENANCE OF SUPPORT SYSTEMS

Income Level:
    Use of social services

Housing

Family Support:
    Provide respite

Losses:
    Counseling for bereavement
    Retirement planning
    Community support

The first step in providing preventive care is to evaluate patients at regular intervals in order to detect early symptoms of illness and to determine whether the patient is at high or low risk for preventable diseases. For example, a 50 year old woman with a definite history of recurrent herpes, who has been highly promiscuous with multiple sexual partners, would require close surveillance for cervical cancer.

In general, women between the ages 50–60 should have a periodic evaluation at a minimum of every 5 years, from 60–70, every 2 years, and at least every year after age 70. In addition, older women should be seen annually for prevention and health maintenance, to include a breast and pelvic examination with hemoccult testing, mammography, Pap smear, vision testing, and other individual evaluations according to risk category.

Scholarly works have compiled arguments which conclude that there is little benefit from a periodic physical examination in asymptomatic adults. In our view, these arguments fail to consider that we are not just lungs to be auscultated or blood pressures to be measured. The interaction between physician and patient at the time of a periodic physical examination offers the opportunity (a unique opportunity, we would argue) for a variety of positive accomplishments, including appropriate historical inquiries and reinforcement of preventive health behaviors.

For periodic health evaluation of asymptomatic women at low medical risk, refer to the chart on the end papers of this book. These recommendations are based on the best current evidence and clinical judgment.

Disease Prevention

Opportunistic Case Finding. As mentioned previously, over 90% of elderly patients and approximately 70% of younger patients make contact with a primary care physician during a 1 year period, providing an excellent opportunity for risk assessment, risk classification, and identification of unreported illnesses. Even during episodic care visits, the physician can capitalize on the doctor-patient relationship and seek information on the key items noted above.

Leading Causes of Death in Women

Heart Diesase	▨▨▨▨▨▨▨▨▨▨
Cancer	▨▨▨▨▨▨▨
Cerebrovascular Disease	▨▨▨
Accidents	▨
Pneumonia/ Influenza	▨
Diabetes	▨

Cardiovascular
Disease

Cardiovascular disease is the most common cause of death in the United States. It includes coronary heart disease, cerebral vascular disease, hypertension, and peripheral vascular disease. Most cardiovascular disease results from atherosclerosis in major vessels. The atherosclerotic process is complex, involving smooth muscle proliferation and lipid deposition with eventual narrowing of the involved arteries. This, of course, eventually results in sufficient compromise in blood supply to produce ischemia and/or organ damage.

Identified risk factors for cardiovascular disease include the following:

Aging
Obesity
Smoking
Hypertension
Cholesterolemia
Diabetes mellitus
Family history of cardiovascular disease

There has been a major decline in coronary heart disease and stroke mortality from 1964 to 1988. Much of this reduction has been attributed to improvement in the detection and treatment of the various risk factors.

Diseases of the heart are the leading cause of death among women in the U.S. and account for 25% of all deaths of women; 250,000 of the 550,000 people in the U.S. who die each year of heart disease are women. (15) About 60% of new coronary heart disease events in women occur in the 20% of women at highest risk. This suggests that preventive measures will be as effective in women as they have been in men.

During the reproductive years women are "protected" from coronary heart disease. The reasons for this are complex, but a significant contribution to this protection can be assigned to the higher high-density lipoprotein (HDL) levels in younger women, an effect of estrogen. Women lag behind men in the incidence of coronary heart disease by 10 years, and for myocardial infarction and sudden death,

39

women have had a 20 year advantage. (16) After menopause, the risk of coronary heart disease doubles for women. In women all the atherogenic lipids rise to about age 60 and then decline. At all ages, HDL-cholesterol values in women are 10 mg/dl higher than in men. When the total cholesterol/HDL-cholesterol ratio exceeds 7.5, women have the same risk as men.

Most research involving the prevention of cardiovascular disease has been performed with male subjects. Although there is some skepticism regarding whether results can be extrapolated from men to women, most of the recommendations for risk intervention are the same for men and women. According to the Framingham data, risk factors have the strongest predictive value in women from ages 50–69. Evidence that risk factor modification in women makes a difference can be derived from the 43% decline in cardiovascular death rates in women in the U.S. from 1963 to 1983.

Black women have a coronary heart disease death rate 5 times higher and a stroke death rate 2.5 times higher than white women. Overall, cardiovascular disease mortality is twice as high in black women compared to white women, and substantially higher in white women compared to non-black women of other races.

Hypertension. Evidence suggests that treatment of hypertension (reviewed more extensively in Chapter 9) has less impact on mortality among women, but that as women age, the effect is more dramatic. The National Health and Nutrition Examination Survey, using a blood pressure of 140/90 as the criterion for hypertension, observed that 26.8% of all women had high blood pressure, and that more than two-thirds of those over 60 were hypertensive. (17) The level of risk for cardiovascular disease is directly related to the level of blood pressure plus association with other risk factors.

Recommendations. The blood pressure should be measured at each visit, and hypertension defined as 140/90 or greater. Hypertension is classified as mild (diastolic 90–104), moderate (diastolic 105–114), and severe (diastolic 115 and above). Specific recommendations for management are in Chapter 9. In general, these involve nonpharmacologic measures (salt restriction, weight reduction, exercise, stress reduction) and pharmacologic treatment with specific drugs. Elevated systolic blood pressure (systolic greater than 160 with a normal diastolic pressure) is predictive of coronary heart disease for women who are older than age 55. The prevalence of isolated systolic hypertension is greater in women compared to men over age 55; however, the efficacy of treatment still awaits clinical study.

Hypercholesterolemia. Elevated blood levels of cholesterol and decreased levels of HDL-cholesterol are independently associated with an increased incidence of coronary heart disease in women. (16) Data from the Framingham study further indicate that an elevation in triglycerides is also an independent risk factor for coronary disease in women. (18) An important observation in this study was the recognition that at all levels of total cholesterol (including those below 200 mg/dl) HDL-cholesterol showed a strong inverse association with the incidence of cardiovascular disease. (19) In women the relation of LDL to cardiovascular risk is less consistent and less striking. (16,20,21) In other words, in women the protective effect of HDL is very important.

Recommendations. All adults should have a screening measurement of total cholesterol and, when appropriate, the lipoproteins. (22) Familial hypercholesterolemia is not always associated with a family history of premature cardiovascular disease. For older women, the total cholesterol should be measured every 5 years. HDL-cholesterol levels should be obtained in women at high risk for heart disease. (23) Abnormal results should be managed according to the guidelines in Chapter 4.

The Normal Cholesterol/Lipoprotein Profile

Total cholesterol	—	Less than 200 mg/dl
HDL-cholesterol	—	Greater than 35 mg/dl
LDL-cholesterol	—	Less than 130 mg/dl
Triglycerides	—	Less than 250 mg/dl

Heart Disease Risk Based on Cholesterol/HDL Ratio

Lowest risk	—	Less than 2.5
Below average risk	—	2.5–3.7
Average risk	—	3.8–5.6
High risk	—	5.7–8.3
Dangerous	—	Greater than 8.3

Dietary modifications are indicated for all patients with total cholesterol levels above 200 mg/dl, and intensive effort should be directed to patients with levels above 240 mg/dl. The goal for the cholesterol/HDL ratio should be 3.7 or below. The HDL-cholesterol level should be at least 35 mg/dl. Regardless of the values for total and HDL-cholesterol levels, a strict dietary program is also recommended if the LDL-cholesterol is greater than 130 mg/dl and triglycerides are greater than 250 mg/dl. In women, drugs should be reserved for those with cholesterol levels greater than 240 mg/dl and/or those associated with other risk factors. There is some concern that a low-fat diet may be less effective in women because it will also lower the protective levels of HDL-cholsterol. (24) When drug therapy is required for high LDL-cholesterol levels, cholesterol-lowering drugs that concomitantly raise HDL-cholesterol are preferred (see Chapter 4). The positive impact of estrogen on HDL makes a powerful argument for hormonal replacement therapy as an important adjunctive treatment (see Chapter 5).

Fiber is the carbohydrate in our diet that cannot be digested. Insoluble fiber provides bulk and is used for the treatment of constipation and diverticular disease Soluble fiber is beneficial in managing diabetes and in lowering cholesterol levels.

Kind of Fiber	Fiber Sources	Effect on Health
Soluble	Oats, legumes (dried beans, peas, lentils), guar gum, psyllium seeds, some fruits and vegetables	Lowers LDL-cholesterol, slows glucose absorption
Insoluble	Whole grains, bran from wheat and corn, whole grain cereals, some fruits and vegetables	Protection against cancer of colon and rectum

SUPER OAT BRAN MUFFINS

2½ cups oat bran Mother Oats
¼ cup safflower oil
3 egg whites
2 tsp baking powder
⅓ cup brown sugar
1 cup pineapple orange juice
1 cup applesauce, pears, or pineapple
    or
2 mashed bananas

Bake at 425° for 18 minutes in muffin tin lightly oiled.
Makes 12.

Smoking. The relationship of cigarette smoking to coronary heart disease, chronic obstructive pulmonary disease, lung cancer, and a number of other chronic diseases is well established. (25) In the Nurses' Health Study, women smokers followed over a 6 year period had a 5-fold increase in myocardial infarction events compared to nonsmokers. (26) It should be emphasized to patients that cessation of cigarette smoking in women decreases their risk of myocardial infarction to that of women who never smoked. (26)

Recommendations. Obtain a smoking history at every visit. Smokers must be repeatedly counseled to quit smoking. Physician persistence pays off! Follow-up visits just for this purpose are worthwhile. The success rate with formal smoking cessation programs increases with repeated usage. Never tire in this crusade, and don't fail to point out that a patient's passive smoke is injurious to others. (27) IT'S NEVER TOO LATE TO STOP! One last point for that dwindling minority of smoking physicians: a recommendation to stop smoking has less impact when it comes from a smoking physician.

Prevention of Cardiovascular Disease

Personal Example

Systematic Follow-up

Alternative Pathways

Realistic Goals

Basic Information

Firm Commitment

Clear Recommendations

Medical Evaluation

Physical Activity. Although data in women are lacking, physical inactivity is well recognized as a coronary artery disease factor in men. (28) There is a significant positive relationship between HDL-cholesterol levels and physical activity in postmenopausal women. (29) Furthermore, in women with low HDL-cholesterol levels, there is a greater increase in HDL-cholesterol with aerobic exercise programs than in women with normal to high levels.

The characteristic marker of beneficial adaptation is the maximal rate of oxygen consumption: Vo_2 max or the aerobic capacity. Because rate of oxygen consumption and the heart rate are linearly related, the heart rate can be used to monitor the response to dynamic exercise. The maximal heart rate for a relatively inactive person can be predicted by the following equation: (30)

$$HR_{max} \text{ (beats/min)} = 198 - (0.63 \times age)$$

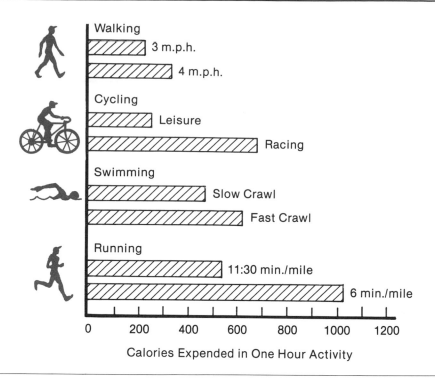

Calories Expended in One Hour Activity

The minimal threshold for a significant training effect is 60% of HR_{max}. (31) The upper limit which can be tolerated by most people is 80% of HR_{max}, therefore the target rate is usually 70–75%. Some form of dynamic exercise is required in order to influence aerobic capacity. This includes swimming, bicycling, running, walking, and cross-country skiing. However, swimming is of questionable effectiveness (due to the buoyant effect of the water) for maintaining bone density. The following precautions should be observed for older women:

1. Include warm-up and cool-down activity (5–10 minutes).

2. Avoid jumping or bouncing (jumping jacks or rapid trunk motions in aerobic dancing).

3. Avoid quick lateral or anteroposterior bending of spine.

Recommendations. For both cardiovascular reasons and protection against osteoporosis, exercise should be strongly encouraged at least 3 times a week. Age should not be a barrier to starting an exercise program; there is no evidence that exercise in moderation is hazardous for the elderly. (32) Risks are minimized by exercising at 70–75% of the maximal heart rate, a level that approximates the threshold for fatigue and tachypnea. Conditioning and protection against osteoporosis can be achieved with regular exercise as follows:

3–5 times per week,
70–75% of maximal heart rate,
50–60 minutes duration each time.

AEROBIC TRAINING GUIDE

45

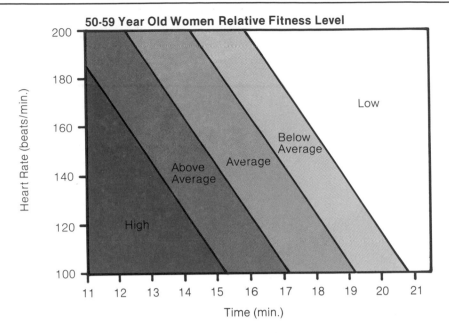

50-59 Year Old Women Relative Fitness Level

Heart Rate (beats/min.)

Time (min.)

Low

Below Average

Average

Above Average

High

Brisk walking provides sufficient exercise for cardiovascular training. Walking for 40 minutes 4 days per week is equivalent to 30 minutes of jogging 3 days per week. A 1 mile walk test can be used to estimate aerobic capacity and guide the prescription of exercise. (33) The following example illustrates how to use the figure:

A 55 year old woman who walks a mile in 17 minutes and has a heart rate at the end of the mile of 130 would be of average fitness, according to the figure, which is based on fitness levels for 50 to 59 year old women. Women can use this figure to chart the progress of their fitness.

Obesity

The incidence of obesity increases 3-fold during adult life in women, leveling off around age 65. (34) Twenty-five percent of white women and 50% of black women between the ages of 18 and 74 are obese, when classified as greater than the 85th percentile of the body mass index (weight in kg divided by height in meters squared). Obesity is a risk factor for diabetes, a low HDL-cholesterol level, and hypertension. As discussed in Chapter 7, the waist:hip ratio has been demonstrated to be more strongly associated with coronary heart disease events than other indices of obesity. There are no data on weight reduction for modification of coronary heart disease risk or in prevention of degenerative arthritis. However, this is considered to be a major health issue for the preventive care of aging women.

Recommendations. Patients should be weighed at each periodic health evaluation. Utilize the body mass index nomogram in Chapter 7 to assess the risk associated with obesity. The waist:hip ratio is a means of estimating the degree of upper (android obesity) to lower body obesity (gynoid obesity). The ratio is obtained by measuring the body diameters at the levels of the umbilicus and the anterior iliac crests. Android obesity (and not gynoid obesity) is associated with an increased risk of cardiovascular disease. Interpretation is as follows:

Greater than 1.2 — Android obesity
From 0.6 to 1.2 — Normal
Less than 0.6 — Gynoid obesity

The physiology of adipose tissue and the clinical management of obesity are discussed in Chapter 7.

Cancer

There are at least 4 important and preventable cancers in women. In order of frequency and importance, they are lung cancer, breast cancer, colon cancer, and uterine cancer (endometrium and cervix). In addition, skin cancer and melanoma may be preventable.

American Cancer Society Statistics for Women (35)

Site	1989 Mortality	% of Cancers	5 Year Survival for Localized Disease
Lung	49,000	11%	13% (all stages)
Breast	43,000	28%	90%
Colon & rectum	31,300	15%	87% (colon) 79% (rectal)
Leukemia/ lymphoma	21,600	7%	33%
Ovary	12,000	4%	85%
Uterus	10,000	9%	80–90% (cervix) 91% (endometrium)
Urinary	7,300	4%	88% (bladder)
Skin	3,000	3%	80% (melanoma)

It has been estimated that over half of the cancers in women are related to lifestyle factors such as infectious diseases, diet, reproduction, and sexual behavior. Therefore both general and specific recommendations can be made.

General Cancer Prevention.

1. Urge the cessation of smoking and the use of tobacco in any form.

2. Recommend alcohol use only in moderation.

3. Have patients evaluate exposure to carcinogens in their work places.

4. Avoid the unnecessary use of drugs that are potentially carcinogenic.

5. Use diagnostic x-rays prudently.

6. Urge susceptible individuals to avoid excessive exposure to sunlight and to utilize appropriate sunscreens for UV light exposure.

7. Use an estrogen-progestin combination for hormone replacement therapy.

8. Condoms should be used for protection against AIDS when sexual partners are at risk.

9. Recommend a diet low in fat and red meat and high in fiber, fresh fruits, and vegetables.

10. Recommend appropriate weight goals and control.

Lung Cancer. The most common cause of lung cancer is cigarette smoking (75% of lung cancer cases among women are due to smoking). This is an easily identifiable factor for reduction of risk. Unfortunately, cessation of smoking is not easy. As emphasized previously, physician persistence is an important key to success, and repeated utilization of cessation programs yields increasing rates of success.

Breast Cancer. The compelling evidence that screening for breast cancer effectively reduces mortality from this cancer is reviewed in Chapter 8. However, it is uncertain when we should stop screening in older women because beyond the age of 74 we have almost no data. Because the risk of breast cancer increases throughout life, we believe women at age 65 should consider continued screening, if not annually, at least every 2 years.

Recommendations.

All women should be taught self-breast examination by age 20. Because of the changes which occur routinely in response to the hormonal sequence of a normal menstrual cycle, breast examination is most effective during the follicular phase of the cycle.

All women over the age of 35 should have an annual breast examination.

A baseline mammogram should be obtained by age 40, or earlier if high risk factors are present.

From ages 40 to 50, mammography should be performed every 2 years in low risk women and every year in women with significant risk factors.

Annual breast examination and annual mammography should be performed in all women over age 50.

SIGNIFICANT HIGH RISK FACTORS

Family history of breast cancer in mother or sister.

Proliferative disease of the breast by biopsy.

First childbirth after age 30.

Dysplasia on mammography.

Relatively low sex hormone binding globulin levels.

Cancer of the Cervix. The annual death rate for cervical cancer is 159 per million in older women compared to 44 per million for younger women. Approximately 40% of the deaths due to invasive cervical cancer occur in women over age 65. It has been estimated that 39% of women over age 75 and 14% of women 65–74 have never had a Pap smear, and an additional 20% report that they have not had regular screening. A single screening Pap smear in an elderly population yields a high prevalence of abnormalities. (36)

The U.S. death rate from uterine cancer has decreased more than 70% over the last 40 years, due mainly to regular examinations and Pap smears. There is no doubt that Pap smear screening for cancer of the cervix effectively reduces the incidence and mortality from this disease. However, the optimal frequency of screening and the appropriate ages to stop continue to be controversial. Women with two negative smears are at low risk for at least 5 years according to clinical data. It has been estimated that screening from age 25–64 at 3 year intervals provides 90% of the maximal protection, requiring 13 tests over a lifetime. Annual screening starting at age 20 yields just over 90% of maximal protection, but requires 35 tests by age 55. Therefore some have recommended a Pap smear every 3 years after 2–3 negatives. We disagree with this recommendation for the following reasons.

High risk patients should definitely have annual Pap smears. Those at high risk for cancer of the cervix are women who have multiple sexual partners or whose sexual partner has had multiple partners. Many of these women have low income and no regular source of medical care. Those with herpes vaginalis or venereal warts are also considered to be at high risk.

Some have recommended that women who have been screened regularly with no abnormality should have screening stopped for cancer of the cervix after age 60. However, there is a problem in trying to be this selective since many women between 50 and 70 have not had adequate screening for cervical cancer and have increasing rates of the disease and mortality. And others have demonstrated that screening low income elderly women is cost effective. (36,37)

Finally, the recommendation to avoid annual Pap smears overlooks the value of the Pap smear in bringing women to a physician. The annual pelvic examination is the only effective means to detect ovarian tumors, a major problem for older women (the incidence peaks at approximately age 70). *Keep in mind that the postmenopausal ovary should be no larger than 2 cm in its largest diameter.* The incidence of vulvar cancer also increases with age, peaking at age 85. And as we have repeatedly mentioned, the annual patient-physician interaction provides the best opportunity for preventive screening and assessment.

Therefore, we recommend that all older women continue to receive annual Pap smears to assure that they have regular cervical cancer screening and to provide additional motivation to the patient for preventive health care.

Colon and Rectal Cancer.   Screening for colon and rectal cancer is not without controversy, but clinical experience favors a mildly aggressive approach. (38) A rectal examination should be part of every annual pelvic examination (required for an adequate evaluation of the cul-de-sac). We recommend that a stool sample be tested for occult blood at each examination. The American Cancer Society suggests that a flexible sigmoidoscopy be performed at age 50, and if negative, every 3–5 years.

Skin Cancer and Melanoma.   The major risk factor for skin cancer and melanoma is UV light exposure. It is recommended that older women avoid tanning booths. When exposed to the sun, appropriate sun screens with an SPF of 15 should be applied as a preventive measure.

Prevention of
Infectious Diseases

Influenza, Tetanus, Pneumonia.   Influenza, tetanus, and pneumonia are discussed in Chapter 18. During influenza epidemics, 80–90% of the deaths attributed to pneumonia and influenza occur in people over 65. We urge the aggressive promotion of the availability, efficacy, and safety of influenza immunization. All women age 65 and older should be immunized every year. Because adults with chronic cardiovascular or pulmonary disorders and older people who are living in chronic care facilities are at high risk for influenza, these should also be immunized annually regardless of age. Because the highest number of unprotected people for tetanus are among those over 60, the tetanus-diphtheria toxoids must be administered to older people with the same frequency as recommended for younger adults (every 10 years). Even though data on the efficacy of pneumococcal vaccine for the elderly are not available, we recommend that the vaccine be offered to all older people because of its safety, inexpensive cost, and the increased incidence of pneumonia with advancing age. It need be given only once. We also recommend post exposure prophylaxis in women exposed to hepatitis A, hepatitis B, tuberculosis, and rabies.

Diseases Related to Overseas Travel.   There are specific recommendations for immunizations to prevent typhoid fever, yellow fever, cholera, hepatitis A, malaria, and other endemic diseases. Since the recommendations vary with the geographic location of the travel, it is worth consulting with one of the guide books such as that produced by the Center for Disease Control. It is extraordinarily important that women traveling to areas endemic for malaria receive appropriate malaria prophylaxis both during the trip and upon return.

Accidents and
Injuries

Accidents are the fifth leading cause of death in the elderly with half of the mortality due to falls. (39) Falls in older women may be due to environmental hazards such as stairs, loose rugs, and poor lighting; chronic diseases including neurologic disorders and cardiac arrhythmias; or the use of medications which cause confusion or hypotension. Two-thirds of falls can be prevented through appropriate intervention. (40) Automobile accidents are another cause for morbidity and mortality among the elderly. When riding or driving in an automobile, only a third of people age 65 and over wear a seat belt most of the time. This is the lowest percentage in any age group. Scalds from hot water are a leading cause of burns among older people; only a third know the water temperature setting on their heaters.

| Iatrogenic Disease | Iatrogenic illness results from medical interventions gone awry. Some common forms include medication misuse, complications of indwelling urinary catheters, deconditioning due to bed rest, and social dependency fostered by families excessively concerned with their elders. Iatrogenic disease should be and is preventable. |

Medications in older women account for a significant portion of iatrogenic problems. Eighty to ninety percent of older individuals take medication. (41) Home surveys have indicated that the average elderly person takes between 2 and 5 prescription medications and 2 to 3 "over the counter" medicines. (42) About one quarter of older people take 4 or more different drugs each day. The more drugs a person is on, the more likely they are to have side effects. In addition to the problem of an excessive number of drugs, proper use and compliance are major issues. Studies have demonstrated that only about half of older patients consume medications according to instructions and as the number of medications increases, compliance decreases. (14)

The first consideration for a clinician evaluating a patient's symptoms should be that the problem may be caused by a drug. Medications are often the cause of confusion in older women. We have the following recommendations.

Recommendations:

1. Avoid unnecessary medications and treatments.

2. Regularly evaluate all drugs used.

3. Avoid premature or early community support when the patient can maintain her own independence.

4. Avoid unnecessary institutionalization and hospitalization.

5. Be wary of complications in the elderly associated with gastrointestinal and intravenous contrast x-rays.

6. Consider iatrogenic disease as a cause for any functional impairment in an older woman.

Hypothyroidism

The prevalence of overt hypothyroidism in older women ranges from 3 to 7% among the various studies.(43) The symptoms and signs are very subtle, but the functional impairment can be great. Since the diagnostic tests have very high sensitivity and specificity combined with low cost, we recommend that older women be screened for both hypothyroidism and hyperthyroidism with the highly sensitive TSH (thyroid stimulating hormone) assay obtained at age 45 and then every 2 years beginning at age 60, or with the appearance of any symptoms suggesting hypothyroidism.

Diabetes Mellitus

Periodic fasting plasma glucose measurements are recommended for women who are markedly obese, those who have a family history of diabetes, and those with a history of gestational diabetes.

| Anemia | We recommend measuring the Hct in women at least once every 10 years after age 40. |

| Excessive Use of Alcohol | It is estimated that alcoholism affects up to 10% of older women, contributing significantly to functional disability. However, the excessive use of alcohol is often overlooked and misdiagnosed. An older woman is at high risk for alcoholism if there is a family history of alcoholism and if there has been personal habitual alcohol use. Empiric evidence suggests that counseling in older patients about excessive use of alcohol can be successful. Heavy drinkers of alcohol have more oral cancer and cancers of the larynx, throat, esophagus, and liver. |

Recommendations:

1. Assess risk, concentrating specifically on family history and habitual use of alcohol.

2. Emphasize that the use of alcohol is best reserved for celebrating.

3. Forcefully remind patients about drinking and driving.

4. Repeatedly promote compliance with recommendations.

5. The CAGE questions are helpful (2 positive answers indicate a problem, and more than 2, probable alcohol dependency):

   C — Have you ever felt the need to *C*ut down on your drinking?

   A — Have you ever felt *A*nnoyed by criticism over your drinking?

   G — Have you ever felt *G*uilty for your drinking?

   E — Do you ever have an *E*ye opener?

Maintenance of Function

Many older people fail to maintain sufficient physical activity to maintain adequate conditioning. Exercise rates among older people are the lowest of any age group; however, physical training programs in older women can improve maximum oxygen consumption, increase muscle strength, improve joint mobility, and improve sense of balance. Regular exercise should be promoted; see the use of the one mile walk outlined earlier in this chapter.

Immobility. Immobility in older women may be due to a number of causes including biomechanical factors, deconditioning, arthritis, and chronic debilitating illness. Many patients will require specific rehabilitation and prescribed therapy to maintain mobility. However, some general reminders can be provided for maintenance of mobility.

Recommendations:

1. Adapt the home environment.

2. Prescribe prosthetic and other devices which can help to maintain function.

3. Avoid overprotection from care givers.

4. Provide home and institutional rehabilitation as needed.

Falls. Falls are a common problem among the elderly, and most fatal injuries are related to falls. The fear of falling can lead to a self-imposed inappropriate reduction of activity. As many as two-thirds of falls are preventable using appropriate medical diagnosis, care with medications, and environmental modifications. (44) Preventing falls requires an appropriate assessment of the factors involved: safety of the home, balance and gait, and a careful review of the circumstances of previous falls.

Recommendations:

1. Avoid sedative medications.

2. Prevent orthostatic hypotension.

3. Remove hazards in the home.

4. Provide adequate light.

5. Insure correct footwear.

6. Appropriately use walking aids.

7. Prevent nocturia.

8. Consider a monitoring alarm system for the home.

Loss of Vision and Hearing. Diminished vision contributes significantly to loss of independence and to accidents. Simple measures, usually not apparent to family, can be advised, such as an improvement in home lighting. Of course, eyeglasses should be provided, and cataract surgery performed when indicated. As many as half of older women have some impairment of hearing. (45) An association with hearing loss has been demonstrated for depression, dementia, and loss of independence. The routine evaluation of hearing can lead to the use of hearing aids and a significant improvement in the quality of life.

Mental Health. Older women are more likely to suffer from simple phobias, including agoraphobia. Cognitive impairment also increases with age. Although more men than women are successful in suicide attempts, 60–70% of those who attempt suicide are women (and 44% of those who commit suicide are over age 44). Prevention of mental illness involves education and anticipatory guidance by health professionals before life crises, and the provision of support systems during the crises which occur with aging. Intervention can shorten episodes, keep disorders from progressing to severe stages, maintain function, and prevent suicide.

It is said that one can tell when one is old by when deaths in friends outnumber the survivors. Losses are inevitable as people get older. These include not only the loss of loved ones, but also the loss of independence and control over one's life.

53

Recommendations:

1. Be aware of life stresses and losses in your patient's life.

2. Be sensitive to the impact of chronic diseases on mood and function.

3. Prevent depression with counseling and assisting in the grieving process.

4. Counteract anxiety and panic with counseling and education.

5. Identify early memory loss and counsel regarding the use of memory aids to maintain function.

Strategies for Changing Health Behavior

A significant part of the success in preventing disease requires people to change their behavior. We are asking people to do things they have not done previously, to stop doing things they have done for years, and to do more of some things and less of others. This contrasts with what we normally do in clinical practice, the active prescribing of something, the giving of something. Even the latter has its problems; compliance with therapeutic regimens is not uniform even when we are offering useful treatment for distressing symptoms.

The identification of a risk behavior is usually not difficult, but effecting a change in that behavior is often frustrating. To change behavior, one must gain the confidence of the patient, and the approach must be consistent with social and cultural assumptions of the patient.

Most clinicians realize that the major causes of death, serious illness, and disability are chronic disease and injuries. And most clinicians can recognize individuals with "suicidal" lifestyle patterns which constitute the major behavioral risks for disease and disability. A major problem is that physicians have not been taught a useful strategy for changing unhealthy behaviors. All too often, this creates frustration and a lack of confidence which then results in no action on important problems (e.g. with cessation of smoking).

The clinician should seek the predisposing factors which have resulted in the behavior. This includes the values and perceptions of the patient. There are also enabling factors which come from peer pressure, family, health education in the community, and work site pressures. All of these potentially change the motivation for behavioral change.

The physician is in an ideal position to influence behavioral change. The physician can identify the risks and with authority point out to the patient the potential important consequences. The physician should at least initiate the modification of unhealthy lifestyles.

There are certain principles which are applicable to most unhealthy behaviors. Most importantly, the physician should provide continuity of personalized medical care, ensuring that clinical services are convenient and empathetic. We recommend a a simple 6 step method based upon the principles of Farquahr. (46)

Step One: Problem Identification:

1. Physician diagnoses or identifies the problem.

2. The patient must recognize it as a problem. Explanations by the physician and educational materials are both important in this vital step which requires a patient to understand why a change is necessary.

Step Two: Building a Commitment to Change:

1. The physician facilitates.

2. The patient chooses to change.

3. A contract is written with the patient. A definite starting date should be entered in this written contract which states the goal the patient wants to accomplish.

Step Three: Teaching Self-Awareness:

1. The physician records history and the patient keeps a diary: note why, where, and the reasons for the behavior.

Step Four: Development of an Action Plan:

1. Outline strategies to change the behavior. A long-range goal is more likely to be achieved through a series of short-term goals.

2. Teach the patient how to overcome the behavior.

3. Teach coping skills and provide support. Support can be drawn from a variety of areas, including family and community resources.

Step Five: Feedback and Evaluation of Success.

Office visits can be and should be a motivating force. Goals, however, may need to be revised to reflect realistic accomplishments.

Step Six: Maintenance of the Change.

Follow-up reinforcement and support are necessary. It is beneficial to involve the entire office staff in this process.

The Secrets of Life

Some people never do learn the secrets of life. The answers are in this book. A positive attitude combined with significant exertion of control over one's life together go a long way toward maximizing health and happiness in life. This is a never-ending effort, and physicians who practice this approach to life have a great deal to offer to their patients.

There is good evidence that risk factors for many diseases and disabilities can be detected early and treatment or prevention can improve outcomes. Unhealthy behaviors account for most of the premature morbidity and mortality in older people. The physician is in an important position to influence health behaviors and to assess risk factors and to provide medical interventions which will effectively prevent premature death and disability.

References

1. **Vital Statistics of the U.S.,** 1980 Life Tables, Vol 11, Sec 6, DHHS Publication No. (PHS)84-1104, U.S. Govt. Printing Office, Washington D.C., 1984.

2. **Levy RL, Moskowitz J,** Cardiovascular research: Decades of progress, decade of promise, Science 217:121, 1982.

3. **Report of the Public Health Service Task Force on Women's Health Issues,** Public Health Reports 100:73, 1985.

4. **Frame PS, Carlson SJ,** A critical review of periodic health screening using specific screening criteria, J Fam Pract 2:29,123,189,283, 1975.

5. **Breslow L, Somers AR,** The lifetime health monitoring program, New Engl J Med 296:601, 1977.

6. **Canadian Task Force on the Periodic Health Examination,** The periodic health examination, Can Med Assoc J 121:1194, 1979.

7. **American Cancer Society,** ACS report on the cancer-related health check-up, CA 30:194, 1980.

8. **AMA Council on Scientific Affairs,** Medical evaluations of healthy persons, JAMA 249:1626, 1983.

9. **Canadian Task Force on the Periodic Health Examination,** The periodic health examination: 1984 update, Can Med Assoc J 130:1278, 1984.

10. **Joint National Committee on the Detection, Evaluation, and Treatment of High Blood Pressure,** The 1984 report, Arch Intern Med 144:1045, 1984.

11. **Report of the U.S. Preventive Services Task Force,** *Guide to Clinical Preventive Services, U.S. Department of Health and Human Services*, 1989.

12. **Belloc NB,** Relationship of health practices to mortality, Prev Med 2:67, 1973.

13. **William EI,** Characteristics of patients aged over 75 not seen during one year in general practice, Brit Med J 288:119, 1984.

14. **Kennie DC, Warshaw G,** in Reichel, W, editor, *Clinical Aspects of Aging*, Williams & Wilkins, Baltimore, 3rd edition, 1989, pp 13–25.

15. **Eaker ED, Packard B, Wenger NK, Clarkson TB, Tyroler HA,** *Coronary Heart Disease in Women*, Haymarket Doyma Inc, New York, 1987.

16. **Kannel WB,** Metabolic risk factors for coronary heart disease in women: Perspective from the Framingham Study, Am Heart J 114:413, 1987.

17. **National Heart, Lung and Blood Institute,** Hypertension prevalence and the status of awareness, treatment and control in the United States, Hypertension Vol 7, 1985.

18. **Kannel WB, Castelli WP, Gordon T,** Serum cholesterol lipoproteins and risk of coronary heart disease, Ann Intern Med 74:1, 1971.

19. **Castelli WP, Garrison RJ, Wilson PWF, Abbott RD, Kalousdian S, Kannel WB,** Incidence of cornary heart disease and lipoprotein cholesterol levels, JAMA 256:2835, 1986.

20. **Bush TL, Barrett-Connor E, Cown LD, et al,** Cardiovascular mortality and noncontraceptive use of estrogen in women: Results from the Lipid Research Clinics' program follow-up study, Circulation 75:1102, 1987.

21. **Burnner D, Weisbort J, Meshulam N, et al,** Relation of serum total cholesterol and high-density lipoprotein cholesterol percentage to the incidence of definite coronary events: Twenty year follow-up of the Donolo-Tel Aviv Prospective Coronary Artery Disease Study, Am J Cardiol 591:1271, 1987.

22. **The National Cholesterol Education Program, National Heart, Lung, and Blood Institute,** Report of the national cholesterol education program expert panel on detection, evaluation, and treatment of high blood cholesterol in adults, Arch Intern Med 148:36, 1988.

23. **Grundy SM, Goodman DW, Rifkind BM, Cleeman JI,** The place of HDL in cholesterol management. A perspective from the National Cholesterol Educational Program, Arch Intern Med 149:505, 1989.

24. **Crouse JR III,** Gender, lipoproteins, diet, and cardiovascular risk, Lancet i:318, 1989.

25. **Willett WC, Hennekens CH, Bain C, et al,** Cigarette smoking in non-myocardial infarction, Am J Epidemiol 113:375, 1981.

26. **Willett WC, Green A, Stampfer MJ, et al,** Relative and absolute excess risk of coronary heart disease among women who smoke cigarettes, New Engl J Med 317:1303, 1987.

27. **Mattson ME, Boyd G, Byar D, Brown C, Callahan JF, Corle D, Cullen JW, Greenblatt J, Haley NJ, Hammond SK, Lewtas J, Reeves W,** Passive smoking on commercial airline flights, JAMA 261:867, 1989.

28. **Curfman GD, Thomas GS, Paffenbarger RS,** Physical activity in primary prevention of cardiovascular disease, Cardiol Clinics 3:203, 1985.

29. **Cauley JA, La Porte RE, Sandler RB, Orchard TJ, Slemenda CW, Petrini AM,** The relationship of physical activity to high density lipoprotein cholesterol in postmenopausal women, J Chron Dis 39:687, 1986.

30. **Jones NL, Makides L, Hitchcock C, et al,** Normal standards for an incremental progressive cycle ergometer test, Am Rev Respir Dis 131:700, 1985.

31. **Idiculla AA, Goldberg G,** Physical fitness for the mature woman, Med Clin No Am 71:135, 1987.

32. **Larson EB, Bruce RA,** Health benefits of exercise in an aging society, Arch Intern Med 147:353, 1987.

33. **Rippe JM, Ward A, Porcari JP, Freedson PS,** Walking for health and fitness, JAMA 259:2720, 1988.

34. **Barrett-Connor E,** Obesity, atherosclerosis, and coronary artery disease, Ann Intern Med 103:1010, 1985.

35. **Silverberg E, Lubera J,** Cancer statistics, 1989, CA 39:3, 1989.

36. **Mandelblatt JS, Fahs MC,** The cost-effectiveness of cervical cancer screening for low income elderly women, JAMA 259:2409, 1988.

37. **Friedman GD, Collen MM, Fireman EH,** Multi-phasic health check up evaluation: A sixteen year follow-up, J Chron Dis 39:453, 1986.

38. **Fleischer DE, Goldberg SB, Browning TH, Cooper JN, Friedman E, Goldner FH, Keeffe EB, Smith LE,** Detection and surveillance of colorectal cancer, JAMA 261:580, 1989.

39. **Rubenstein LZ,** Falls in the elderly: A clinical approach, West J Med 138:273, 1983.

40. **Stults BM,** Preventive health care for the elderly, West J Med 141:832, 1984.

41. **Ostrom JR, Hammarlund ER, Christensen DB, Plein JB, Keithley AJ,** Medication use in the elderly poplation, Med Care 23:157, 1985.

42. **Wandless I, et al,** Compliance with prescribed medications: A study of elderly patients in the community. J Roy College Gen Pract 29:391, 1979.

43. **Robuschi G, Safran M, Braverman LE, Gnudi A, Roti E,** Hypothyroidism in the elderly, Endocrine Rev 8:142, 1987.

44. **Tinetti ME, Speechley M,** Prevention of falls among the elderly, New Engl J Med 320:1055, 1989.

45. **Salomon G,** Hearing problems and the elderly, Danish Med Bull 33:Suppl 3, 1986.

46. **Farquahr JW,** *The American Way of Life Need Not Be Hazardous to Your Health*, Addison-Wesley Publishing Co., Inc., Reading, MA, 1987.

4

The Cholesterol-Lipoprotein Profile: A Risk Factor for Cardiovascular Disease

Cardiovascular diseases are the predominant cause of death in American women, accounting for about 500,000 deaths per year. Fifty percent of American women die from atherosclerotic diseases, primarily myocardial infarction and stroke. Coronary heart disease alone accounts for nearly 28% of all deaths in women. Twice as many women die of cardiovascular disease than cancer, and the number of deaths due to cardiovascular disease far exceeds those due to gynecologic cancers. (1)

Although coronary heart disease is uncommon in premenopausal women, after the menopause, women develop coronary disease at the same rate as men, but 6–10 years later. (2) Most epidemiologic studies of cardiovascular disease as well as intervention trials have studied middle aged to older men. It is now apparent, however, that the major risk factors identified for men are shared by women, although there are some important sex-related differences.

Lipoproteins and Cholesterol

Cholesterol is the basic building block in steroidogenesis. All steroid-producing organs except the placenta can synthesize cholesterol from acetate. Progestins, androgens, and estrogens, therefore, can be synthesized in situ from the 2-carbon acetate molecule via cholesterol as the common steroid precursor. However, the major resource is blood cholesterol, which can be inserted into the biosynthetic pathway or stored in esterified form for later use. The cellular entry of cholesterol is mediated via a cell membrane receptor for low-density lipoprotein (LDL), the bloodstream carrier for cholesterol.

Lipoproteins are large molecules that facilitate the transport of nonpolar fats in a polar solvent, the blood plasma. There are 5 major categories of lipoproteins according to their charge and density (flotation during ultracentrifugation). They are derived from each other in the following cascade of decreasing size and increasing density:

Chylomicrons. Large, cholesterol (10%) and triglyceride (90%) carrying particles formed in the intestine after a fatty meal.

59

Very Low-Density Lipoproteins (VLDL). Also carry cholesterol, but mostly triglycerides; more dense than chylomicrons.

Intermediate-Density Lipoproteins (IDL). Formed from VLDL (for a transient existence) by the removal of some of the triglyceride from the interior of the VLDL particle.

Low-Density Lipoproteins (LDL). The end products of VLDL catabolism, formed after further removal of triglyceride leaving approximately 50% cholesterol; the major carriers (⅔) of cholesterol in the plasma and thus a strong relationship exists between elevated LDL levels and cardiovascular disease.

High-Density Lipoproteins (HDL). The smallest and most dense of the lipoproteins with the highest protein and phospholipid content; HDL levels are inversely associated with atherosclerosis (high levels are protective).

The lipoproteins contain 4 ingredients: 1) cholesterol in two forms: free cholesterol on the surface of the spherical lipoprotein molecule, and esterified cholesterol in the molecule's interior; 2) triglycerides in the interior of the sphere; 3) phospholipids; and 4) protein: electrically charged substances on the surface of the sphere and responsible for miscibility with plasma. The surface proteins, called *apoproteins*, constitute the sites which bind to the lipoprotein receptor molecules on the cell surfaces. The principal protein of LDL is apoprotein B, and apoprotein A-I is the principal apoprotein of HDL. These protein moieties of the lipoprotein particles are strongly related to the risk of cardiovascular disease, and genetic abnormalities in their synthesis or structure can result in atherogenic conditions. (3)

The distribution of the lipoproteins within the LDL and HDL categories indicates subpeaks or subfractions. HDL_2 is a fraction with more lipid than protein, and with less density. HDL_2 is strongly associated with cardiovascular disease.

The lipoproteins are a major reason for the disparity in arteriosclerosis risk between men and women. Throughout adulthood, the blood HDL-cholesterol level is about 10 mg/dl higher in women, and this difference continues through the postmenopausal years. Total and LDL-cholesterol levels are lower in premenopausal women than in men, but after menopause they rise rapidly.

LDL is removed from the blood by organ (mainly liver) receptors which recognize one of the surface apoproteins. The liver is the favored site for this process because it contains the largest number of LDL receptors as well as a unique high-affinity receptor for one of the apoproteins, apoprotein E. The lipoprotein bound to the cell membrane receptor is internalized and degradated. The number of LDL receptors in liver cells is increased (up regulated) when the concentration of intracellular cholesterol declines, and decreased (down regulated) when intracellular cholesterol increases. This explains why excessive dietary cholesterol can increase the circulating levels of cholesterol.

When LDL receptors are saturated or deficient, LDL is taken up by "scavenger" cells (most likely derived from macrophages) in other tissues, most notably the arterial intima. Thus these cells can become the nidus for atherosclerotic plaques.

The protective nature of HDL is due to its ability to pick up free cholesterol from cells or other circulating lipoproteins. In so doing, HDL acquires apoprotein E and this apoprotein E-rich, lipid-rich HDL is known as HDL_c. Thus HDL converts lipid-rich scavenger cells back to their low-lipid state, and carries the excess cholesterol to sites (mainly liver) where it can be metabolized.

Another method by which HDL removes cholesterol from the body focuses on the uptake of free cholesterol from cell membranes. The free cholesterol is esterified and moves to the core of the HDL particle. This lipid-rich particle is the HDL_2 subfraction. Thus both HDL_2 and HDL_c can remove cholesterol by delivering cholesterol to sites for utilization (steroid-producing cells) or metabolism and excretion (liver).

Understanding the role of the cell surface receptors for the homeostasis of cholesterol, the work of the 1985 Nobel laureates M.S. Brown and J.L. Goldstein, revolutionized our concepts of cholesterol, lipoprotein metabolism, and hormonal action at the cell membrane. (4) In their Nobel lecture, Brown and Goldstein paid tribute to cholesterol as the most highly decorated small molecule in biology.

The Normal Cholesterol/Lipoprotein Profile

Total cholesterol	— Less than 200 mg/dl
HDL-cholesterol	— Greater than 35 mg/dl
LDL-cholesterol	— Less than 130 mg/dl
Triglycerides	— Less than 250 mg/dl

The relationship between cholesterol levels and death from cardiovascular disease is strong and continuous, i.e., increasing risk with increasing levels. (5) Levels of cholesterol less than 200 mg/dl are associated with a lower risk of atherosclerosis. When LDL-cholesterol levels are below 100 mg/dl (equivalent to an approximate total cholesterol level of 170 mg/dl), heart attacks are rare. LDL-cholesterol levels rise above 100 mg/dl only in people who eat a diet rich in saturated animal fats and cholesterol. Cholesterol, smoking, and hypertension are additive or even multiplicative risk factors for coronary heart disease. Adding one of these risk factors to the other decreases the age at which a critical degree of coronary atherosclerosis is achieved by about 10 years. (6)

An important NIH angiographic study demonstrated that lowering of total cholesterol levels and improving the ratio of total cholesterol to HDL correlated with lack of progression of coronary atherosclerosis. (7) In a clinical trial using cholestyramine to lower LDL levels in men, there was a 2% decrease in risk of first heart attacks for every 1% fall in total cholesterol levels. (8,9) The benefit could be attributed to both a lowering of LDL-cholesterol and an increase in HDL levels.

The Framingham Study report confirmed that total cholesterol and HDL-cholesterol levels are strongly related to the development of cardiovascular disease in both men and women. (10) An important observation in this report was the recognition that at all levels of total cholesterol (including those below 200 mg/dl) HDL-cholesterol showed a strong inverse association with the incidence of cardiovascular disease.

For good cardiovascular health, the blood concentration of cholesterol must be kept low and its escape from the bloodstream must be prevented. The problem of cholesterol transport is solved by esterifying the cholesterol and packaging the ester within the cores of plasma lipoproteins. The delivery of cholesterol to cells is in turn solved by lipoprotein receptors. After binding the lipoprotein with its package of esterified cholesterol, the complex is delivered into the cell by receptor-mediated endocytosis, where the lysosomes liberate cholesterol for use by the cell.

Major protection against atherosclerosis depends upon the high affinity of the receptor for LDL and the ability of the receptor to recycle multiple times, thus allowing large amounts of cholesterol to be delivered while maintaining a healthy low blood level of LDL. Cells can control their uptake of cholesterol by increasing or decreasing the number of LDL receptors according to the intracellular cholesterol levels.

There are 3 important clinical points:

1. Atherosclerotic disease is related to increased LDL and decreased HDL-cholesterol concentrations.

2. Lowering LDL levels and raising HDL levels can reduce the incidence of atherosclerotic disease.

3. Atherosclerosis is not a disease limited to aging people. It begins in early childhood, and its manifestation later in life can be influenced by health care behavior during younger years.

Risk Factors for CV Disease

Risk factors for cardiovascular disease include the following:

1. Cigarette smoking.

2. Hypertension.

3. Diabetes mellitus.

4. Low HDL-cholesterol.

5. Significant obesity.

6. Age.

7. Family history of premature coronary heart disease.

8. Cerebrovascular or peripheral vascular disease.

9. Sedentary lifestyle.

In addition, the cholesterol-lipoprotein profile is significantly related to the risk of cardiovascular disease, and this profile undergoes considerable change after menopause. Coronary heart disease rates increase tenfold for women 55 years or older compared to women 35 to 54 years old. (11) In women, blood lipids, including total cholesterol, LDL-cholesterol, and VLDL-cholesterol, rise with age. Total cholesterol levels in 20–30 year old women are generally less than 200 mg/dl. Between 45 and 55 years of age, average cholesterol levels in U.S. women increase sharply to above 230 mg/dl, and after age 55, are often greater than 240 mg/dl. The LDL-cholesterol averages about 10 mg/dl lower in women than in men ages 50–54, and thereafter, the LDL-cholesterol level exceeds those for men through ages 75–79.

Nine prospective studies have documented the strong association between total cholesterol and coronary heart disease in women. (11–15) Coronary heart disease risk appears at higher total cholesterol levels for women than for men. Women with total cholesterol concentrations greater than 265 mg/dl have rates of coronary heart disease 3 times those of women with low levels. Even in elderly women, a high total cholesterol remains a significant predictor of heart disease.

Risk of Coronary Heart Disease: The Framingham Study (5)

Total Cholesterol	Age-Adjusted Rate per 1000			
	Men		Women	
	Ages 35–64	65–94	35–64	65–94
84–204 mg/dl	8	22	4	11
205–234	13	24	5	15
235–264	14	26	4	17
265–294	15	23	7	17
>294	26	38	10	21

The strongest predictor of coronary heart disease in women is a low HDL-cholesterol. The average HDL-cholesterol in women is approximately 55 mg/dl, about 10 mg/dl higher than in men. A decrease in HDL-cholesterol of 10 mg/dl increases coronary heart disease risk by 40–50%. Women with very high HDL-cholesterol levels (over 55–60 mg/dl) have virtually no increased risk of heart disease even in the presence of elevated concentrations of total cholesterol. In some studies, elevated LDL-cholesterol has been identified as a predictor of coronary heart disease in women, but in others it has not. It should be emphasized that modest elevations in blood pressure markedly increase the risk associated with an elevated LDL-cholesterol or a low HDL-cholesterol.

Triglycerides are also an important risk factor for coronary heart disease in women. If the triglyceride level is greater than 250 mg/dl and the HDL-cholesterol is less than 45 mg/dl, the risk of heart disease is substantially increased. Patients with an elevated triglyceride level and a positive family history for heart disease most likely have an autosomal dominant disorder classified as familial combined hyperlipidemia. This disorder accounts for most myocardial infarctions in women less than 40 years old. (2)

The proportion of HDL-cholesterol in the total cholesterol decreases with age in women and results in an age-related increase in the ratio of total cholesterol to HDL-cholesterol, from 3.4 at ages 25–34 years to 4.7 at ages 75–89 years. When the ratio exceeds 7.5, women have the same coronary heart disease risk as men. The optimal ratio is about 3.5, and risk increases significantly above 5.0. *For ease of remembering, consider anything below 4.5 as good and any ratio above 4.5 as unhealthy.*

It should be remembered, however, that a low HDL-cholesterol and a high total cholesterol are independent risk factors. Each needs to be considered independently in evaluating risk and treatment in women.

Risk of Coronary Heart Disease over the Age of 50: The Framingham Study (13)

Cholesterol/HDL Ratio	Age-Adjusted Rate per 1000	
	Men	Women
Less than 3.5	70	34
3.5–5.4	95	56
5.5–7.4	152	78
7.5–9.4	176	171
Greater than 9.5	275	281

Although the risk of coronary heart disease in women appears to occur at higher levels of total cholesterol compared to men, the National Cholesterol Education Program and the National Cholesterol Consensus Conference have concluded that the same levels of total cholesterol and HDL-cholesterol should be used in assigning risk in both women and men. (16)

Sex Hormones and the Lipid Profile

Women have low rates of coronary heart disease during the premenopausal years, and subsequently after menopause have an increase in coronary disease and death with advancing age. In addition, early menopause (natural or surgical) increases the risk of coronary heart disease in young women. This obviously points to an important role for the hormone changes associated with menopause. The cholesterol profile is linked to testosterone and estrogen dominance in men and women. Total cholesterol and LDL-cholesterol are higher in men than in premenopausal women, while HDL-cholesterol levels are 6–10 mg/dl higher in women prior to menopause.

Nevertheless, observational studies and clinical trials indicate that the major determinants of blood lipid levels are the same for both sexes. A diet high in saturated fatty acids and dietary cholesterol unfavorably increases blood lipids. Excessive caloric intake and obesity decrease HDL-cholesterol and increase total cholesterol, LDL-cholesterol, and triglycerides. Smoking decreases HDL-cholesterol (and also produces lower estrogen levels and an earlier menopause). Finally, genetic defects of receptor-mediated cholesterol uptake account for only a small percentage of hyperlipidemia in men and women.

The cessation of estrogen secretion at the time of menopause correlates with a moderate increase in total and LDL-cholesterol, while

64

at the same time, HDL-cholesterol decreases. Thus estrogen deficiency is associated with an adverse profile in terms of risk for cardiovascular disease. The protective effect of estrogen treatment is discussed in Chapter 5.

Clinical Guidelines

A U.S. consensus has been reached regarding the evaluation and treatment of elevated cholesterol levels. (16,17) This strategy is heavily influenced by the fact that the American population has a high average total cholesterol level induced largely by the dietary intake of saturated fat and cholesterol.

1. Every woman 20 years and older should learn her total cholesterol level as a routine part of an encounter with a health professional.

2. A total cholesterol less than 200 mg/dl indicates a low risk. Re-screening should be performed in 5 years.

3. A total cholesterol of 240 mg/dl or greater indicates significant risk of cardiovascular disease. Immediate relatives, including parents, siblings, and children, should also be tested.

4. A total cholesterol in the range of 200–239 mg/dl is considered borderline. Estimation of risk must include consideration of other factors, including low HDL-cholesterol, hypertension, smoking, diabetes mellitus, family history of premature cardiovascular disease, obesity, and presence of peripheral vascular disease.

5. Total cholesterol from 200 to 239 mg/dl along with two other associated risk factors indicates increased risk of cardiovascular disease.

6. Total cholesterol above 200 mg/dl on two occasions requires a fasting lipid profile to estimate the HDL-cholesterol and calculate the LDL-cholesterol.

7. HDL-cholesterol less than 35 mg/dl indicates high risk for cardiovascular disease.

8. LDL-cholesterol greater than 160 mg/dl indicates high risk for cardiovascular disease.

9. LDL-cholesterol from 130 to 159 mg/dl along with two other associated risk factors indicates increased risk for cardiovascular disease.

10. Triglyceride levels in the range of 250–500 mg/dl require treatment only when associated with a strong family history of coronary heart disease, an elevated LDL-cholesterol, or a low HDL-cholesterol. Levels greater than 500 mg/dl deserve drug treatment; there is a definite risk of pancreatitis.

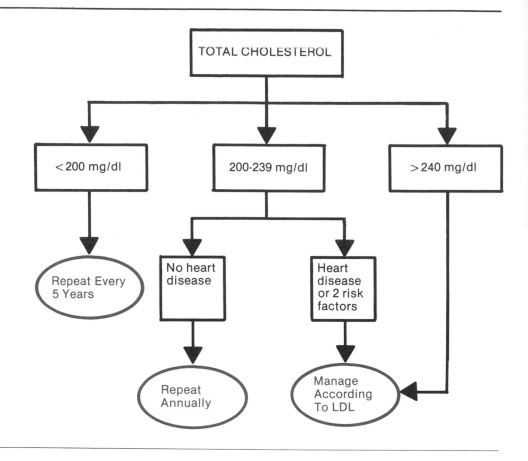

Because HDL-cholesterol is such an important predictor in women, the following information is important. If the ratio of total cholesterol to HDL-cholesterol is greater than 4.5, intervention is required. If the ratio is unfavorable and the LDL-cholesterol is 160 mg/dl or greater, drug treatment is indicated. Some would argue that the HDL-cholesterol level in women should be at least 45 mg/dl.

If the LDL-cholesterol is 160 mg/dl or greater, intervention is necessary, and if other risk factors are present, the goal should be to lower the LDL-cholesterol to under 130 mg/dl. When the HDL-cholesterol level is 55 mg/dl or greater, only those women with very high LDL-cholesterol levels (greater than 190 mg/dl) or with a strong family history should be treated.

Clinical trials in men have definitely shown that the risk of coronary heart disease can be altered by lowering the total cholesterol level. It is likely that similar results will be obtained in women by modifying the cholesterol-lipoprotein profile. However, it will take considerable time to accumulate this evidence. In the meantime, clinicians must make decisions now. It is our opinion that the U.S. national guidelines should be applied to women. A more conservative approach in proceeding from diet modification to drug therapy may be appropriate, reserving drug therapy only for those women at highest risk.

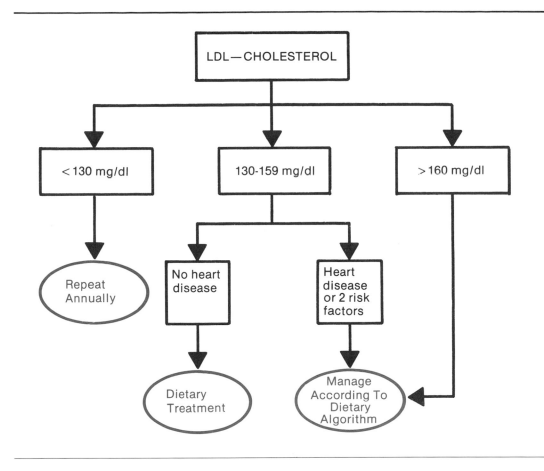

Other Causes for Hypercholesterolemia. Remember that other conditions can cause secondary hyperlipoproteinemia. These include hypothyroidism, nephrotic syndrome, diabetes mellitus, obstructive liver disease, and some drugs, especially anabolic steroids. Therefore, the evaluation of hypercholesterolemia should include a complete blood count, urinalysis, routine blood chemistries, and a screen of thyroid function.

We have sufficient evidence to recommend treatment of women with hypercholesterolemia. In those women with an elevated total cholesterol and LDL-cholesterol, diet therapy should be initiated and the effects periodically assessed. Patients with an abnormal cholesterol-lipoprotein profile combined with other risk factors, or combined with a poor cholesterol/HDL-cholesterol ratio should be considered for drug treatment.

Diet Treatment. The American Heart Association Step I diet consists of:

Fat: total not to exceed more than 30% of the daily caloric intake (the current U.S. fat intake is about 40%), with saturated fat less than 10% of calories. Fat intake should consist of equal proportions of monounsaturated and polyunsaturated fat.

Cholesterol: less than 250–300 mg/day.

Carbohydrates: 55% of daily caloric intake.

Proteins: 15% of daily caloric intake.

Intervention studies have demonstrated that diet modification can significantly reduce the levels of total cholesterol and LDL-cholesterol. (18,19) For individuals whose LDL-cholesterol levels remain elevated despite the Step I diet, the more vigorous Step II diet is recommended in which the daily intake of cholesterol is limited to less than 200 mg/day and saturated fats are limited to less than 7% of calories. Expert help from a dietitian will be necessary for effective implementation of the Step II diet.

The nature of the fat intake is also important. Keep in mind that there is no requirement for cholesterol or saturated fat; the body can make all it needs. Women who consume a low polyunsaturated to saturated fat ratio (approximately 0.3) demonstrate a decrease in HDL-cholesterol levels. When the ratio of polyunsaturated fat to saturated fat approximates 1.0, no significant change occurs in HDL-cholesterol.

Saturated Fats. Saturated fats are fats which are generally solid at room temperature. They increase LDL-cholesterol, and consist of animal fats, butterfat products, and the following vegetable oils: coconut, cocoa, palm, palm kernel, and other vegetable oils when they are hydrogenated. Saturated fats in the diet are the most important determinant of the circulating LDL-cholesterol level. Many foods promoted as containing no cholesterol contain saturated fats.

Monounsaturated Fats. Monounsaturated fats have no significant impact on the cholesterol profile (a slight decrease in LDL-cholesterol), and consist mainly of olive oil and peanut oil.

Polyunsaturated Fats. The polyunsaturated fats are the essential fatty acids; they reduce cholesterol and LDL-cholesterol. Most vegetable oils are polyunsaturated fats, including soybean, cottonseed, corn, sunflower, and safflower.

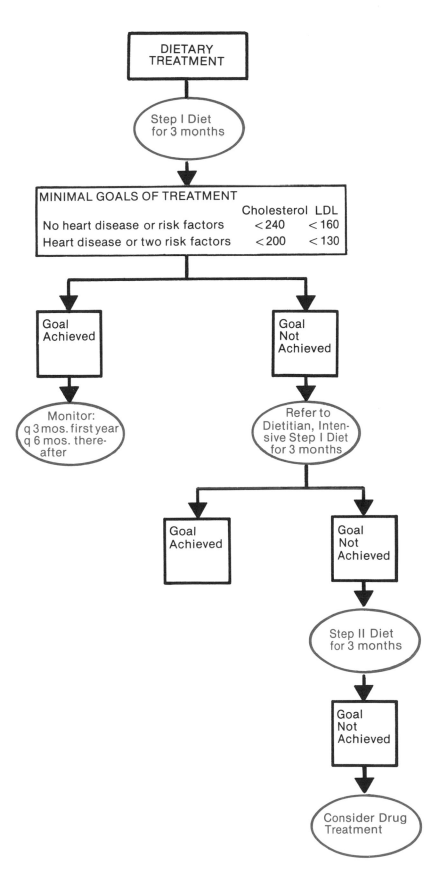

DIETARY TREATMENT

Step I Diet for 3 months

MINIMAL GOALS OF TREATMENT

	Cholesterol	LDL
No heart disease or risk factors	< 240	< 160
Heart disease or two risk factors	< 200	< 130

Goal Achieved

Goal Not Achieved

Monitor: q 3 mos. first year q 6 mos. thereafter

Refer to Dietitian, Intensive Step I Diet for 3 months

Goal Achieved

Goal Not Achieved

Step II Diet for 3 months

Goal Not Achieved

Consider Drug Treatment

Fish Oils. Fish oils are a special class of polyunsaturated fats, and they lower cholesterol and triglyccridcs.

Most diets designed to lower cholesterol levels must limit butterfat; milk fat contributes more to the increase in cholesterol than other fats because of the high amount of saturated fatty acids in milk. Whole milk contains about 45% of calories as fat. Low fat milk (2%) still has 30% of calories as fat. Only skim milk (nonfat milk) does not contain excessive concentrations of fat. Most cheeses are very high in fat and even low fat cheeses contain high concentrations of saturated fatty acids. Of course eggs are a problem; an egg yolk contains the entire daily allowance of cholesterol (250–300 mg). While chicken and turkey contain less saturated fatty acids, the skin of these birds is high in undesirable fat, and unfortunately, fast food chicken preparations (chicken nuggets) contain significant amounts of skin.

To substitute for the decrease in fat, more fruits, vegetables, and grains should be eaten. Avocados and nuts are high in fat, but it is unsaturated fat with little impact on cholesterol. The unacceptable saturated fats include butter, lard, tallow and plant oils such as coconut oil and palm oil. A Mediterranean type of diet limits the frequency of coronary heart disease: olive oil on the salads, pastas, fish, vegetables, and grains.

Clinical evidence indicates that soluble and insoluble fiber, oat bran, or psyllium (1 teasp tid) lower total and LDL-cholesterol 5–15%. They can be recommended as useful adjuvants in patients not responding to diet alone before proceeding to drug treatment.

Drug Treatment. A maximal effort at dietary therapy should be initiated prior to drug treatment, and should be continued even if drug treatment is required. There are 3 situations which are most likely to respond to lipid-lowering drugs:

1. An LDL-cholesterol level at 160 mg/dl or greater in the presence of coronary disease.

2. An LDL-cholesterol level at 160 mg/dl or greater in the presence of two other risk factors.

3. A cholesterol/HDL-cholesterol ratio greater than 4.5 or an LDL-cholesterol at 190 mg/dl or greater.

Drugs for consideration include bile acid sequestrants (cholestyramine and colestipol), nicotinic acid (niacin), HMG CoA reductase inhibitors, and gemfibrozil. Considerable patient education is necessary to achieve and maintain good compliance.

We have considered 5 important features in making recommendations about these drugs: lipid-modifying effects, proven efficacy, long-term safety, convenience, and side effects. The bile acid sequestrants and niacin are considered the drugs of first choice. Both cholestyramine and niacin have been shown to lower coronary heart disease risk in clinical trials with men, and their long-term safety has been established. Lovastatin acts as an HMG CoA reductase inhibitor and dramatically lowers LDL-cholesterol; however, the effect on actual

Lipid-Lowering Drugs

Drug	Dosage	Action	Side Effects
Cholestyramine Colestipol	8–12 g bid 10–15 g bid	Bind bile and increase LDL receptors	GI distress, nausea, constipation
Niacin	0.5–1.5 g bid	Inhibits secretion of lipoproteins	Flushing, skin rash, GI distress, hepatic dysfunction
Lovastatin	20–40 g bid	Inhibits cholesterol synthesis	GI distress, insomnia, hepatitis
Gemfibrozil	600 mg bid	Increases VLDL breakdown	Hepatic dysfunction

coronary disease and the long-term safety have not been established, and cost is an important consideration. One of the major mechanisms by which gemfibrozil lowers coronary heart disease mortality is its action to raise HDL-cholesterol levels. It is an important drug to consider when treating patients with an elevated LDL-cholesterol and a low HDL-cholesterol, or if one is treating a patient with high triglycerides. The long-term (lifelong) tolerance of the newer drugs is not yet certain.

Specific Lipid Effects and Potency

Drug	LDL-Cholesterol	HDL-Cholesterol	Triglycerides
Bile sequestrants	15–25% decrease	5% increase	10% increase
Niacin	15–20% decrease	30–35% increase	25–30% decrease
Lovastatin	20–45% decrease	10% increase	20% decrease
Gemfibrozil	15% decrease	15–20% increase	35–50% decrease

The bile acid resins and gemfibrozil have approximately equivalent LDL-cholesterol lowering effects, while lovastatin is about twice as effective. Niacin and gemfibrozil increase HDL-cholesterol the most, lovastatin has an intermediate effect, and the bile sequestrants have a modest effect. Niacin, gemfibrozil, and lovastatin all lower triglycerides, but the binding resins elevate triglycerides. The drugs can be used in combination, except for gemfibrozil with lovastatin (there has been a 5% incidence of acute myositis).

Bile Acid Sequestrants. Bile acid sequestrants should be considered for patients with elevated cholesterol and normal triglycerides. The drugs are not absorbed into the blood stream, and thus they bind bile acids in the small intestine. This in turn stimulates the production of new bile acids which consume intrahepatic cholesterol. The liver responds to the decrease in intracellular cholesterol by making more cell surface receptors to remove cholesterol from the blood. Cholestyramine and colestipol are equally effective, achieving maximal results when taken before or immediately after meals. About 10% of patients experience the major side effect, constipation. The drugs may also cause heartburn, abdominal discomfort, bloating and belching, diarrhea, nausea, and vomiting, but the side effects decrease with continued use. A stool softener should be prescribed for the initial treatment period. Bile acid sequestrants interfere with the absorption of other drugs, and other medication should be taken 1 hour before or 4 hours after these drugs. Cholesterol lowering effects can be seen in as little as 3 weeks, but the optimal effects usually occur in 6–8 weeks.

Nicotinic Acid (Niacin). Niacin (vitamin B_3) can be used for high cholesterols with or without elevated triglycerides. High doses inhibit the release of fatty acids from fat tissues and decrease the liver secretion of triglyceride-rich VLDL. Niacin is an "over the counter" medication, available in tablets containing 50, 100, 250, and 500 mg which must be taken tid. Timed release capsules containing 250, 400, and 500 mg can be taken bid. The drug must be initiated in low doses with a gradual titration to higher doses. The usual starting dose is 100 mg tid, followed by a weekly increase of 50–100 mg until the usual lipid-lowering dose of 1500–2000 mg per day is reached. The maximal dose is considered to be 6000 mg per day. Utilizing this program, it may take 3 months to reach therapeutic level. Side effects are common, but none is permanent or irreversible. The most common side effect, prostaglandin-mediated skin flushing, occurs 30–60 minutes after taking the drug. This can be minimized by taking the medication after meals and adding a single aspirin tablet 15–30 minutes before each dose. After several months, flushing tends to disappear. If several doses are missed, the patient may need to return to lower doses and build up to the regular level. The time release capsules are associated with less flushing but more gastrointestinal side effects. Other side effects include a rise in blood sugar and uric acid, and abnormalities in liver function; all require periodic monitoring. The drug should not be given to patients with diabetes, gout, peptic ulcer disease (which can be aggravated), or liver disease. Other minor side effects include pruritus, skin rashes, fatigue, abdominal pain, anorexia, nausea, and vomiting.

Lovastatin. Lovastatin inhibits the cholesterol synthesizing enzyme, thus depleting intrahepatic cholesterol concentrations, stimulating the liver to extract more cholesterol from the blood stream. An asymptomatic increase in liver enzymes occurs in 2% of patients. All patients must have baseline liver function tests, and liver function should be monitored every 4–6 weeks during the first year of treatment and periodically thereafter. Lovastatin should not be given to patients with liver disease or to women who plan on becoming pregnant or to women who are breast feeding (animal studies with large doses have demonstrated teratogenicity). The observation of cataracts in beagle dogs taking large doses of lovastatin has led to the recommendation that patients undergo slit examination of the lens annually. The most common side effects are flatulence, diarrhea, and sleep disorders. The usual starting dose is 20 mg with dinner, gradually increased to 20–40 mg bid.

Gemfibrozil. Gemfibrozil, a fibric acid derivative, can have a dramatic effect on triglycerides, lowering them by as much as 40% while increasing HDL-cholesterol. The drug increases the clearance of VLDL from the blood and the secretion of cholesterol into bile. The drug is very easy to take with infrequent side effects. The most common side effects are abdominal pain, diarrhea, nausea, vomiting, and gas. The drug should not be used in patients with kidney or liver disease, and probably not in patients known to have gall stones. Periodic monitoring of the liver and the complete blood count is recommended.

**Other
Factors**

Other factors which should not be underrated include obesity, exercise, and smoking. Obesity has an adverse effect on the cholesterol-lipoprotein profile, and the treatment program should include caloric restriction and exercise in order to achieve ideal body weight. Although some studies have found no effect of exercise, in general women runners have lower total cholesterol and LDL-cholesterol levels and higher HDL-cholesterol. (20) An adverse impact on the lipoprotein profile is only one of the many detrimental effects of smoking. (21)

**Monitoring the
Profile**

In order to monitor the impact of interventions or drug therapy, a periodic assessment of the cholesterol-lipoprotein profile is necessary. It is important to recognize that in some laboratories, total cholesterol may vary by as much as 10%, and HDL-cholesterol even more. One must be conservative in making decisions about whether the lipids are being affected. Furthermore, a long period of observation is necessary for an accurate appraisal. We believe that it is worthwhile to measure the fasting cholesterol-lipoprotein profile on an annual basis.

References

1. **Vital Statistics of the United States, 1981,** Mortality, Part A, The National Center for Health Statistics, Hyattsville, Maryland, 1986.

2. **Castelli, WP,** Cardiovascular disease in women, Am J Obstet Gynecol, 158:1553, 1988.

3. **Freedman DS, Srinivasan SR, Shear CL, Franklin FA, Webber LS, Berenson GS,** The relation of apolipoproteins A-I and B in children to parental myocardial infarction, New Engl J Med 315:721, 1986.

4. **Brown MS, Goldstein JL,** A receptor-mediated pathway for cholesterol homeostasis, Science 232:34, 1986.

5. **Stamler J, Wentworth D, Neaton JD,** Is relationship between serum cholesterol and risk of premature death from coronary heart disease continuous and graded? JAMA 256:2823, 1986.

6. **Grundy SM,** Cholesterol and coronary heart disease, JAMA 256:2849, 1986.

7. **Levy RI, Brensike JF, Epstein SE, et al,** The influence of changes in lipid values induced by cholestyramine and diet on progression of coronary artery disease: results of the NHLBI Type II coronary intervention study, Circulation 69:325, 1984.

8. **The Lipid Research Clinics Program,** The Lipid Research Clinics Coronary Primary Prevention Trial Results: I. Reduction in the incidence of coronary heart disease, JAMA 251:351, 1984.

9. **The Lipid Research Clinics Program,** The Lipid Research Clinics Coronary primary prevention trial results: II. The relationship of reduction in incidence of coronary heart disease to cholesterol lowering, JAMA 251:365, 1984.

10. **Casteli WP, Garrison RJ, Wilson PWF, Abbott RD, Kalousdian S, Kannel WB,** Incidence of coronary heart disease and lipoprotein cholesterol levels, JAMA 256:2835, 1986.

11. **Lerner DJ, Kannel WB,** Patterns of coronary heart disease morbidity and mortality in the sexes: A 26-year follow-up of the Framingham population, Am Heart J 111:383, 1988.

12. **Bush TL, Fried LP, Barrett-Connor E,** Cholesterol, lipoproteins, and coronary heart disease in women, Clin Chem 34:B60, 1988.

13. **Kannel WB,** Metabolic risk factors for coronary heart disease in women: Perspective from the Framingham Study, Am Heart J 114:413, 1987.

14. **Brunner D, Weisbort J, Meshulam N, Schwartz S, Gross J, Saltz-Rennert H, Alman S, Loebel K,** Relation to serum total cholesterol and high-density lipoprotein percentage to the incidence of definite coronary advance: Twenty-year follow-up of the Donolo Tel Aviv prospective coronary heart disease study, Am J Cardiol 59:1271, 1987.

15. **Focus on women and coronary heart disease: Lipids, sex hormones and risk,** Lipid Digest 2:12B, 1989.

16. **The National Cholesterol Education Program, National Heart, Lung, and Blood Institute,** Report of the National Cholesterol Education Program expert panel on detection, evaluation, and treatment of high blood cholesterol in adults, Arch Intern Med 148:36, 1988.

17. **Blum CB, Levy RI,** Current therapy for hypercholesterolemia, JAMA 261:3582, 1989.

18. **Ernst N, Fisher M, Bowen P, Schaefer J, Levy RI,** Changes in plasma lipids in lipoproteins after modified fat diet, Lancet ii:111, 1980.

19. **Jones BY, Judd JT, Taylor PR, Campbell WS, Nair PP,** Influence of caloric contribution in saturation of dietary fat on plasma lipids in premenopausal women, Am J Clin Nutr 45:1451, 1987.

20. **Wood PD, Haskell WL, Stern MP, Lewis S, Perry C,** Plasma lipoprotein distribution in male and female runners, Ann NY Acad Sci 301:748, 1977.

21. **Craig WY, Palomaki GE, Haddow HE,** Cigarette smoking and serum lipid and lipoprotein concentrations: an analysis of published data, Br Med J 298:784, 1989.

5 Menopause and Hormone Replacement

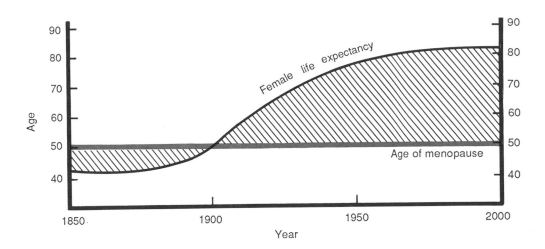

At approximately 40 years of age, the frequency of ovulation decreases. This initiates a period of waning ovarian function called the climacteric, which will last as long as 20 years, and will carry a woman through decreased fertility, menopause, and manifestations of progressive tissue atrophy and aging. The major factor in this evolving picture is the decrease in estrogen production associated with this period of life. A single point in time is the menopause, when insufficient ovarian follicle maturation results in inadequate estrogen and no menses.

Menopause occurs in American women between the ages 48 and 55, with the median age being approximately 50. (1) An earlier menopause is associated with cigarette smoking and living at high altitudes. (2) There is reason to believe that premature ovarian failure can occur in women who have previously undergone abdominal hysterectomy, presumably because ovarian vasculature has been compromised. (3) About 1% of women will experience menopause before the age of 40. (4) In contrast to a decline in the age of menarche during modern times, a review of medieval sources has indicated that the age of menopause has not changed significantly since early Greek days. (5)

The population of postmenopausal women is increasing. Current American census figures indicate that in the 1990's we will approach a figure of 40 million women over 50 years of age. An American woman at the age of 50 can expect to live another 30 years; therefore, women in our country now live approximately one-third of their lives after ovarian failure. The problems of the postmenopausal period, by virtue of the older population size alone, have achieved the status of a major public health concern.

There is a concern at the individual level as well. For some women, menopause signals the beginning of an era of aging with its connotations of diminishing abilities and competence. The menopause, however, should and can mark the beginning of a new and promising period of life, relatively free from previous obligations, ready for new career choices, more education, and new ventures. Good medical practice dictates that the concerned physician should support patients in a positive outlook for this period of time, a period of time which is growing in length and should be increasingly productive and rewarding.

"We are living in the bodies of our ancestors in a world they never dreamed would exist."

—Robert S. Eliot

Hormone Production After Menopause

Shortly after the menopause, one can safely say that there are no remaining ovarian follicles. (6) Prior to menopause, the remaining follicles begin to perform less well. During the perimenopausal period, women who are having regular periods can have lower estradiol levels and higher levels of FSH, and the cycle begins to change, mainly because of a shortening of the follicular phase. (7) This is a time period during which postmenopausal levels of FSH (greater than 40 mIU/ml) can be seen despite continued menstrual bleeding, while LH levels usually still remain in the normal range. It is likely that the elevated FSH levels reflect a declining regulation by the negative feedback action of a nonsteroidal substance produced by the granulosa cells, a peptide called inhibin. Occasionally corpus luteum formation and function occur, and the perimenopausal woman is not totally safe from the threat of an unplanned and unexpected pregnancy until elevated levels of both FSH and LH can be demonstrated. A woman from Portland, Oregon, holds the modern record for the oldest pregnancy, conceiving when 57 years and 120 days old.

As cycles become irregular, vaginal bleeding occurs at the end of an inadequate luteal phase or after a peak of estradiol without subsequent ovulation or corpus luteum formation. Eventually there is a 10–20-fold increase in FSH and approximately a 3-fold increase in LH, reaching a maximal level 1–3 years after menopause, after which there is a gradual, but slight, decline in both gonadotropins. Elevated levels of both FSH and LH at this time in life are conclusive evidence of ovarian failure. FSH levels are higher than LH because LH is cleared from the blood so much faster (half-lives are about 30 minutes for LH and 4 hours for FSH).

After menopause, the circulating level of androstenedione is about one half that seen prior to menopause. (8) Most of this postmenopausal androstenedione is derived from the adrenal gland, with only a small amount secreted from the ovary. Testosterone levels do not fall appreciably, and, in fact, the postmenopausal ovary in most women, but not all, secretes more testosterone than the premenopausal ovary. With the disappearance of follicles and estrogen, the elevated gonadotropins probably drive the remaining stromal tissue in the ovary to a level of increased testosterone secretion. The total amount of testosterone produced, however, is decreased because the amount of the primary source, peripheral conversion of androstenedione, is reduced.

The circulating estradiol level after menopause is approximately 10–20 pg/ml, most of which is derived from peripheral conversion of estrone. (8,9) The circulating level of estrone in postmenopausal women is higher than that of estradiol, the mean level being approximately 30–70 pg/ml. The average production rate of estrogen is approximately 45 μg/24 hours; almost all, if not all, being estrogen derived from the peripheral conversion of androstenedione. The androgen/estrogen ratio changes drastically after menopause because of the more marked decline in estrogen, and an onset of hirsutism is common, reflecting this marked shift in the sex hormone ratio. With increasing age, a decrease can be measured in the circulating levels of dehydroepiandrosterone (DHA) and its sulfate (DHAS), whereas the circulating postmenopausal levels of androstenedione, testosterone, and estrogen remain relatively constant.

Blood Production Rates of Steroids (10)

	Reproductive Age	Postmenopausal	Oophorectomized
Androstenedione	2–3 mg/day	0.5–1.0 mg/day	0.4–0.8 mg/day
Dehydroepiandrosterone	6–8	1.5–4.0	1.5-4.0
Dehydroepiandrosterone sulfate	8–16	4–9	4–9
Testosterone	0.2–0.25	0.05–0.1	0.02–0.07
Estrogen	0.350	0.045	0.045

Although estrogen does not wane in a straight line function, its progressive diminution over time leads to a sequential loss of estrogen-dependent functions: ovulation, menstrual function, vaginal and vulvar tissue strength, and finally, generalized atrophy of all estrogen-sensitive tissues.

This estrogen loss is due to the continued attrition in the numbers of residual follicle units in the 5th decade of life. Because fewer follicles are available, less and less estrogen production is possible. It must be remembered that these oldest follicle units have perhaps remained in the ovary unstimulated by gonadotropins not entirely by chance, but possibly due to their inherent refractoriness to otherwise appropriate gonadotropin stimulation. When these are finally activated, the degree of differentiation each is likely to experience is limited. Thus each follicle growth period will be increasingly blunted, with less estrogen produced. Eventually even the older and sluggish follicles are exhausted, and estrogen production is now at a low level, resulting almost entirely from indirect resources, the peripheral conversion in nonendocrine tissue sites of ovarian and adrenal precursors to active estrogen.

Estrogen production by the ovaries does not continue beyond the menopause; however, estrogen levels in postmenopausal women can be significant, principally due to the extraglandular conversion of androstenedione and testosterone to estrogen. The clinical impact of this estrogen will vary from one postmenopausal woman to another, depending upon the degree of extraglandular production, modified by a variety of factors.

77

The percent conversion of androstenedione to estrogen correlates with body weight. Increased production of estrogen from androstenedione with increasing body weight is probably due to the ability of fat to aromatize androgens. This fact and a decrease in the levels of sex hormone binding globulin (which results in increased free estrogen concentrations) are the basis for the well-known association between obesity and the development of endometrial cancer. Body weight, therefore, has a positive correlation with the circulating levels of estrone and estradiol. Aromatization of androgens to estrogens is not limited to adipose tissue, however, as almost every tissue tested has shown this activity.

Eventually, the ovarian stroma is exhausted and, despite huge reactive increments in FSH and LH, no further steroidogenesis of importance results from gonadal activity. With increasing age, the adrenal contribution of precursors for estrogen production proves inadequate. In this final stage of estrogen availability, levels are insufficient to sustain secondary sex tissues.

The symptoms frequently seen and related to estrogen loss in this protracted climacteric are:

1. Disturbances in menstrual pattern, including anovulation and reduced fertility, decreased flow or hypermenorrhea, and irregular frequency of menses.

2. Vasomotor instability (hot flushes and sweats). Hot flushes are not well understood, but apparently are the result of instability between the hypothalamus and the autonomic nervous system, brought about by a decline in estrogen. They are especially disturbing at night, perhaps because the hypothalamus is relatively unoccupied.

3. Psychological symptoms, including anxiety, increased tension, mood depression, and irritability, although a direct cause and effect relationship between these symptoms and estrogen is hard to establish.

4. Atrophic conditions: atrophy of vaginal epithelium, formation of urethral caruncles, dyspareunia and pruritus due to vulvar, introital, and vaginal atrophy, general skin atrophy, urinary difficulties such as urgency and abacterial urethritis and cystitis.

5. A variety of complaints such as headaches, insomnia, myalgia, and changes in libido.

6. Health problems secondary to long-term deprivation of estrogen: the consequences of osteoporosis and cardiovascular disease.

A precise understanding of the symptom complex the individual patient may display is often difficult to achieve. Some patients will experience severe multiple reactions that may be disabling. Others will show no reactions, or minimal reactions, which go unnoticed until careful medical evaluation. The majority of women (50–60%) require medical assistance and support for intermittent difficulties of moderate severity.

It is helpful to classify the hormonal problems in 3 categories:

1. Those associated with *estrogen deprivation* such as flushes, atrophic vaginitis, urethritis, and osteoporosis.

2. Those associated with relative *estrogen excess* such as dysfunctional uterine bleeding, endometrial hyperplasia, and endometrial cancer.

3. Those associated with *estrogen-progestin replacement therapy*.

The Problems of Postmenopausal Estrogen Deprivation

Altered Menstrual Function

Oligomenorrhea followed by amenorrhea is usually the first clinical evidence of the female climacteric, although fertility has declined since age 30, and many premenopausal women note the transient presence of hot flushes prior to the cessation of menses. The diagnosis of permanent loss of menses requires sufficient follow-up time for retrospective confirmation. Usually 6–12 months of amenorrhea in a woman over 45 years of age is the commonly accepted rule of thumb for diagnosis of menopause. Only rarely will vaginal bleeding reappear; when it does, organic pathology must be ruled out. Many women will insist that pregnancy be ruled out and confirmation of postmenopausal status be obtained by measurement of FSH and LH levels.

Vasomotor Symptoms

The vasomotor flush is viewed as the hallmark of the female climacteric, experienced to some degree by at least 85% of postmenopausal women. The term "hot flush" is descriptive of a sudden onset of reddening of the skin over the head, neck and chest, accompanied by a feeling of intense body heat and concluded by sometimes profuse perspiration. Their duration varies from a few seconds to several minutes, and rarely for an hour. Their frequency may be rare to recurrent every 10–30 minutes. Finally, flushes are more frequent and severe at night (when a woman is often awakened from sleep) or during times of stress. Although the flush can occur in the premenopause, it is a major feature of postmenopause, lasting in most women for 1–2 years, but, in some (as many as 25–50%) for longer than 5 years.

Although the hot flush is the most common problem of the postmenopause, it presents no inherent health hazard. The flush coincides with a surge of LH (not FSH) and is preceded by a subjective prodromal awareness that a flush is beginning. (11) This aura is followed by measurable increased heat over the entire body surface. Core temperature falls. In short, the flush is not a release of accumulated body heat but is a sudden inappropriate excitation of heat release mechanisms. Its relationship to the LH surge and temperature change within the brain is not understood. The observation that flushes occur after hypophysectomy indicates that the mechanism is not dependent or due directly to LH release. In other words, the same hypothalamic event that causes flushes also stimulates gonadotropin releasing hormone (GnRH) secretion and elevates LH.

79

The correlation between the onset of flushes and estrogen reduction is clinically supported by the effectiveness of estrogen replacement therapy and the absence of flushes in hypoestrogen states, such as gonadal dysgenesis. Only after estrogen is administered and withdrawn do hypogonadal women experience the hot flush. Curiously, control of this symptom can require estrogen doses in excess of premenopausal physiologic levels. Although the clinical impression is widely held that premenopausal surgical castrates suffer more severe vasomotor reactions, this is not borne out in objective study. (12)

Osteoporosis

Osteoporosis, a change of bone structure characterized by a reduction in quantity rather than chemical composition, results in mechanical fragility with subsequent fracture. This is the most prevalent form of postmenopausal bone loss and is discussed in detail in Chapter 17.

Loss of estrogen is a major factor affecting the risk of osteoporosis for postmenopausal women; 75% or more of the bone loss which occurs in women during the first 20 years after menopause is attributable to estrogen deficiency rather than to aging itself. (13,14) Vertebral bone is especially vulnerable, beginning to decline as early as 20 years of age. (15) A study of the premenopausal daughters of women with osteoporosis revealed a reduction in bone mass, suggesting either a genetic influence or the sharing of a lifestyle which produces a relatively low peak bone mass. (16) The risk of fracture depends upon 2 factors: the bone mass achieved at maturity and the subsequent rate of bone loss. The bone density which is the threshold for vertebral fractures is only slightly below the lower limit of normal for premenopausal women. (17)

With estrogen replacement treatment, one can expect a 50 to 60% decrease in fractures of the arm and hip (18–20), and when estrogen is supplemented with calcium, an 80% reduction in vertebral compression fractures can be observed. (21) It should be noted that the addition of vitamin D, or its active metabolite, has no impact on the fracture rate, and some women develop hypercalcemia with a risk of renal stone formation. (21,22) The addition of fluoride, a potent stimulator of bone formation, does offer some benefit; however, a high rate of side effects (40%) is encountered, including joint and tendon inflammation, anemia, and gastrointestinal disturbances. Therefore, the optimal regimen is a combination of sex steroids and calcium.

An analysis of aging women's calcium needs indicated a greater requirement than previously appreciated. (23) In order to remain in zero calcium balance, women on estrogen replacement require a total of 1,000 mg elemental calcium per day. Since the average woman receives only 500 mg of calcium in her diet, the minimal daily supplement equals an additional 500 mg. Women not on estrogen replacement require a daily supplement of at least 1,000 mg. Unfortunately, in the absence of estrogen there is significant impairment of calcium absorption. Even with the commonly used therapeutic doses of calcium, nearly 40% of postmenopausal women will have inefficient absorption. (24) Therefore estrogen improves calcium absorption and makes it possible to utilize supplemental calcium in effective doses without the side effects associated with higher doses (constipation and flatulence) which diminish compliance.

Despite the important role for calcium, older women cannot totally substitute for the effectiveness of estrogen by compensatory increases in calcium supplementation. In the absence of estrogen, calcium, even in supplemental doses of 2000 mg/day, has only a little impact on trabecular bone and a minor impact on compact bone. (25,26) Furthermore, studies have been unable to detect any impact of dietary calcium intake (high or low) on the bone density of women in the early postmenopausal period. (27) Thus only a minimal level of calcium supplementation is necessary with hormonal replacement, and high calcium intake neither replaces hormone therapy nor adds to its impact.

Because progestational agents are anti-estrogenic, it is not illogical to question whether the addition of a progestin to an estrogen program counters the beneficial impact of estrogen on the bone. Fortunately, progestational agents independently reduce bone resorption in a manner similar to estrogen, and when such agents are added to estrogen, no loss of protection against osteoporosis occurs. (28–31)

The positive impact of hormone replacement therapy on bone has been demonstrated to take place even in women over age 65. (30,32) This is a strong argument in favor of treating very old women who have never been on estrogen. Estrogen use between the ages of 65 and 74 has been documented to protect against hip fractures. (20)

The precise mechanism of action for sex steroid protection of bones remains unknown. It is apparent that the beneficial impact is achieved without significant changes in the blood levels of the various calcium regulating hormones. In addition, data do not support a role for calcitonin in postmenopausal osteoporosis. (33) Increased efficiency of calcium absorption and a still to be determined role for the estrogen receptors in the osteoblasts are likely important factors. (34,35)

The protection of estrogen is maintained only while women are maintained on the replacement hormone. In the 3 to 5 year period following loss of estrogen, whether after menopause or after cessation of estrogen therapy, there is an accelerated loss of bone. (36,37) While this was not confirmed in one study (38), a careful analysis points out that bone mineral must be measured in the same exact sites because of differences in composition. When this is done an effect of estrogen is seen only in current users, and prior users have a prevalence rate of vertebral osteoporosis similar to women who have never taken estrogen. (39) For the greatest impact on fractures, it is vital that estrogen-progestin replacement be initiated as close to the menopause as possible, and it must be maintained long-term, if not life long.

Cigarette smoking is associated with an earlier menopause and an increased risk of osteoporosis. Because estrogen blood levels are lower in smokers who are on estrogen when compared to nonsmokers, it is concluded that smoking increases liver metabolism of estrogen. (40) Others have documented that smoking induces 2-hydroxylation of estradiol; the metabolic products, 2-hydroxyestrogens, have minimal estrogenic activity and are cleared rapidly from the circulation. (41) In addition, constituents of cigarette smoke inhibit granulosa cell aromatase, providing a further explanation for an earlier menopause in smokers. (42) Lower blood levels of estrogen in smokers have been correlated with a reduced bone density, and therefore, estrogen replacement does not totally counteract the predisposition toward osteoporosis in smokers.

Patients who already have clinically significant osteoporosis should be treated more vigorously. In addition to hormone replacement, treatment should include the active metabolite of vitamin D, and either fluoride or calcitonin or both, depending upon the severity of the condition. Calcitonin inhibits osteoclast activity, and when compared to estrogen in postmenopausal women, it is just as effective in reducing vertebral bone loss. (43)

Physical activity (weight-bearing), as little as 30 minutes a day, 3 times a week, will increase the mineral content of bone in older women. (44) The exercise need not be extreme. Walking 1.5 miles and ordinary calisthenics will suffice. The impact of exercise on vertebral trabecular bone is significantly less, however, and women require the full combination of hormone replacement, calcium supplementation, and exercise in order to fully minimize the risk of vertebral compression fractures.

An aggressive approach is necessary for two reasons. First, therapy is more effective the closer it is initiated to menopause, and second, once significant amounts of bone have been lost, complete retrieval can never be achieved.

Cardiovascular Effects

In the United States, diseases of the heart and the circulation are now the leading causes of death.

Conditions Possibly Affected by Estrogen

Condition	Cumulative Mortality Ages 50–75 per 100,000
Ischemic heart disease	10,500
Breast cancer	1,875
Osteoporotic fractures	938
Endometrial cancer	188

A protective effect of replacement estrogen on heart disease, if real, would be a significant benefit of therapy. A review of the literature finds overwhelming support for a reduced risk of cardiovascular disease in estrogen users. In 10 case-control studies, only one failed to show a decreased relative risk of cardiovascular disease, a study which included only 17 cases, most of whom were smokers and all under age 50. (46–55)

One unique and large case-control study (1444 cases and 744 controls) compared postmenopausal women undergoing coronary arteriography, and therefore utilized an objective endpoint for coronary disease. (54) The relative risk of coronary disease was reduced overall by 56% in estrogen users after adjustment for age, cigarette smoking, diabetes, cholesterol, and hypertension. Even women over age 70 demonstrated a 44% reduction in risk. Two other observations were especially noteworthy. Estrogen protection was increased at high cholesterol levels, and while smokers were protected, the degree of protection was less compared to nonsmokers.

82

Estrogen Use and Risk of Coronary Artery Disease (54)

	Cholesterol < 235	Cholesterol > 235
Nonsmokers	69% reduction	88% reduction
Smokers	33% reduction	72% reduction

In another study of women undergoing angiography a comparison of coronary artery occlusion in users and nonusers of estrogen indicated a significant protective effect of postmenopausal estrogen. (55) A higher rate of myocardial infarction was also noted in the nonusers of estrogen. The only significant lipid difference between users and nonusers consisted of elevated HDL-cholesterol levels in users of estrogen. Notably, there were no differences in LDL-cholesterol or triglycerides.

In 8 cohort studies, 5 showed a reduced risk of ischemic heart disease in estrogen users; the 3 others produced conflicting data. (56–63) The Walnut Creek Study (59), one of the 3 with conflicting data, had only 26 women with infarctions, and only 9 were estrogen users.

The Framingham Study presented data in 1978 and 1985 which argued that there was a 50% increased risk for cardiovascular disease among estrogen users, although there was no difference in fatality rates between users and non-users. (58,62) Because of the respect the Framingham Study carries, its impact is significant. There are, however, major criticisms of the Framingham report. First, the patient numbers are relatively small (302 postmenopausal women on estrogen) in comparison to the patient numbers in other studies on this particular issue. Furthermore, the effect of dose and duration of treatment cannot be ascertained; they were not recorded. Finally and most conclusively, a subsequent reanalysis of the Framingham data by the authors of the study reversed their conclusion. (64) The early reports from the Framingham Study, therefore, stand in lonely opposition to overwhelming evidence that appropriately low doses of estrogen protect postmenopausal women against cardiovascular disease.

The Nurses' Health Study surveyed 121,964 nurses; 32,317 postmenopausal women were free of coronary heart disease when initially evaluated, and subsequently 90 had either nonfatal or fatal disease. (63) The age-adjusted relative risk of coronary disease in ever-users showed a 50% reduction, and current users showed a 70% reduction!

The Lipid Research Clinics Follow-Up Study (a prospective 8.5 year follow-up of 2270 women) has demonstrated a 63% reduction in the relative risk of fatal cardiovascular disease in current estrogen users, including a protective effect in current and exsmokers. (60) A longitudinal study in a retirement community (under relatively controlled and accurate conditions), begun in 1981, had, by 1987, demonstrated a 20% decrease in death from all causes in estrogen users, and a 41% decrease in death from acute myocardial infarctions (53% decrease in current users). (45)

Sophisticated assessment and analysis (using the methods of information synthesis and meta-analysis) indicate that the effect of estrogen on heart disease is not controversial or ambiguous, but there clearly exists a protective benefit. (65) The public health importance of the impact of estrogen on cardiovascular disease is very significant, outranking even osteoporosis.

The bulk of evidence, when controlled for age and cigarette smoking, indicates that women who undergo a natural menopause do not have an appreciable increase in the risk of coronary heart disease as compared with premenopausal women until 10–12 years into the postmenopausal period. (66) In contrast, bilateral oophorectomy, especially relatively early in life, quickly increases the risk of heart disease.

The protective effect of estrogen is achieved by specific pharmacologic consequences. Approximately 75% of the overall reduction in mortality in estrogen ever-users is due to protection against heart disease. The mechanism of this protection appears to be due in significant part (about 50% of the protective effect) to a pharmacologic effect of estrogen on lipoprotein levels. (60)

The lipoproteins which carry cholesterol in the blood affect the risk of cardiovascular disease. The low-density lipoprotein carrier of cholesterol (LDL-cholesterol) is the fraction which is most atherogenic. Particularly in older people, an inverse relationship exists between the high-density lipoprotein (HDL-cholesterol) and coronary mortality. The mechanism of change due to sex steroids involves a plasma enzyme, hepatic lipase, which catalyzes the hydrolysis of phospholipids on the surface of the lipoproteins, allowing the lipoproteins to be irreversibly degraded. Androgens increase this enzyme activity, and estrogen decreases it. (67) Thus the elevated levels of HDL-cholesterol associated with estrogen replacement, and protection against heart disease, consist of the subfraction of HDL-cholesterol which is most strongly associated with both estrogen and risk of cardiovascular disease. The small increase in triglyceride often seen with estrogen is of no consequence except in individuals with genetic disorders of triglyceride metabolism.

The impact of estrogen therapy on the lipid profile is maintained as long as women remain on the estrogen. A higher HDL-cholesterol and lower LDL-cholesterol have been documented to persist through at least 10 years of postmenopausal treatment. (68) Here too is another argument in favor of physical exercise. There is a significant positive relationship between HDL-cholesterol levels and physical activity in postmenopausal women. (69)

An important study in monkeys has supported the protective action of estrogen against atherosclerosis, but by a mechanism independent of the cholesterol profile. Oral administration of a combination of estrogen and and a high dose of progestin to monkeys fed a high cholesterol diet decreased the extent of coronary atherosclerosis despite a reduction in HDL-cholesterol levels. (70) In a somewhat similar experiment, estrogen treatment markedly prevented arterial lesion development in rabbits without significant differences in cholesterol or lipoprotein patterns. (71) This suggests that women with already favorable cholesterol profiles may benefit through this additional action.

Because the public health benefit of estrogen replacement on cardiovascular disease is of such enormous impact, it is vital that we know whether the addition of monthly progestin has an adverse effect on the lipid profile, and ultimately on cardiovascular disease. A review of the literature on this question suggests a dose-response relationship. (72–79)

A decrease in HDL-cholesterol has been noted with 10 day monthly treatment with norethindrone (5 mg), megestrol acetate (5 mg), levonorgestrel (250 μg), and even medroxyprogesterone acetate (10 mg). No significant change was noted with micronized progesterone (200 mg). It is probable that there is a dose-response relationship between progestins and their effect on the lipoproteins. The lack of an effect noted with micronized progesterone was observed with a dose (200 mg daily) which yields a normal luteal phase blood level of progesterone. A similar "physiologic" dose of synthetic progestins may be free of an adverse impact on HDL-cholesterol. In at least one study, a small amount of synthetic progestin (30 μg levonorgestrel) had no effect on LDL-cholesterol and HDL-cholesterol. (78) It is imperative that clinical studies determine the long-term relationship between various progestins and the lipoproteins as soon as possible. This underscores the need to determine the lowest progestational dose which safely maintains endometrial protection (and perhaps the breast) as well. One 3 year study of the usual sequential program with the utilization of 10 mg medroxyprogesterone acetate for 10 days every month concluded that a favorable lipoprotein profile was maintained. (80)

Barrett-Connor and colleagues have been studying the adult residents of Rancho Bernardo, California. In a recent report, the women using both estrogen and progestin demonstrated the same favorable impact on cardiovascular risk factors as estrogen-only users, when compared to the non-users. (81) It will be a long time before the gold standard, a randomized clinical trial, will provide us with answers in this important area. Until then, in our view, it is wise to measure the cholesterol-lipoprotein profile on an annual basis in women receiving estrogen-progestin replacement therapy. In our practice, this assessment has been very reassuring, indicating that patients on estrogen-progestin combinations are able to maintain favorable levels of cholesterol, LDL-cholesterol, and HDL-cholesterol.

Stroke.   In a prospective cohort study, estrogen replacement therapy was associated with a 46% overall reduction in the risk of death from stroke, with a 79% reduction in recent users. (82) This protection was present in both women with hypertension and those without, and in both smokers and nonsmokers. This level of protection was similar to that observed in this same population for estrogen protection against deaths due to myocardial infarction. (45) It is likely that the mechanism for this protection goes beyond the estrogen impact on the cholesterol-lipoprotein profile, and multiple effects are probable.

Hypertension.   Hypertension is both a risk factor for cardiovascular mortality and a common problem in older people. It is important, therefore, to know that no relationship has been established between hypertension and the doses of estrogen used for replacement therapy. Studies have either shown no effect or a small, but statistically significant, decrease in blood pressure due to estrogen treatment.(83–87) This has been the case in both normotensive and hypertensive women. The very rare cases of increased blood pressure due to estrogen replacement therapy truly represent idiosyncratic reactions. Because of the protective impact of appropriate estrogen replacement on the risk of cardiovascular disease, it can be argued that a woman with controlled hypertension is in need of that specific benefit of estrogen.

The blood pressure impact of the addition of a progestational agent to an estrogen replacement program is yet unknown, although clinical experience and early reports (87) thus far indicate that current low doses have no effect on blood pressure. Here again, until this information is documented long-term, there is no reason to change the current practice or to withhold an estrogen-progestin program from women with controlled hypertension; however, close monitoring of the blood pressure makes good clinical sense.

Atrophic Change

With extremely low estrogen production in the late postmenopausal age, or many years after castration, atrophy of all mucosal surfaces takes place, accompanied by vaginitis, pruritus, dyspareunia, and stenosis. Genitourinary atrophy leads to a variety of symptoms which affect the ease and quality of living. Urethritis with dysuria, urgency incontinence, and urinary frequency are further results of mucosal thinning, in this instance, of the urethra and bladder. Vaginal relaxation with cystocele, rectocele, and uterine prolapse, and vulvar dystrophies are not a consequence of estrogen deprivation. Although it is argued that genuine stress incontinence will not be affected by treatment with estrogen, others contend that estrogen treatment improves or cures genuine stress incontinence in over 50% of patients due to a direct effect on the urethral mucosa. (88,89) However, most cases of urinary incontinence in elderly women are a mixed problem with a significant component of urge incontinence which definitely can be improved by estrogen therapy.

Unless dermatologic conditions exist masquerading as menopausal atrophy, estrogen replacement is invariably successful in reversing these atrophic problems. Relief from these problems often results in significant improvements in general well-being.

Dyspareunia seldom brings older women to our offices. A basic reluctance to discuss sexual behavior still permeates our society, especially among older patients and physicians. Gentle questioning may lead to estrogen treatment of atrophy and enhancement of sexual enjoyment.

Objective measurements have demonstrated that vaginal factors which influence the enjoyment of sexual intercourse can be maintained by appropriate doses of estrogen. (90) Both patient and physician should be aware that a significant response can be expected by one month but it takes a long time to fully restore the genitourinary tract (6–12 months), and physicians and patients should not be discouraged by an apparent lack of immediate response. Furthermore sexual activity by itself supports the circulatory response of the vaginal tissues and enhances the therapeutic effects of estrogen. Therefore sexually active older women will have less atrophy of the vagina even without estrogen replacement.

One of the features of aging in men and women is a steady reduction in muscular strength. Many factors affect this decline, including height, weight, and level of physical activity. However, women currently using estrogen replacement do not demonstrate this age-related decline in muscular competence (as measured by handgrip strength). (91) This can be viewed as another substantial benefit of estrogen replacement, with potential protective consequences against fractures, as well as a benefit due to the ability to maintain vigorous physical exercise. In addition, there is evidence that estrogen replacement before the onset of joint disease is associated with protection against rheumatoid arthritis. (92)

The Menopausal Syndrome

There are additional problems encountered in the early postmenopause that are seen frequently, but their causal relation with estrogen is uncertain. Called the menopausal syndrome, these problems include fatigue, nervousness, headaches, insomnia, depression, irritability, joint and muscle pain, dizziness, and palpitations. Attempts to study the effects of estrogen on these problems have been hampered by the subjectivity of the complaints (high placebo responses) and the "domino effect" of what reduction of hot flushes does to the frequency of the symptoms. Using a double-blind crossover prospective study format, Campbell and Whitehead (93) have concluded that many symptomatic "improvements" ascribed to estrogen therapy result from relief of hot flushes—a domino effect. On the other hand, a tonic effect (improvement in memory and reduction of anxiety) was also noted in these observations. Fatigue, irritability, headache, and depression are not thought to be estrogen-related phenomena.

Emotional stability during the perimenopausal period may be disrupted by poor sleep patterns. Estrogen therapy improves the quality of sleep, decreasing the time to onset of sleep, and increasing the rapid eye movement (REM) sleep time. (94) Perhaps flushing may be insufficient to awaken a woman, but sufficient to affect the quality of sleep, thereby diminishing the ability to handle the next day's problems and stresses.

There is a general clinical consensus that certain physical changes (redistribution of fat deposits and loss of elastic tissue of the skin with wrinkling) are due to aging rather than to estrogen deprivation.

Problems of Excess Estrogen

Not all climacteric women experience symptoms or signs of estrogen deprivation. Some actually manifest estrogen excess via the presence of uterine bleeding (dysfunctional uterine bleeding).

Throughout the usual period of life identified with perimenopause (ages 40–60), there is a significant incidence of dysfunctional uterine bleeding. Although the greatest concern provoked by this symptom is endometrial neoplasia, the usual finding is non-neoplastic tissue displaying estrogen effects unopposed by progesterone. This results from anovulation in the premenopausal women and from extragonadal endogenous estrogen production or estrogen administration in the postmenopausal woman.

There are 4 mechanisms which could result in increased endogenous estrogen levels:

1. Increased precursor androgen (functional and nonfunctional endocrine tumors, liver disease, stress).

2. Increased aromatization (obesity, hyperthyroidism, liver disease).

3. Increased direct secretion of estrogen (ovarian tumors).

4. Decreased levels of SHBG (sex hormone binding globulin) leading to increased levels of free estrogen.

In all women, whether premenopausal or postmenopausal, whether on or off hormone therapy, specific organic causes (neoplasia, complications of unexpected pregnancy, or bleeding from extrauterine sites) must be ruled out. In addition to careful history and physical examination, dysfunctional uterine bleeding should be evaluated by aspiration endometrial biopsy. If the uterus is normal to examination, for reasons of both accuracy and cost effectiveness, the method of biopsy should be an office aspiration curettage, NOT the traditional, more costly and risky, in-hospital dilatation and curettage (D&C). (95)

We recommend the use of the plastic endometrial suction device (Pipelle from Unimar, Wilton, Connecticut, or the Z-Sampler from Zinnanti, Chatsworth, California). It is easy to use, requires no cervical dilatation (3 mm diameter), and is virtually painless. This device is as efficacious as the Vabra aspirator. (96) Insertion should first be attempted without the use of a tenaculum. In many patients, this is feasible and avoids the sensation of the tenaculum grasping the cervix. Once the suction is applied, the endometrial cavity should be thoroughly curetted in all directions, just as one would with a sharp curette during a D&C. If the cannula fills up with tissue, a second and even a third cannula should be inserted until tissue is no longer obtained. Although most patients report no problems with cramps or pain, the application of suction in some patients stimulates cramping which usually passes within 5–10 minutes. Because cramping occurs in such a small minority of patients, it is not our practice to routinely give an inhibitor of prostaglandin synthesis. For repeat biopsies, in patients known to cramp, it would be useful to use such an agent at least 20 minutes before the procedure.

Less than 10% of postmenopausal women cannot be adequately evaluated by office biopsy. Most commonly, the reason is the inability to enter the uterine cavity. In such instances, an in-hospital D&C is in order. *Furthermore, if the uterus is not normal on pelvic examination, the office endometrial biopsy must yield to an in-hospital D&C in order to achieve accuracy of diagnosis.*

If vulva, vagina, and cervix appear normal to inspection, perimenopausal bleeding can be assumed to be intrauterine in origin. Confirmation requires the absence of abnormal cytology on the Pap smear. The principal symptom of endometrial cancer is abnormal vaginal bleeding, but carcinoma will be encountered in only about 2% of postmenopausal endometrial biopsies. (97) Normal endometrium is found over half the time, polyps in about 3%, and endometrial hyperplasia about 15% of the time. Postmenopausal bleeding should always be taken seriously.

Additional procedures include the following:

Colposcopy and cervical biopsy for abnormal cytology or obvious lesions.

Endocervical assessment by curettage for abnormal cytology (the endocervix must always be kept in mind as a source for abnormal cytology).

Hysterogram or hysteroscopy if bleeding persists to determine the presence of endometrial polyps or submucosal fibroids.

Keep in mind that the pathologic reading, "tissue insufficient for diagnosis," when a patient is on estrogen-progestin treatment, represents atrophic, decidualized endometrium that yields little to the exploring curet. The clinician must be confident in his or her technique, knowing that a full investigation of the intrauterine cavity has been accomplished—then this reading can be interpreted as comforting and benign, the absence of pathology.

In postmenopausal women, one must view any adnexal mass as cancer until proven otherwise. Surgical intervention is usually necessary, and appropriate consultation must be obtained not only for the surgical procedure but also for suitable preoperative evaluation and preparation. Cysts which are less than 5 cm in diameter and without septations or solid components have a very low potential for malignant disease and may be managed with serial ultrasound surveillance. (98)

In the absence of organic disease, appropriate management is dependent upon the age of the woman and endometrial tissue findings. In the perimenopausal woman with dysfunctional uterine bleeding associated with proliferative or hyperplastic endometrium (uncomplicated by atypia or dysplastic constituents), periodic oral progestin therapy is mandatory, such as 10 mg medroxyprogesterone acetate given daily the first 10 days of each month. If hyperplasia is present, follow-up aspiration curettage after 3–4 months is required, and if progestin is ineffective and histological regression is not observed, formal curettage is an essential preliminary to alternate therapeutic surgical choices.

When monthly progestin therapy reverses hyperplastic changes (which it does in 95–98% of cases) and controls irregular bleeding, treatment should be continued until withdrawal bleeding ceases. This is a reliable sign (in effect, a bioassay) indicating the onset of estrogen deprivation and the need for the addition of estrogen. If vasomotor disturbances begin before the cessation of menstrual bleeding, the combined estrogen-progestin program can be initiated as needed to control the flushes.

Problems of Estrogen-Progestin Therapy

General and Metabolic

The increased incidence of thromboembolism and hypertension and the altered carbohydrate metabolism during use of the older high dose oral contraceptives is well documented. Because of the lower dosage in a hormone replacement program, these metabolic effects are not seen in postmenopausal therapy. Postmenopausal women on estrogen therapy are NOT at risk for myocardial infarction, thromboembolism, or breast tumors. As with oral contraception, estrogen replacement therapy may carry a 1.5–2.0-fold increased risk of gall bladder disease. (99) However, at least two other case-control studies concluded that estrogen use is not a risk factor for gall stone disease in postmenopausal women. (100,101) The routine, periodic use of blood chemistries is not cost effective, and careful monitoring for the appearance of the symptoms and signs of biliary tract disease will suffice.

Patients with high risk factors need special attention when a decision for estrogen therapy is debated. Metabolic contraindications to estrogen replacement therapy include chronically impaired liver function, acute vascular thrombosis (with or without emboli), and neuroophthalmologic vascular disease. Estrogens may have adverse effects on some patients with seizure disorders, familial hyperlipidemias (very high triglycerides), and migraine headaches. The risk in women with a past history of thromboembolism is not known, and a careful assessment of the risk-benefit balance may justify treatment of such patients.

Endometrial Neoplasia

Estrogen normally promotes mitotic growth of the endometrium. Abnormal progression of growth through cystic hyperplasia, adenomatous hyperplasia, atypia, and early carcinoma has been associated with unopposed estrogen activity. Some 10% of women with adenomatous hyperplasia progress to frank cancer, and adenomatous hyperplasia is observed to antedate adenocarcinoma in 25–30% of cases. Retrospective studies have estimated that the risk of endometrial cancer in women on estrogen replacement therapy (unopposed by a progestational agent) is increased by a factor of somewhere from 2 to 10 times the normal incidence of 1 per 1,000 postmenopausal women per year. The risk increases with duration of exposure and dose of estrogen and lingers for up to 10 years after estrogen is discontinued, and the risk of cancer that has already spread beyond the uterus is increased 3-fold in women who have used estrogen a year or longer. (102,103)

It is now apparent, however, that this risk can be reduced by the addition of a progestational agent to the program. Whereas estrogen promotes the growth of endometrium, progestins inhibit that growth. This counter effect is accomplished by progestin reduction in cellular receptors for estrogen, and by induction of target cell enzymes that convert estradiol to an excreted metabolite, estrone sulfate. As a result, the number of estrogen receptor complexes that are retained in the endometrial nuclei is decreased, as is the overall intracellular availability of the powerful estradiol.

Reports of the clinical impact of adding progestin in sequence with estrogen include both the reversal of hyperplasia and a diminished incidence of endometrial cancer. (104–107) The protective action of progestational agents operates via a mechanism which requires time in order to reach its maximal effect. For that reason, the duration of exposure to the progestin each month is critical. The optimal number of days for progestin administration remains somewhat controversial. While one standard method has incorporated the addition of a progestational agent for the last 10 days of estrogen exposure, some have argued in favor of 12 or 14 days. Clinical data to resolve this debate are not available; however, a study from London is noteworthy. (108) A total of 398 women are being treated with a variety of estrogens and progestins, with a duration of progestin exposure that varies from 7 to 21 days per month. These women have received an endometrial curettage under general anesthesia every year since 1976. By 1985, not one woman who received 10 or more days of progestin had developed hyperplasia, and there have been no cases of adenomatous hyperplasia or cancer. About 2% of the women developed cystic hyperplasia when progestin was administered for only 7 days. Until new data argue to the contrary, it is appropriate to adhere to the standard of 10 days as a minimal requirement for monthly progestational exposure.

It is likely that the daily dose of the progestational agent is associated with a threshold level below which endometrial protection can be insufficient. Currently, the sequential program utilizes 10 mg of medroxyprogesterone acetate and the combined, daily method uses 2.5 mg. Although lower doses of progestational agents are effective in achieving target tissue responses (such as reducing the nuclear concentration of estrogen receptors), the long-term impact on endometrial histology has not yet been firmly established. The question of dose is an issue of major importance, especially in terms of the cardiovascular system.

Although adenocarcinoma of the endometrium is an estrogen-dependent neoplasm, experience in providing estrogen replacement to women who have completed therapy for all grades of Stage I disease does not show an increased risk of recurrence. (109) Prudent judgment would strongly suggest that combined treatment with a progestational agent is the method of choice.

Breast Cancer

The possibility that estrogen use increases the risk of breast cancer must be intensively scrutinized. The American epidemiologic data on the scope of human female breast cancer are astonishing: 1 of every 10 women will develop breast cancer in her lifetime. In America, breast cancer is the leading type of cancer in women (28%) and now second to lung cancer as the leading cause of cancer death in women (18%), about 10 times the number of deaths from endometrial cancer.

Unlike endometrial cancer, the incidence of breast cancer continues to rise progressively throughout life. Factors which increase the relative risk of breast cancer have a common theme: prolonged accumulated exposure to unopposed estrogen. These factors include low parity, first childbirth after age 30, obesity, anovulation, early menarche, and late menopause. Early studies on estrogen use and breast cancer indicated higher risks in special subcategories, such as women with benign breast disease or natural versus surgical menopause. One prospective cohort study and two large case-control studies are now available, and they do not show an increased risk for breast cancer associated with the postmenopausal use of estrogen. (110–112) These studies are large enough to have reliable results in various subcategories, and an absence of an effect was evident in all of the following designations: parity, age at first pregnancy, early or late menopause, menopause by hysterectomy or oophorectomy, family history of breast cancer, presence of benign breast disease, use for many years, and use of high doses. Therefore this absence of an increase in relative risk is not modified by the other known breast cancer risk factors. In the prospective cohort study, the absence of risk in women who developed breast cancer was present for up to 5 years' duration of use. *This is strong evidence that treatment does not accelerate subclinical growth which might be present during the period of estrogen use.*

In addition, a recent case-control study from Australia which attempted to control for secular trends in estrogen use, type of menopause, and duration of estrogen use concluded that that there was no evidence for an association between estrogen use and the risk of breast cancer in postmenopausal women. (113) An Australian meta-analysis of 23 studies of estrogen use and breast cancer concluded "unequivocally" that estrogen use did not alter the risk of breast cancer. (114)

In a retrospective cohort study of women who underwent biopsy for benign breast disease, the use of exogenous estrogen appeared to lower the risk of developing breast cancer. (115) In women with atypical hyperplasia on biopsy, the risk of developing breast cancer in women not taking estrogen was increased 4.5 times, but in women on estrogen the risk was increased only 3-fold. The importance of this observation is that this evidence indicates that benign breast disease does not represent a contraindication to estrogen replacement treatment.

There is reason to believe that exposure to progestational agents offers protection against breast cancer. It is logical to expect that the same mechanism of estrogen receptor depletion should operate in both the endometrium and the breast, and that protection against abnormal mitotic activity should exist in both target tissues. However, this remains to be definitely demonstrated. Only two reports have claimed that the addition of a progestational agent protects against breast cancer; the first, although it is the only randomized, placebo-controlled trial, was hampered by small numbers, and the second was limited by bias in treatment selection. (116,117) This probability has led to the recommendation that the combined estrogen-progestin program be utilized even in the absence of a uterus.

There are two recent studies on breast cancer and hormone replacement treatment which deserve some discussion. Bergkvist and colleagues from Uppsala, Sweden, in a case-cohort study concluded that estrogen use was associated with a slight increase (10%) in the risk of breast cancer, that there was a relationship with duration of use, and that the risk was increased among those women who took a combination of estradiol and progestin. (118) Besides method problems which introduced the possibility of selection bias and surveillance bias, there is reason to be skeptical regarding the significance of the data. The authors correctly indicate that there was a *trend* toward increasing relative risk with duration of use (in other words, it was not statistically significant), and that the indication of increased risk was based on small numbers of women with breast cancer. A case-control study from Denmark which utilized questionnaires to obtain information from both the cases and controls also indicated a slightly increased risk of breast cancer associated with hormonal replacement therapy. (119) This study contains limitations similar to the Uppsala study (e.g. the relative risk associated with estrogen-progestin use was 1.36 but the confidence interval did not cross 1.0).

Balancing the information available involving all of the health issues affected by hormone replacement therapy, a combined estrogen-progestin program in appropriate doses continues to offer significant benefits for postmenopausal women. As time goes on, more studies and greater duration of use should provide us with better answers to many of our questions. By virtue of the magnitude of the postmenopausal female population, these questions deserve continuing biologic and epidemiologic research from both the public health and individual points of view.

Postmenopausal Estrogen-Progestin Replacement Therapy

In view of the above considerations, our opinion is as follows: There is little question that women who suffer from hot flushes or atrophy of reproductive tract tissues can and should be relieved of their problems by use of estrogens. It also is now definite that the long-term disabilities of osteoporosis can be largely prevented by therapy with estrogen and progestin. It is very probable that appropriate doses of estrogen have a beneficial impact on the lipid profile and the risk of cardiovascular disease. We suggest treatment with estrogen for all women showing any stigmata of hormone deprivation, and advocate hormonal prophylaxis against osteoporosis and cardiovascular disease. The decision to use or not to use estrogen belongs to the patient, and it should be based upon the information available in this chapter. The recommendation that replacement therapy be given for the shortest period of time appears to be shortsighted in view of the impressive evidence that therapy has a profound impact on osteoporosis and cardiovascular disease, and that there are more beneficial than potentially harmful effects.

Women Under the Age of 40 (Castrates and Women with Gonadal Dysgenesis)

In these women, the duration of estrogen deprivation is prolonged and the loss of estrogen acute. The cyclic use of estrogen is recommended for short-term reduction of vasomotor symptoms and for long-term prophylaxis against cardiovascular disease, osteoporosis, and target organ atrophy. In many young patients, 0.625 mg conjugated estrogens are insufficient to allow menstrual bleeding. Because women of this age ordinarily are exposed to estrogen levels which stimulate endometrial growth and withdrawal bleeding, and for psychological reasons, a higher dose should be used to maintain withdrawal bleeding until the menopausal time of life. The standard sequential program is utilized. In those patients castrated because of endometriosis, recurrence of endometriosis has very rarely been a problem with estrogen replacement, but because endometrial cancer has been reported to occur in remaining endometriosis exposed to unopposed estrogen, the estrogen and progestin daily combination is recommended.

Perimenopausal Dysfunctional Uterine Bleeding

After exclusion of other gynecologic causes, dysfunctional bleeding is treated by progestin therapy, and if necessary, biopsy surveillance. Vasomotor reactions appearing in women despite the presence of menstrual bleeding (presumably the flushes are due to a relative decrease in estrogen) should be treated by the usual estrogen-progestin regimen. A perimenopausal, menstruating woman suffering with hot flushes should not be made to wait for therapy.

| The Early Postmenopause | In anovulatory, menstruating women, progestin therapy is administered periodically (every month) until withdrawal bleeding does not occur. If vasomotor reactions begin, then estrogen is added regardless of the presence of menstrual bleeding. The long-term postmenopausal use of hormone therapy depends heavily upon a woman's own informed assessment, a process which should occur at this point in life. An understanding of hormone replacement is an important component in any preventive health program directed toward the postmenopausal years. At the low doses of estrogen recommended for replacement, increased growth of uterine fibroids, endometriosis, and breast reactions are rarely seen. |

As a result of immediate responses in early climacteric symptoms, the patient enters the climacteric more confident of herself emotionally, sexually, and physically. In our view, this establishes or cements good patient-physician interchange and relations. The follow-up of the patient on effective estrogen-progestin replacement is more secure and certain. The practitioner offering estrogen-progestin replacement has a better and more reliable opportunity to act as primary physician for these aging women. All monitoring of health systems will be improved as a result of this single involvement.

The Late Postmenopause

Atrophic conditions can be effectively treated with local or oral therapy in low maintenance doses. If there is no apparent basis for osteoporosis other than aging and ovarian failure, estrogen-progestin therapy and calcium supplementation are advisable even for very old women. Further loss of bone can be slowed, and the risk of fractures reduced. In these older women, a higher dose of estrogen (1.25 mg conjugated estrogens or equivalent) may be necessary; an assessment of progress can be obtained by measuring bone density, using either photon absorptiometry or CT scanning.

Method of Management

Which Drug Should Be Used? There currently is no evidence that one form of estrogen is superior to another. The specific estrogen is not as important as the duration, dose, and the presence or absence of a progestin. Which estrogen is administered is not as important as the method with which it is used.

The dose of estrogen which is effective in maintaining the axial and peripheral bone mass is equivalent to 0.625 mg conjugated estrogens. (120,121) The relative potencies of commercially available estrogens become of great importance when prescribing estrogen.

Relative Estrogen Potencies (122,123)

Estrogen	FSH Levels	Liver Proteins	Bone Density
Piperazine estrone sulfate	1.0 mg	2.0 mg	—
Micronized estradiol	1.0 mg	1.0 mg	1.0 mg
Conjugated estrogens	1.0 mg	0.625 mg	0.625 mg
Ethinyl estradiol	5.0 µg	2–10 µg	5–10 µg

The dose-response effect of ethinyl estradiol on bone has not been sufficiently studied, and it is probable that the dose equivalent to 0.625 mg conjugated estrogens approximates 5–10 µg. The 17α-ethinyl group of ethinyl estradiol appears to be responsible for a specific hepatic effect, for no matter by which route it is administered, liver metabolism is affected. (124) The same is true for conjugated equine estrogens. Contrary to the case with estradiol, the liver appears to preferentially extract ethinyl estradiol and conjugated equine estrogens no matter what the route of administration. Thus the route of administration appears to influence the metabolic responses only in the case of specific estrogens, most notably estradiol.

At one time, the consequence of the first pass through the liver of estrogens other than ethinyl estradiol and conjugated equine estrogens was thought to be of great importance in terms of HDL-cholesterol. Initial reports of transdermal application, subdermal implants, and cutaneous administration of estradiol all demonstrated profound impacts on hot flushes and vaginal cytology, but only a limited impact on lipoproteins. (125–128) These were short-term studies, however, and while oral therapy is associated with an immediate impact on the lipoprotein profile, percutaneous administration achieves significant changes in lipids and lipoproteins only after 6 months of treatment. After 12 months of percutaneous *high dose* estrogen therapy, there is a significant reduction in the serum levels of total cholesterol and LDL-cholesterol, and after 24 months, HDL-cholesterol levels are increased by percutaneous estrogen combined with cyclic micronized progesterone. (129) The blood level of estradiol achieved in this study was significantly elevated (3–5 times those associated with transdermal estradiol), and the standard dose required to produce a favorable lipoprotein profile remains to be established for each method of administration other than the oral route. It is likely that the dose administered is more critical than "first pass" through the liver.

One would not expect the route of administration to influence the effect on postmenopausal bone loss, and indeed this may be the case. Percutaneous as well as oral estrogen therapy offers effective protection against osteoporosis. (130) But once again effective dosage for long-term protection against osteoporosis is established only for the oral route of administration. Until dose-response studies are available indicating the range which without question provides the desired benefits for vaginal, parenteral, and transdermal types of administration, the oral program must be followed in the interests of patient safety and health.

The Sequential Method of Treatment.   There are two sequential methods which have been in general use. In one, estrogens are administered from the 1st through the 25th of each month, as a convenient aid to remembering the routine. For the last 10 days of estrogen administration, a daily dose of 10 mg of medroxyprogesterone acetate is added. In the other sequential method (more popular in Europe), estrogen is taken every day throughout the month and the progestational agent is administered daily for the first 14 days of the month.

Some patients develop unwanted reactions to this dose of progestin: weight gain, fluid retention, breast tenderness, and/or depression. A lower dose (5 mg) usually solves this problem. The lowest effective dose of medroxyprogesterone acetate has not been established, and for this reason, the starting dose remains at 10 mg. Studies with endometrium, however, indicate that lower doses are effective in reducing the target tissue content of estrogen receptors. (131) Future studies may reveal that lower doses protect the endometrium (and perhaps the breast) and maintain the advantage of elevated HDL-cholesterol levels. Unfortunately, the great majority of women (90%) on this regimen experience withdrawal menstrual bleeding. (132)

In the absence of a uterus, some do not see the need to use cyclic administration of a progestin. However, in view of a possible impact on the breast, a schedule including the use of a progestin can be considered.

The dose of estrogen utilized is that which will provide sufficient estrogen to sustain physiologic functions. For early climacteric where there is still considerable endogenous estrogen present, the usual effective dose is 0.625 mg conjugated estrogens per day. In late climacteric where endogenous estrogen is very low, a higher dose, 1.25 mg, may be necessary. Unfortunately, there are no studies available which have utilized very old women. For optimal protection against osteoporosis, the hormonal regimen is supplemented with 500 mg calcium daily.

The Continuous/Combined Method of Treatment. Manipulation of the standard sequential regimen was often necessary in order to maintain patient compliance in the presence of bleeding and other symptoms. One approach for the problem of bleeding has been to reduce the daily dose of estrogen. It is useful to note that bone density remains stable with a daily dose of 0.3 mg conjugated estrogens if the daily calcium supplementation is increased to 1,500 mg, although this response may also be dependent upon the inclusion of monthly exposure to a progestational agent as well. (26)

More recently we and others have advocated the continuous daily use of an estrogen-progestin combination. (76,133–138) We have used combinations of the following estrogens and progestins:

Daily Estrogen: 0.625 mg conjugated estrogen, or
                      1.0 mg micronized estradol

Daily Progestin: 2.5 mg medroxyprogesterone acetate, or
                      0.35 mg norethindrone

After 4–6 months of such continuous treatment, bleeding usually ceases and essentially all biopsies show atrophic endometrium. While one study has reported a decrease in HDL-cholesterol, another demonstrated a favorable impact on the cholesterol-lipoprotein profile. (76,135) In our own experience, this continuous approach maintains a beneficial lipoprotein pattern and increases the bone density in the spinal column in the first year of use to a level which is then maintained, while others have noted an increasing bone density for at least 18 months. (31) Also of note, we and others have encountered no adverse effects on blood pressure. (87,139)

Clinical trials are essential to ascertain the effects of various doses and formulations on the lipoprotein profile and the risk of cardiovascular disease, beyond the obvious need for a safe impact on bones and the endometrium. Until such data are available, annual assessment of the lipoprotein profile is worthwhile to detect any adverse effects.

Contraindications to Hormone Replacement. Estrogen sensitive cancer stands out as the most logical and convincing contraindication to hormone replacement therapy. However, ethical, as well as logistic, considerations prevent the proper study of this issue. Therefore, decisions regarding the two major cancers sensitive to estrogen, breast cancer and endometrial cancer, must be based upon medical-legal fears and the knowledge reviewed in this chapter.

It has been demonstrated that patients who have had Stage I adenocarcinoma of the endometrium can take estrogen replacement without fear of recurrence. (109) Nothing is known about the risk in patients with more advanced disease. Because the latent period with endometrial cancer is relatively short, a period of time (5 years) without evidence of recurrence would increase the liklihood of safety on an estrogen program. The combination of estrogen-progestin is recommended in view of the potential protective action of the progestational agent. A similar approach makes sense for patients previously treated for endometrioid tumors of the ovary. In view of the fact that adenocarcinoma has been reported in patients with pelvic endometriosis and on unopposed estrogen, the combined estrogen-progestin program is advised in patients with a past history of endometriosis. (139)

A decision regarding hormone replacement is even more difficult in women with a previous history of breast cancer. The benefits of hormone replacement may outweigh the risks if one considers the lack of evidence connecting estrogen replacement and an increased risk of developing breast cancer, the lack of an adverse impact of a pregnancy on the prognosis of breast cancer, and no specific harm evident in women with breast cancer who subsequently become pregnant. (140) On the other hand, the possible risk in a woman with an estrogen receptor positive breast cancer and positive nodes seems excessive. And at the same time, perhaps women years removed from treatment of node free, estrogen receptor negative disease may represent a reasonable risk.

One approach to symptomatic (mainly hot flushes) women who have had breast cancer is to utilize daily progestin (10 mg medroxyprogesterone acetate). This treatment will relieve hot flushes and offer (along with 1000 mg calcium supplementation daily) protection against osteoporosis. Unfortunately, vaginal dryness and dyspareunia may be made worse. A patient and physician may elect (knowing there exists an unknown risk) to add the use of vaginal estrogen, in a minimal self-titrated dose to enhance sexual enjoyment. This approach can be associated with a decrease in HDL-cholesterol, and surveillance of the lipoprotein profile is indicated.

Another area which remains unstudied is the problem case of a woman who wishes to use hormone replacement but has a previous history of a cardiovascular event, such as a myocardial infarction, stroke, or embolism. While it is known that the doses of estrogen used for replacement have no significant impact on the clotting mechanism and no increased risks for thrombotic clinical events have been demonstrated, these findings are derived from women without previous events. Does the woman with a previous event represent a different risk? And again, on the other hand, the woman with a previous event may be the very woman who needs the protection of estrogen against cardiovascular disease. This, too, is a difficult decision requiring unknown risk taking by both physician and patient. In our opinion, estrogen treatment is appropriate for these patients.

Metabolic contraindications to estrogen include impaired liver function and acute vascular disease (including embolus and thrombosis). Close surveillance is indicated for some patients with seizure disorders, familial hyperlipidemias (elevated triglycerides), and migraine headaches. Patients with migraine headaches often improve if a daily, continuous method of treatment is used, eliminating a cyclic change in hormone levels which can serve to trigger headaches.

Conditions which do not represent contraindications include controlled hypertension, diabetes mellitus, varicose veins, and gall stones. The belief that estrogen is potentially harmful with each of these clinical situations is derived from old studies of high dose birth control pills. Estrogen in appropriate doses is acceptable in the presence of these conditions.

Fibroid tumors of the uterus are almost never stimulated to grow by replacement doses of estrogen. Nevertheless, pelvic examination surveillance is a wise course. No other cancers (besides those mentioned above) are known to be adversely affected by hormone replacement.

Other Considerations. High dose calcium supplementation can unmask asymptomatic hyperparathyroidism. Women receiving calcium supplementation in excess of 500 mg daily should have their blood levels of calcium and phosphorus measured yearly for the first 2 years. If normal, no further surveillance is necessary.

A striking and consistent finding in most studies dealing with menopause and hormonal replacement is a marked placebo response in a variety of symptoms, including flushing. A significant clinical problem encountered in our referral practice is the following scenario: A woman will occasionally undergo an apparent beneficial response to estrogen, only to have the response wear off in several months. This leads to a sequence of periodic visits to the physician and ever-increasing doses of estrogen therapy. When a patient reaches a point of requiring large doses of estrogen (2.5 mg conjugated estrogens), a careful inquiry must be undertaken for a basic psychoneurotic problem.

Veralipride (100 mg/day), a strong blocker of dopamine receptors in the hypothalamus, prevents hot flushes very effectively. (141) The main side effect is galactorrhea. Clonidine has also been found to reduce the frequency of flushes, but it is less effective than either estrogen or progestin, and the dose required is associated with a high rate of side effects. Propranolol and similar agents are ineffective.

Hormonal treatment for decreased libido should be discouraged. Psychosocial reasons are usually to blame. However, we have found that occasionally the addition of androgen (methyltestosterone, up to 5 mg daily), in addition to the estrogen, may provide an increased sense of well-being, along with an increase in libido, and this has been supported by well-designed, controlled studies. (142) A commercial preparation is available in the U.S. (Estratest HS), containing 0.625 mg esterified estrogens and 1.25 mg methyltestosterone. The patient should be cautioned that hirsutism can develop. The long-term effect on the lipid profile is unknown, and the lipoprotein profile should be monitored. In addition, the estrogen-androgen combination does not prevent endometrial hyperplasia, and the addition of a progestational agent is still necessary.

We find no need to monitor dosage by any means other than symptoms and bleeding; assessing vaginal cytology is not useful.

We believe that the benefits of estrogen-progestin replacement therapy make it worthwhile to offer this preventive health care program to almost all women. It is not cost effective to attempt to select a high risk group (e.g. bone density measurements to select those at high risk for osteoporosis). (143) Such efforts are useful when an individual woman requires the information in order to make an informed decision regarding hormone replacement. Because smokers have lower estrogen levels on estrogen therapy, it might be worthwhile to document the impact of treatment on bone density in order to consider whether dosage is adequate. The method of choice, in terms of accuracy and sensitivity, is either dual-photon absorptiometry or a quantitative CT scan of the metabolically active trabecular bone in the spine. There is an increased risk of fracture when the bone density is less than 1 g of mineral/cm^2 by dual photon absorptiometry or below 110 mg/cm^3 by CT scan.

When To Biopsy?.   The cost effectiveness of routine endometrial biopsies can be argued. It has been estimated that over 3,000 biopsies are necessary in order to detect a single case of an atypical lesion in an asymptomatic woman. A reasonable economic moderation would be to limit biopsies (using the plastic endometrial suction device in the office) to patients at higher risk for endometrial changes: those women with conditions associated with chronic estrogen exposure (obesity, dysfunctional uterine bleeding, anovulation and infertility, hirsutism, high alcohol intake, hepatic disease, metabolic problems such as diabetes mellitus and hypothyroidism) and those women in whom irregular bleeding occurs while on estrogen-progestin therapy. In the absence of abnormal bleeding, a certain amount of trust in the protective effects of the progestin is justified, and routine, periodic biopsies are not necessary.

References

1. **Krailo MD, Pike MC,** Estimation of the distribution of age at natural menopause from prevalence data, Am J Epidemiol 117:356, 1983.

2. **McKinlay SM, Bifano NL, McKinlay JB,** Smoking and age at menopause in women, Ann Intern Med 103:350, 1985.

3. **Siddle N, Sarrel P, Whitehead M,** The effect of hysterectomy on the age at ovarian failure: identification of a subgroup of women with premature loss of ovarian function and literature review, Fertil Steril 47:94, 1987.

4. **Coulam CB, Adamson SC, Annegers JF,** Incidence of premature ovarian failure, Obstet Gynecol 67:604, 1986.

5. **Amundsen DW, Diers CJ,** The age of menopause in medieval Europe, Hum Biol 45:605, 1973.

6. **Gosden RG,** Follicular status at menopause, Human Reprod 2:617, 1987.

7. **Sherman BM, West JH, Korenman SG,** The menopausal transition: analysis of LH, FSH, estradiol, and progesterone concentrations during menstrual cycles of older women, J Clin Endocrinol Metab 42:629, 1976.

8. **Meldrum DR, Davidson BJ, Tataryn IV, Judd HL,** Changes in circulating steroids with aging in postmenopausal women, Obstet Gynecol 57:624, 1981.

9. **Judd HL, Shamonki IM, Frumar AM, Lagasse LD,** Origin of serum estradiol in postmenopausal women, Obstet Gynecol 59:680, 1982.

10. **Longcope C, Jaffee W, Griffing G,** Production rates of androgens and oestrogens in post-menopausal women, Maturitas 3:215, 1981.

11. **Meldrum DR,** The pathophysiology of postmenopausal symptoms, Seminars Reprod Endocrinol 1:11, 1983.

12. **Aksel S, Schomberg DW, Tyrey L, Hammond CB,** Vasomotor symptoms, serum estrogens and gonadotropin levels in surgical menopause, Am J Obstet Gynecol 126:165, 1976.

13. **Richelson LS, Wahner HW, Melton LJ III, Riggs BL,** Relative contributions of aging and estrogen deficiency to postmenopausal bone loss, New Engl J Med 311:1273, 1984.

14. **Nilas L, Christiansen C,** Bone mass and its relationship to age and the menopause, J Clin Endocrinol Metab 65:697, 1987.

15. **Avioli LV,** Calcium and osteoporosis, Annu Rev Nutr 4:471, 1984.

16. **Seeman E, Hopper JL, Bach LA, Cooper ME, Parkinson E, McKay J, Jerums G,** Reduced bone mass in daughters of women with osteoporosis, New Engl J Med 320:554, 1989.

17. **Riggs BL, Wahner HW, Dunn WL, Mazess RB, Offord KP, Melton LJ III,** Differential changes in bone mineral density of the appendicular and axial skeleton with aging: Relationship to spinal osteoporosis, J Clin Invest 67:328, 1981.

18. **Weiss NC, Ure CL, Ballard JH, Williams AR, Daling JR,** Estimated incidence of fractures of the lower forearm and hip in postmenopausal women, New Engl J Med 303:1195, 1980.

19. **Ettinger B, Genant HK, Cann CE,** Long-term estrogen replacement therapy prevents bone loss and fractures, Ann Intern Med 102:319, 1985.

20. **Kiel DP, Felson DT, Anderson JJ, Wilson PWF, Moskowitz MA,** Hip fracture and the use of estrogens in postmenopausal women: The Framingham Study, New Engl J Med 317:1169, 1987.

21. **Riggs BL, Seeman E, Hodgson SF, Taves DR, O'Fallon WM,** Effect of the fluoride/calcium regimen on vertebral fracture occurrence in postmenopausal osteoporosis, New Engl J Med 306:446, 1982.

22. **Jensen GF, Christiansen C, Transbol I,** Treatment of postmenopausal osteoporosis. A controlled therapeutic trial comparing oestrogen/gestagen, 1,25-dihydroxy-vitamin D3, and calcium, Clin Endocrinol 16:515, 1982.

23. **Heaney RP, Recker RR, Saville PD,** Menopausal changes in calcium balance performance, Lab Clin Med 92:953, 1978.

24. **Heaney RP, Recker RR,** Distribution of calcium absorption in middle-aged women, Am J Clin Nutrition 43:299, 1986.

25. **Riis B, Thomsen K, Christiansen C,** Does calcium supplementation prevent postmenopausal bone loss? New Engl J Med 316:173, 1987.

26. **Ettinger B, Genant HK, Cann CE,** Postmenopausal bone loss is prevented by treatment with low-dosage estrogen with calcium, Ann Intern Med 106:40, 1987.

27. **Stevenson JC, Whitehead MI, Padwick M, Endacott JA, Sutton C, Banks LM, Freemantle C, Spinks TJ, Hesp R,** Dietary intake of calcium and postmenopausal bone loss, Brit Med J 297:15, 1988.

28. **Abdalla HI, Hart DM, Lindsay R, Leggate I, Hooke A,** Prevention of bone mineral loss in postmenopausal women by norethisterone, Obstet Gynecol 66:789, 1985.

29. **Selby PL, Peacock M, Barkworth SA, Brown WB, Taylor GA,** Early effects of ethinyl oestradiol and norethisterone treatment in postmenopausal women on bone resorption and calcium regulating hormones, Clin Sci 69:265, 1985.

30. **Christiansen C, Nilas L, Riis BJ, Rodbro P, Deftos L,** Uncoupling of bone formation and resorption by combined oestrogen and progestagen therapy in postmenopausal osteoporosis, Lancet ii:800, 1985.

31. **Munk-Jensen N, Nielsen SP, Obel EB, Eriksen PB,** Reversal of postmenopausal vertebral bone loss by oestrogen and progestogen: A double blind placebo controlled study, Brit Med J 296:1150, 1988.

32. **Quigley MET, Martin PL, Burnier AM, Brooks P,** Estrogen therapy arrests bone loss in elderly women, Am J Obstet Gynecol 156:1516, 1987.

33. **Tiegs RD, Body JJ, Wahner HW, Barta J, Riggs BL, Heath H,** Calcitonin secretion in postmenopausal osteoporosis, New Engl J Med 312:1097, 1985.

34. **Komm BSD, Terpening CM, Benz DJ, Graeme KA, Gallegos A, Korc M, Greene GL, O'Malley BW, Haussler MR,** Estrogen binding, receptor mRNA, and biologic response in osteoblast-like osteosarcoma cells, Science 241:81, 1988.

35. **Eriksen EF, Colvard DS, Berg NJ, Graham ML, Mann KG, Speisberg TC, Riggs BL,** Evidence of estrogen receptors in normal human osteoblast-like cells, Science 241:84, 1988.

36. **Lindsay R, MacLean A, Kraszewski A, Clark AC, Garwood J,** Bone response to termination of estrogen treatment, Lancet i:1325, 1978.

37. **Horsman A, Nordin BEC, Crilly RG,** Effect on bone of withdrawal of estrogen therapy, Lancet ii:33, 1979.

38. **Christiansen C, Christiansen MS, Transbol IB,** Bone mass in postmenopausal women after withdrawal of oestrogen/gestagen replacement therapy, Lancet i:459, 1981.

39. **Wasnich R, Yano K, Vogel J,** Postmenopausal bone loss at multiple skeletal sites: Relationship to estrogen use, J Chron Dis 36:781, 1983.

40. **Jensen J, Christiansen C, Rodbro P,** Cigarette smoking, serum estrogens, and bone loss during hormone replacement therapy early after menopause, New Engl J Med 313:973, 1985.

41. **Michnovicz JJ, Hershcopf RJ, Naganuma H, Bradlow HL, Fishman J,** Increased 2-hydroxylation of estradiol as a possible mechanism for the anti-estrogenic effect of cigarette smoking, New Engl J Med 315:1305, 1986.

42. **Barbieri RL, McShane PM, Ryan KJ,** Constituents of cigarette smoke inhibit human granulosa cell aromatase, Fertil Steril 46:232, 1986.

43. **MacIntyre I, Stevenson JC, Whitehead MI, Wimalawansa SJ, et al,** Calcitonin for prevention of postmenopausal bone loss, Lancet i:900, 1988.

44. **Chow RK, Harrison JE, Brown CF, Hajek V,** Physical fitness effect on bone mass in postmenopausal women, Arch Phys Med Rehabil 67:231, 1986.

45. **Henderson BE, Paganini-Hill A, Ross RK,** Estrogen replacement therapy and protection from acute myocardial infarction, Am J Obstet Gynecol 159:312, 1988.

46. **Rosenberg L, Armstrong B, Jick H,** Myocardial infarction and estrogen therapy in postmenopausal women, New Engl J Med 294:1256, 1976.

47. **Pfeffer RI, Whipple GH, Kurosake TT, Chapman JM,** Coronary risk and estrogen use in postmenopausal women, Am J Epidemiol 107:479, 1978.

48. **Jick H, Dinan B, Rothman KJ,** Noncontraceptive estrogens and non-fatal myocardial infarction, JAMA 239:1407, 1978.

49. **Rosenberg L, Sloane D, Shapiro S, Kaufman D, Stolley PD, Miethinen OS,** Noncontraceptive estrogens and myocardial infarction in young women, JAMA 224:339, 1980.

50. **Ross RK, Paganini-Hill A, Mack TM, Arthur M, Henderson BE,** Menopausal oestrogen therapy and protection from death from ischaemic heart disease, Lancet i:585, 1981.

51. **Bain C, Willett W, Hennekens CH, Rosner B, Belanger C, Speizer FE,** Use of postmenopausal hormones and risk of myocardial infarction, Circulation 64:42, 1981.

52. **Adam S, Williams V, Vessey MP,** Cardiovascular disease and hormone replacement treatment: A pilot case-control study, Brit Med J 282:1277, 1981.

53. **Szklo M, Tonascia J, Gordis L, Bloom I,** Estrogen use and myocardial infarction risk: A case-control study, Prevent Med 13:510, 1984.

54. **Sullivan JM, Vander Zwaag R, Lemp GF, Hughes JP, Maddock V, Kroetz FW, Ramanathan KB, Mirvis DM,** Postmenopausal estrogen use and coronary atherosclerosis, Ann Intern Med 108:358, 1988.

55. **Gruchow HW, Anderson AJ, Barboriak JJ, Sobocinski KA,** Postmenopausal use of estrogen and occlusion of coronary arteries, Am Heart J 115:954, 1988.

56. **Burch JC, Byrd BF, Vaughn WK,** The effects of long-term estrogen on hysterectomized women, Am J Obstet Gynecol 118:778, 1974.

57. **Hammond CB, Jelovsek FR, Lee KL, Creasman WT, Parker RT,** Effects of long-term estrogen replacement therapy: I. Metabolic effects, Am J Obstet Gynecol 133:525, 1979.

58. **Gordon T, Kannel WB, Hjortland MC, McNamara PM,** Menopause and coronary heart disease: The Framingham Study, Ann Intern Med 89:157, 1978.

59. **Petitti DB, Wingerd J, Pellegrin F, Ramcharan S,** Risk of vascular disease in women: smoking, oral contraceptives, non-contraceptive estrogens, and other factors, JAMA 242:1150, 1979.

60. **Bush TL, Barrett-Connor E, Cowan DK, Criqui MH, Wallace RB, Suchindran CM, Tyroler HA, Rifkind BM,** Cardiovascular mortality and noncontraceptive use of estrogen in women: Results from the Lipid Research Clinics Program Follow-up Study, Circulation 75:1102, 1987.

61. **Lafferty FW, Helmuth DO,** Postmenopausal estrogen replacement: The prevention of osteoporosis and systemic effects, Maturitas 7:147, 1985.

62. **Wilson PWF, Garrison RJ, Castelli WP,** Postmenopausal estrogen use, cigarette smoking, and cardiovascular morbidity in women over 50. The Framingham Study, New Engl J Med 313:1038, 1985.

63. **Stampfer MJ, Willett WC, Colditz GA, Rosner B, Speizer FE, Hennekens CH,** A prospective study of postmenopausal estrogen therapy and coronary heart disease, New Engl J Med 313:1044, 1985.

64. **Eaker ED, Castelli WP,** Coronary heart disease and its risk factors among women in the Framingham Study, in Eaker ED, Packard B, Wenger NG, editors, *Coronary Heart Disease in Women*, Haymarket Doyma Inc, New York, 1987, pp 122-130.

65. **Speroff T, Dawson N, Speroff L,** Is postmenopausal estrogen use risky? Results from a methodologic review and information synthesis, Clin Res 35:362A, 1987.

66. **Colditz GA, Willett WC, Stampfer MJ, Rosner B, Speizer FE, Hennekens CG,** Menopause and the risk of coronary heart disease in women, New Engl J Med 316:1105, 1987.

67. **Sorva R, Kuusi T, Dunkel L, Taskinen M-R,** Effects of endogenous sex steroids on serum lipoproteins and postheparin plasma lipolytic enzymes, J Clin Endocrinol Metab 66:408, 1988.

68. **Hart DM, Farish E, Fletcher DC, Howie C, Kitchener H,** Ten years postmenopausal hormone replacement therapy—effect on lipoproteins, Maturitas 5:271, 1984.

69. **Cauley JA, La Porte RE, Sandler RB, Orchard TJ, Slemenda CW, Petrini AM,** The relationship of physical activity to high density lipoprotein cholesterol in postmenopausal women, J Chron Dis 39:687, 1986.

70. **Adams MR, Clarkson TB, Koritnik DR, Nash HA,** Contraceptive steroids and coronary artery atherosclerosis in cynomolgus macaques, Fertil Steril 47:1010, 1987.

71. **Hough JL, Zilversmit DB,** Effect of 17 beta estradiol on aortic cholesterol content and metabolism in cholesterol-fed rabbits, Arteriosclerosis 6:57, 1986.

72. **Hirvonen E, Malkonen M, Manninen V,** Effects of different progestogens on lipoproteins during postmenopausal therapy, New Engl J Med 304:560, 1981.

73. **Mattsson L, Cullberg LG, Samsioe G,** Influence of esterified estrogens and medroxyprogesterone on lipid metabolism and sex steroids. A study in oophorectomized women, Hormone Metab Res 14:602, 1982.

74. **Silferstolpe G, Gustafsson A, Samsioe G, Syanborg A,** Lipid metabolic studies in oophorectomized women: Effects on serum lipids and lipoproteins of three synthetic progestogens, Maturitas 4:103, 1983.

75. **Ylostalo P, Kauppila A, Kivinen S, Tuimala R, Vihkoo R,** Endocrine and metabolic effects of low-dose estrogen-progestin treatment in climacteric women, Obstet Gynecol 62:682, 1983.

76. **Mattsson L, Cullberg G, Samsioe G,** A continuous estrogen-progestogen regimen for climacteric complaints, Acta Obstet Gynecol Scand 63:673, 1984.

77. **Ottosson UB, Carlstrom K, Damber JE, von Schoultz B,** Serum levels of progesterone and some of its metabolites including deoxycorticosterone after oral and parenteral administration, Brit J Obstet Gynecol 91:1111, 1984.

78. **Wren B, Garrett D,** The effect of low-dose piperazine oestrogen sulphate and low-dose levonorgestrel on blood lipid levels in postmenopausal women, Maturitas 7:141, 1985.

79. **Ottosson UB, Johansson BG, von Schoultz B,** Subfractions of high-density lipoprotein cholesterol during estrogen replacement therapy: A comparison between progestogens and natural progesterone, Am J Obstet Gynecol 151:746, 1985.

80. **Ravnikar V, Murin V, Nutkik J, Ryan KJ, Schiff I,** Blood lipid levels in postmenopausal women on hormone replacement therapy, 35th Annual Meeting, Soc Gynecol Invest, Abstract No. 422, 1988.

81. **Barrett-Connor E, Wingard DL, Criqui MH,** Postmenopausal estrogen use and heart disease risk factors in the 1980s, JAMA 261:2095, 1989.

82. **Paganini-Hill A, Ross RK, Henderson BE,** Postmenopausal oestrogen treatment and stroke: A prospective study, Brit Med J 297:519, 1988.

83. **Lind T, Cameron EC, Hunter WM, Leon C, Moran PF, Oxley A, Gerrard J, Lind UCG,** A prospective, controlled trial of six forms of hormone replacement therapy given to postmenopausal women, Brit J Obstet Gynaecol (Suppl 3) 86:1, 1979.

84. **Pfeffer RI, Kurosaki TT, Charlton SK,** Estrogen use and blood pressure in later life, Am J Epidemiol 110:469, 1979.

85. **Lutola H,** Blood pressure and hemodynamics in postmenopausal women during estradiol-17β substitution, Ann Clin Res (Suppl 38) 15:9, 1983.

86. **Wren BG, Routledge AD,** The effect of type and dose of oestrogen on the blood pressure of postmenopausal women, Maturitas 5:135, 1983.

87. **Hassager C, Christiansen C,** Blood pressure during oestrogen/progestogen substitution therapy in healthy post-menopausal women, Maturitas 9:315, 1988.

88. **Wilson PD, Faragher B, Butler B, Bullock D, Robinson EL, Brown ADG,** Treatment with oral piperazine oestrone sulphate for genuine stress incontinence in postmenopausal women, Brit J Obstet Gynaecol 94:568, 1987.

89. **Bhatia NN, Bergman A, Karram MM,** Effects of estrogen on urethral function in women with urinary incontinence, Obstet Gynecol 160:176, 1989.

90. **Semmens JP, Wagner G,** Effects of estrogen therapy on vaginal physiology during menopause, Obstet Gynecol 66:15, 1985.

91. **Cauley JA, Petrini AM, LaPorte RE, Sandler RB, Bayles CM, Robertson RJ, Slemenda CW,** The decline of grip strength in the menopause: Relationship to physical activity, estrogen use and anthropometric factors, J Chron Dis 40:115, 1987.

92. **Vandenbroucke JP, Witteman JCM, Valkenburg HA, Boersma JW, Cats A, Festen JJM, Hartman AP, Huber-Bruning O, Rasker JJ, Weber J,** Noncontraceptive hormones and rheumatoid arthritis in perimenopausal and postmenopausal women, JAMA 255:1299, 1986.

93. **Campbell S, Whitehead M,** Estrogen therapy and the menopausal syndrome, Clin Obstet Gynecol 4:31, 1977.

94. **Schiff I, Regestein Q, Tulchinsky D, Ryan KJ,** Effects of estrogens on sleep and psychological state of hypogonadal women, JAMA 242:2405, 1979.

95. **Grimes DA,** Diagnostic dilation and curettage: A reappraisal, Am J Obstet Gynecol 142:1, 1982.

96. **Kaunitz AM, Masciello A, Ostrowski M, Rovira EZ,** Comparison of endometrial biopsy with the endometrial Pipelle and Vabra aspirator, J Reprod Med 33:427, 1988.

97. **Einerth Y,** Vacuum curettage by the Vabra method. A simple procedure for endometrial diagnosis, Acta Obstet Gynecol Scand 61:373, 1982.

98. **Goldstein SR, Subramanyam B, Snyder JR, Beller U, et al,** The postmenopausal cystic adnexal mass: The potential role of ultrasound in conservative management, Obstet Gynecol 73:8, 1989.

99. **Boston Collaborative Drug Surveillance Program,** Surgically confirmed gallbladder disease, venous thromboembolism, and breast tumors in relation to postmenopausal estrogen therapy, New Engl J Med 290:15, 1974.

100. **Scagg RKR, McMichael AJ, Seamark RF,** Oral contraceptive, pregnancy and endogenous estrogen in gallstone disease—a case-control study, Brit Med J 288:1795, 1984.

101. **Kakar F, Weiss NS, Strite SA,** Non-contraceptive estrogen use and the risk of gallstone disease in women, Am J Pub Health 78:564, 1988.

102. **Shapiro S, Kelly JP, Rosenberg L, Kaufman DW, Helmrich SP, Rosenshein NB, Lewis JL Jr, Knapp RC, Stolley PD, Schottenfeld D,** Risk of localized and widespread endometrial cancer in relation to recent and discontinued use of conjugated estrogens, New Engl J Med 313:969, 1985.

103. **Paganini-Hill, Ross RK, Henderson BE,** Endometrial cancer and patterns of use of oestrogen replacement therapy: A cohort study, Brit J Cancer 59:445, 1989.

104. **Thom MH, White PJ, Williams RM, Sturdee PW, Paterson MEL, Wade-Evans T, Studd JWW,** Prevention and treatment of endometrial disease in climacteric women receiving estrogen, Lancet ii:455, 1979.

105. **Whitehead MI, Townsend PT, Pryse-Davies J, Ryder TA, King RJB,** Effects of estrogen and progestins on the biochemistry and morphology of the postmenopausal endometrium, New Engl J Med 305:1599, 1981.

106. **Gambrell RD Jr, Babgnell CA, Greenblatt RB,** Role of estrogens and progesterone in the etiology and prevention of endometrial cancer: A review, Am J Obstet Gynecol 146:696, 1983

107. **Persson I, Adami H-O, Bergkvist L, Lindgren A, Pettersson, Hoover R, Schairer C,** Risk of endometrial cancer after treatment with oestrogens alone or in conjunction with progestogens: Results of a prospective study, Brit Med J 298:147, 1989.

108. **Varma TR,** Effect of long-term therapy with estrogen and progesterone on the endometrium of postmenopausal women, Acta Obstet Gynecol Scand 64:41, 1985.

109. **Creasman WT, Henderson D, Hinshaw W, Clarke-Pearson DL,** Estrogen replacment therapy in the patient treated for endometrial cancer, Obstet Gynecol 67:326, 1986.

110. **Kaufman DW, Miller DR, Rosenberg L, Helmrich SP, Stolley P, Schottenfeld D, Shapiro S,** Noncontraceptive estrogen use and the risk of breast cancer, JAMA 252:63, 1984.

111. **Wingo PA, Layde PM, Lee NC, Rubin G, Ory HW,** The risk of breast cancer in postmenopausal women who have used estrogen replacement therapy, JAMA 257:209, 1987.

112. **Buring JE, Hennekens CH, Lipnick RJ, Willett W, Stampfer MJ, Rosner B, Peto R, Speizer FE,** A prospective cohort study of postmenopausal hormone use and risk of breast cancer in U.S. women, Am J Epidemiol 125:939, 1987.

113. **Rohan TE, McMichael AJ,** Non-contraceptive exogenous oestrogen therapy and breast cancer, Med J Aust 148:217, 1988.

114. **Armstrong BK,** Oestrogen therapy after the menopause—boon or bane? Med J Aust 148:213, 1988.

115. **Dupont WD, Page DL, Rogers LW, Parl FF,** Influence of exogenous estrogens, proliferative breast disease, and other variables on breast cancer risk, Cancer 63:948, 1989.

116. **Nachtigall LE, Nachtigall RH, Nachtigall RD, Beckman EM,** Estrogen replacement therapy. II. A prospective study in the relationship to carcinoma and cardiovascular and metabolic problems, Obstet Gynecol 54:74, 1979.

117. **Gambrell RD Jr, Maier R, Sancers BI,** Decreased incidence of breast cancer in postmenopausal estrogen-progestogen users, Obstet Gynecol 62:435, 1983.

118. **Bergkvist L, Hans-Olov A, Persson I, Hoover R, Schairer C,** The risk of breast cancer after estrogen and estrogen-progestin replacement, New Engl J Med 321:293, 1989.

119. **Ewertz M,** Influence of non-contraceptive exogenous and endogenous sex hormones on breast cancer risk in Denmark, Int J Cancer 42:832, 1988.

120. **Genant HK, Cann CE, Ettinger B, Gordan GS,** Quantitative computed tomography of vertebral spongiosa: A sensitive method for detecting early bone loss after oophorectomy, Ann Intern Med 97:699, 1982.

121. **Lindsay R, Hart M, Clark DM,** The minimum effective dose of estrogen for prevention of postmenopausal bone loss, Obstet Gynecol 63:759, 1984.

122. **Mashchak CA, Lobo RA, Dozono-Takano R, Eggena P, Nakamura RM, Brenner PF, Mishell DR Jr,** Comparison of pharmacodynamic properties of various estrogen formulations, Am J Obstet Gynecol 144:511, 1982.

123. **Horsman A, Jones M, Francis R, Nordin C,** The effect of estrogen dose on postmenopausal bone loss, New Engl J Med 309:1405, 1983.

124. **Goebelsmann U, Mashchak CA, Mishell DR Jr,** Comparison of hepatic impact of oral and vaginal administration of ethinyl estradiol, Am J Obstet Gynecol 151:868, 1985.

125. **Laufer LR, DeFazio JL, Lu JKH, Meldrum DR, Eggena P, Sambhi MP, Hershman JM, Judd HL,** Estrogen replacement therapy by transdermal estradiol administration, Am J Obstet Gynecol 146:533, 1983.

126. **Fahraeus L, Larsson-Cohn U, Wallentin L,** Lipoproteins during oral and cutaneous administration of oestradiol-17β to menopausal women, Acta Endocrinol 101:597, 1982.

127. **Fahraeus L, Wallentin L,** High density lipoprotein subfraction during oral and cutaneous administration of 17β-estradiol to menopausal women, J Clin Endocrinol Metab 56:797, 1983.

128. **Fletcher CD, Farish E, Hart DM, Barlow DH, Gray CE, Conaghan CJ,** Long-term hormone implant therapy—effects on lipoproteins and steroid levels in post-menopausal women, Acta Endocrinol 111:419, 1986.

129. **Jensen J, Riis BJ, Strom V, Nilas L, Christiansen C,** Long-term effects of percutaneous estrogens and oral progesterone on serum lipoproteins in postmenopausal women, Am J Obstet Gynecol 156:66, 1987.

130. **Riis BJ, Thomsen K, Strom V, Christiansen, C,** The effect of percutaneous estradiol and natural progesterone on postmenopausal bone loss, Am J Obstet Gynecol 156:61, 1987.

131. **Gibbons WE, Moyer DL, Lobo RA, Roy S, Mishell DR Jr,** Biochemical and histologic effects of sequential estrogen/progestin therapy on the endometrium of postmenopausal women, Am J Obstet Gynecol 154:456, 1986.

132. **Strickland DM, Hammond TL,** Postmenopausal estrogen replacement in a large gynecologic practice, Am J Gynecol Health 2:33, 1988.

133. **Mattsson L, Cullberg G, Samsioe G,** Evaluation of a continuous oestrogen-progestogen regimen for climacteric complaints, Maturitas 4:95, 1982.

134. **Magos AL, Brincat M, Studd JWW, Wardle P, Schlesinger P, O'Dowd T,** Amenorrhea and endometrial atrophy with continuous oral estrogen and progestogen therapy in postmenopausal women, Obstet Gynecol 65:496, 1985.

135. **Jensen J, Riis BJ, Strom V, Christiansen C,** Continuous oestrogen-progestogen treatment and serum lipoproteins in postmenopausal women, Brit J Obstet Gynaecol 94:130, 1987.

136. **Prough SG, Aksel S, Wiebe RH, Shepherd J,** Continuous estrogen/progestin therapy in menopause, Am J Obstet Gynecol 157:1449, 1987.

137. **Riis BJ, Johansen J, Christiansen C,** Continuous oestrogen-progestogen treatment and bone metabolism in post-menopausal women, Maturitas 10:51, 1988.

138. **Williams SR, Frenchek B, Speroff T, Speroff L,** A study of combined continuous ethinyl estradiol and norethindrone acetate for postmenopausal hormone replacement, Am J Obstet Gynecol 162:438, 1990.

139. **Reimnitz C, Brand E, Nieberg RK, Hacker NF,** Malignancy arising in endometriosis associated with unopposed estrogen replacement, Obstet Gynecol 71:444, 1988.

140. **Wile AG, DiSaia PJ,** Hormones and breast cancer, Am J Surg 157:438, 1989.

141. **David A, Don R, Tajchner G, Wessglas L,** Veralipride: Alternative antidopaminergic treatment for menopausal symptoms, Am J Obstet Gynecol 158:1107, 1988.

142. **Sherwin BB, Gelfand MM, Brender W,** Androgen enhances sexual motivation in females: A prospective, crossover study of sex steroid administration in the surgical menopause, Psychosom Med 47:339, 1985.

143. **Hall FM, Davis MA, Baran DT,** Bone mineral screening for osteoporosis, New Engl J Med 316:212, 1987.

6 Sexuality in the Older Years

What is sexuality is a simple question, but there are many answers. We recommend the following suggestions, quoted from a very helpful book, *Sex Is Not Simple*, by Stephen Levine: (1)

1. "Sexuality is a vehicle within each of us for pleasure, self-discovery, and attachment to others."

2. "Sexuality is a personal, multidimensional experience consisting of gender identity, orientation, intention, desire, arousal, and orgasm."

3. "Sexuality is a resource requiring thoughtful management. Its challenge is to realize physical and emotional pleasure as well as self- and partner-love. Its major dangers are personal and partner despair, premature or unvalued pregnancy, and venereal disease."

4. "Sexuality is the intimate physical interaction with partners and the complex meanings that we, our partners, and society give to this behavior."

5. "Sexuality is a type of voice, a running dialogue in our privacy that sheds light on our psychological selves at every stage of life. This voice speaks to us of our needs for attachment to others and our comfort in being intimate. The voice blurts out unsociable and unkind truths that, when occurring with persistent repetition, motivate us to make changes in ourselves and our relationships."

6. "Sexuality is a repair mechanism with the power to cut loose our painful pasts and allow us to experience our bodies and our psychological selves (they are ultimately inseparable) as good and loved, even though as children we might have been uncertain about ourselves. This repair mechanism does not work for everybody—many peoples' adult sexual lives are constricted by severe problems."

7. "Sexuality is an ever-changing natural force like the wind, a force whose basic nature and origins are mysterious. We still do not know many of the biological foundations of sexuality. Although there has been an explosion of information about sex during the last two decades, there is much to be learned about the basic anatomy and physiology of sexuality."

8. ''Sexuality is another vantage point from which to study how our minds work. It is an introduction to the psychology of intimacy. Intimacy is often held up as a goal for long-term relationships without sufficient appreciation for what it is and how difficult it is to achieve and maintain.''

Sexuality is a life-long behavior with evolving change and development. It begins with birth (maybe before) and ends with death. The notion that it ends with aging is inherently illogical. The need for closeness, caring, and companionship is life-long. Old people today live longer, are healthier, have more education and leisure time, and have had their consciousness raised in regard to sexuality.

Masters and Johnson pointed out that one of the last bastions of culturally enforced ignorance is the area of sexuality in older people.(2) Since old age is a relatively new phenomenon, it is not surprising that understanding and appreciating sexuality in older life are new requirements for all of us. But the situation is changing. The early 1980s saw a flurry of medical articles emphasizing the sexuality of older people. It is no longer necessary to raise medical consciousness on this issue; now it is time to deal with it.

The aging woman finds herself in an uncomfortable societal position. Chances are excellent that she has outlived her spouse. She, therefore, finds herself experiencing sexual feelings without an available partner in an environment that provides little encouragement. The physician can become the resource for information, education, and coping strategies.

Sexual Changes with Aging

The female sexual response, as first described by Masters and Johnson, applies to women of all ages. This description, now an accepted classic, divides the sexual response into 4 phases:

1. **The Excitement Phase.** This phase is marked by vaginal lubrication, increased muscle tension, an increase in heart rate and blood pressure, engorgement of the breasts and the labia, and erection of the clitoris and the nipples. The production of vaginal lubrication is the female counterpart of the male's erection.

2. **The Plateau Phase.** During this phase, there is increased venous congestion throughout the body and lengthening of the vagina with dilatation of the upper two-thirds.

3. **The Orgasm Phase.** A release of sexual tension is accompanied by muscle contractions throughout the body, including the uterus.

4. **The Resolution Phase.** This phase is marked by a rapid decrease in vasocongestion and muscle tension.

There are two main sexual changes in the aging woman not on hormone replacement. There is a reduction in the rate of production and volume of vaginal lubricating fluid, and there is some loss of vaginal elasticity, and thus the ability to tolerate deep thrusting or long-continuing thrusting. The dyspareunia associated with postmenopausal urogenital atrophy includes a feeling of dryness and tightness, vaginal irritation and burning with coitus, and postcoital spotting and soreness.

110

Coital activity is not correlated with blood levels of estradiol, testosterone, androstenedione, follicle-stimulating hormone (FSH), or luteinizing hormone (LH). (3) Less vaginal atrophy is noted in sexually active women compared to inactive women; presumably the activity maintains vaginal vasculature and circulation. However, objective measurements of the degree of lubrication have demonstrated that the vaginal factors which influence the enjoyment of sexual intercourse can be maintained by estrogen replacement therapy. (4) There have been no studies of sexuality and estrogen replacement in the very old.

In the man, there are 4 changes associated with aging.

1. In response to sexual stimulation, it takes longer to achieve full engorgement. The spontaneity of the erectile process may be replaced with a response that relies on direct partner involvement.

2. There is a decrease in the expulsive pressure of the ejaculate.

3. There is a reduction in the volume of seminal fluid in the ejaculate.

4. There is a reduction or loss of ejaculatory demand. The familiar subjective demand for release of sexual tension is either reduced or absent. The refractory period between ejaculations extends to hours and even days with aging.

Unlike women at menopause, men do not experience an abrupt loss of sex hormones. Total and free blood testosterone levels decline with age as gonadotropins increase; however, the majority of men over age 80 still have testosterone levels within the normal range. (5) Indeed, no difference can be found in sperm counts and sperm morphology between young and old men. Despite a small decrease in endocrine reserve, there is no decline in the fertilizing capacity in men if they sustain sexual activity. (6)

The changes in older men are of importance not only to men, but knowledge of these changes is important to the female partner as well. A woman may react to these changes by questioning her own sexuality, and the result may be unfounded fears and reactions. Here is a logical thought: better sex education during adolescence might lead to better sexual functioning with aging.

Aging and Sexual Attitudes

Younger people, especially physicians, underrate the extent of sexual interest in older people. In a random sample of women ages 50 to 82 in Madison, Wisconsin, nearly one-half of the women reported an on-going sexual relationship. (7) In the famous Duke longitudinal study on aging, 70% of men in the 67 to 77 age group were sexually active, and 80% reported continuing sexual interest, while 50% of all older women were still interested in sex. (8)

The two most important influences on older sexual interaction are the strength of a relationship and the physical condition of each partner. The single most significant determinant of sexual activity for older women, therefore, is the unavailability of partners due to divorce and the fact that women are outliving men. Adding to this problem is the persistence of cultural taboos regarding sex, especially for older women. Many older women today have lived through a

111

period of differing cultural and social values. They may find themselves with a problem that their physician may not understand.

The decline in sexual activity with aging is influenced more by culture and attitudes than by nature and physiology. Given the availability of a partner, the same general high or low rate of sexual activity can be maintained throughout life. (9) No important relationships can be found between the amount of sexual activity and features of the marital history, the sexual attractiveness of wives, sexual attitudes, or current marital adjustment. The major factor is the rate of sexual activity earlier in life, which persists into old age.

Longitudinal studies indicate that the level of sexual activity is more stable over time than previously suggested. (10–12) Both men and women attribute the decrease in sexual activity with age to the male partner. Sexual attitudes and behavior in old age are a continuation of lifelong patterns, and the main reason for declining sexuality in older women is the unavailability of a healthy and willing partner. Sexual desire remains intact. (3) Sexuality is an integral component of everyone's quality of life. Even if the desire or ability to have sexual intercourse is no longer present, the desire to be affectionate and intimate persists.

The problems of aging people include changing relationships within their families, loneliness, dealing with death and dying, and changes in sexual expression. Happy older life requires human friendships (or with animal pets), caring, sharing, being needed, being respected, and receiving and giving affection. It is important to let older women know that sexual fantasies, desires, and dreams are normal as long as we live. There is no reason for guilt, discomfort, or shame. The elderly, sick or well, need to be hugged and cared for as much as young people (maybe more).

Little is known about the sexual activity of elderly lesbians. Older homosexual people can be even more troubled. There are no children or grandchildren, and chances are greater that there is no partner. Will older women without partners be more accepting of homosexuality to satisfy their needs?

Institutionalized elderly have another source of difficulty. Staff attitudes and beliefs are the central problem for institutionalized elderly who are categorized as having sexual problems. (13) These most often include exposure of genitalia, masturbation, and sexual talk. These "sexual problems" indicate the need for closeness, tenderness, and warmth. Sexual segregation in institutional homes is nothing but a barrier to natural and comfortable relationships. The elderly do not lose their capacity for sexual pleasure, especially the need to be touched and to touch. A controlling and limiting environment denies this human need. Advise patients and families to look for nursing homes where living is more family-like, conducive to normal relationships. The key is a staff that understands and supports sexuality, especially the components of loving and feeling.

Illness and Sex

It will not be uncommon to encounter women who have had surgery that affects sexuality. The list includes hysterectomy, vulvectomy, coronary bypass surgery, and surgery of the breast. Sexual problems are not limited, however, to surgical procedures and illnesses of the genitalia. Altered self image can occur with diseases of any site.

Sexual counseling, to be effective, must be provided to couples both before and after surgery. It is not unexpected that the surgeon may not be fully capable of providing this counseling. A major contribution from an older woman's primary physician is to arrange for competent and experienced sexual counseling. Unfortunately most physicians operate on the principle that if no questions are raised there is no problem. The expert surgeon should be grateful for the help of experts in psychosexual therapy. Seek out the potential for post-treatment sexual morbidity before the treatment. Assess the patient's abilities for coping, her sense of body image. Consider the quality of the patient's relationship, and be sensitive to the absence of a relationship. This entire effort may take some time. The normal state of presurgical anxiety, fear, and denial hampers good communication.

Hysterectomy. Conventional wisdom dictates that the only purpose of the uterus is reproduction. It is more accurate to admit that the conventional wisdom is limited by what is definitely known. For some women, the cervix and uterine corpus may contribute to sexual pleasure, either by movement or by contractions. This may explain why some women do report decreased sexual response after hysterectomy. (14) On the other hand, the majority of women experience no sexual loss after hysterectomy. This is an area deserving of more study. Unanswered questions include the following: What is the precise contribution of cervix and corpus to sexuality? To what degree is posthysterectomy sexual change due to preoperative problems? A physician, whether surgeon or not, should at least take time to provide patients and partners education regarding anatomy and physiology, and dispel misconceptions and fears based on ignorance (even in patients who seem highly sophisticated).

Vulvectomy. Unfortunately there continues to be a significant amount of misconception and unfamiliarity in women regarding the external genitalia. It is not surprising that there is a considerable reduction in coitus and masturbation after vulvectomy, but in a powerful statement regarding the importance of sexuality, it is remarkable that even without adequate counseling about one-third of couples are able to maintain satisfactory sexual function postoperatively. (15) A careful and thorough preoperative counseling program should be an essential part of this major surgical procedure. Postoperatively, patients and partners may need to be taught to discover new forms of sexual pleasure.

Breast Cancer. Approximately 25% of mastectomy patients undergo significant emotional disruption and sexual dysfunction which persist for up to one year after surgery. (16) The importance of conserving a woman's breast should not be underrated, since recent studies support the conclusion that the less extensive operative procedures produce fewer psychological problems. Although the primary consideration for the extent of surgery should be the prognosis with the procedure, there is now good evidence that in some patients less extensive surgery has equivalent therapeutic efficacy. Conservation preserves body image, protects feelings of sexual attractiveness and desirability, and influences a woman's perceptions of her sexual partner's reactions. The issue of sexuality should be addressed promptly after treatment of breast cancer. The quality of the first sexual experience after treatment strongly influences later sexual adjustment. Women most likely to have problems are those with infertility, a history of psychologic reactions, and single women. Attention to sexual function following breast cancer treatment should be an integral part of the medical care.

Hormone replacement after breast cancer is a difficult issue. There are no data to help patients and physicians. Even in the face of a tumor negative for estrogen receptors, we do not know the risk of estrogen treatment. Because of the long latent period associated with breast cancer, we do not know if duration since treatment can be considered a safety factor for estrogen replacement. It has been our practice to use oral medroxyprogesterone acetate (10–20 mg daily) to relieve vasomotor symptoms and to provide a beneficial impact on calcium balance. When estrogen is not administered, calcium should be supplemented at the rate of 1000 mg per day. Unfortunately, vaginal atrophy is not improved with progestin treatment, and dyspareunia due to dryness can even be intensified. The use of vaginal estrogen can be considered by patient and physician, balancing the sexual benefit with the unknown risk. The dose of the vaginal estrogen should be titrated by the patient to produce relief with the lowest dose possible. In addition, the daily use of a progestin can be associated with a decrease in HDL-cholesterol, and surveillance of the cholesterol-lipoprotein profile is recommended.

Coronary Bypass Surgery.   Women undergoing coronary bypass surgery do not demonstrate a significant decline in frequency of intercourse one year after surgery. (17) A good key, as with all older people, is the level of activity prior to surgery. If high, the patient and partner should be encouraged and counseled to resume sexual activity.

Myocardial Infarction.   Women (and men) do not receive satisfactory sexual counseling following heart attacks. Approximately one-half of women and husbands expressed fear of resumption of sexual activity following myocardial infarction, and only 45% received sexual counseling (in only 18% did the physician raise the subject). (18) Simply giving sexual instructions did not relieve the fear involved with resumption of activity; distributing printed material is not enough. In those couples who do not resume sexual activity, there is a deterioration of their emotional relationships.

Women receive less sexual counseling after acute coronary heart disease than do men. (19) One cannot make assumptions about the level of sexual activity or interest based on marital status or (hopefully after reading this chapter) age. Health care professionals need to be educated, not only patients.

Most patients can resume sexual activity several months after myocardial infarction. The risk of death during sexual intercourse after a heart attack is very low. The cardiovascular changes during sexual activity are similar to those encountered with ordinary activities. Studies of postcoronary patients have indicated that physical conditioning both improves the quality of sexual activity and reduces the symptoms subsequently experienced. (20)

114

Other Conditions. The most common identifiable cause of impotency in older men is diabetes mellitus. Impotency due to diabetes involves neuropathic and vascular changes. While men lose their capacity for an erection, women become nonorgasmic. However, sexual interest and desire remain, and the physician can help the couple to expand their repertoire of sexual and pleasure-giving activities.

Most men fully recover from prostate surgery within a few months and are able to resume sexual activity.

Antihypertensive agents are frequently responsible for male sexual dysfunction, but little information is available regarding female sexual function. (21) However, remember that vaginal lubrication is the female counterpart to the male erection, and therefore, vaginal dryness is a likely consequence. Adrenergic blocking agents are especially noted to affect libido and potency in men. Similarly, psychotropic drugs of all categories have been associated with inhibition of sexual function in men. Finally, one should always suspect alcoholism when patients complain of sexual dysfunction.

Management

Incorporating a brief sexual history into the general history gives a message to the patient: sexuality is important and a natural part of life. Because subsequent sexual activity is so heavily determined by the previous level of activity, some knowledge of the previous patterns is useful for the physician. An appreciation for the extent of the patient's knowledge and feelings regarding masturbation is also important. An additional important consideration: noncoital sex can be a satisfying method to achieve and maintain intimacy.

Some Key Questions:

1. Are you sexually active?

2. Do you have a healthy partner?

3. Is there any change in your level of desire?

4. Is there any discomfort with your sexual activity?

5. Is vaginal dryness a problem?

6. Is there any difficulty achieving orgasm?

What can the physician do? The following 5 items are most important:

1. Recognize and validate the patient's sexuality.

2. Give information and education.

3. Respond to the patient's concerns and questions.

4. Be nonjudgmental.

5. Be aware of the influence of drugs.

The use of referral resources is encouraged but not aggressively. A patient's own physician is better, and further fragmentation of care is to be avoided with older people. An important job for the physician is to promote for the patient the idea of pleasure and enjoyment for whatever pattern of sexual activity the patient wants or likes. One way for physicians to learn about these things (and to be more effective) is to talk with some selected older patients with whom they have a special relationship. Learn from your patients and look inward. If a physician cannot believe that sexuality is appropriate at all ages without guilt or shame, then referral is necessary.

Older people can respond to sexual counseling and change old attitudes. (12) Even more formal sex education for older people, their families, and people who work with the aged increases knowledge regarding sexuality and aging, and yields more permissive attitudes. (22)

Signs that signal a need for referral include the following:

1. Significant psychiatric illness unresponsive to your treatment.

2. When the continuation of an on-going relationship is threatened.

3. When sexual counseling efforts have failed.

Special Issues

1. Because the excitement phase is less intense in both men and women, longer, slower, and more direct stimulation may be necessary.

2. Depression is often a major reason for decreased sexuality in older people. Attention to this problem and pharmacologic treatment can yield a satisfying increase in sexual desire and activity.

3. Estrogen replacement is invariably successful in reversing atrophic problems. Vaginal lubrication and a nonfragile mucosa can be restored. Both patient and physician should be aware that a significant response can be expected by one month, but it takes a long time to fully restore the genitourinary tract (6–12 months). Couples should not be discouraged by an apparent lack of immediate response. Steege gives a nicely balanced view: sexual changes, estrogen deficiency, and mental status are overlapping and interacting. (23) Improvements in each area can help the others.

4. A form of vaginismus occurs in older women: involuntary vaginal muscle contractions because of painful intercourse. Estrogen treatment and appropriate explanation during a pelvic examination are helpful. Teaching a woman to voluntarily contract and relax the introitus can rapidly improve a woman's ability to control vaginal relaxation. (23) The woman can practice this with a finger in the introitus, then with her partner. Entry by the partner should be by stages, limiting deep penetration until the woman is sexually aroused.

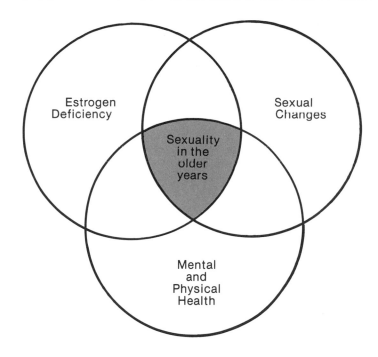

Estrogen
Deficiency

Sexual
Changes

Sexuality
in the
older
years

Mental
and
Physical
Health

after Steege (23)

5. It should be kept in mind that all individuals are susceptible to dysfunction when they resume sexual activity after a period of abstinence, and this is even more of a problem with the elderly. Perhaps the most important ingredient in reversing this problem is the cooperation and understanding of a patient partner. If there has been a pleasurable previous sexual life, this period of dysfunction responds readily if addressed promptly. If allowed to continue, it may be difficult to salvage.

6. It is worth asking women with pelvic relaxation (including cystocele, rectocele, and prolapse of the uterus) whether there is any problem with sexual response. One of the benefits of surgical repair can be a more enjoyable sexual experience for both partners.

7. Occasionally hormonal treatment for decreased libido can be helpful. The addition of androgen to an estrogen replacement program provides an increased sense of well-being in addition to the increase in libido. (24,25) A commercial preparation is available in the U.S. (Estratest HS) containing 0.625 mg esterified estrogens and 1.25 mg methyltestosterone. Hirsutism can develop, and the long-term effect on the cholesterol-lipoprotein profile is unknown. In addition, the estrogen-androgen combination does not prevent endometrial hyperplasia, and the addition of a progestational agent is still necessary.

8. Vaginal penetration with a not-so-firm erection can be aided by position changes and by the woman's hands.

9. A physician has an obligation to see to the provision of privacy for institutionalized patients, to allow at least a minimum of intimate interchange.

Masturbation Revisited. For some older people, masturbation may be the only convenient and available form of sexual activity. When we are young, orgasm contributes to our well-being (and often relieves anxiety). It is appropriate to suggest this method of satisfaction and relief to older patients. Masturbation (either manual or with the use of a mechanical device) can provide a sexual release; however, for some women it may increase the feelings of loneliness and anguish over the absence of shared intimacy. A physician should be cautious with this subject.

Abstinence. While sexuality in the aged is a subject of appropriate concern, we must be careful not to go to an extreme and impose upon those who are quite satisfied with their level of sexual activity or even total abstinence.

Final Thoughts

Sexuality is not the answer to all life's problems; we can live without sex. Other things in life are sensual: travel, gardening, the enjoyment of nature. Sexuality is just another pleasure of life, not the only one.

Pleasuring is a worthwhile objective for older people. Pleasuring can be defined as any sensual experience that feels good. This opens sexuality up to many different forms of contact and intimacy. And it doesn't require an erection. Unfortunately, the male erection still holds sway over the potential for gentle pleasure and intimacy.

We can expect future generations of elderly people to be more forthcoming with a different set of expectations, derived from their early years in a time of greater sexual openness and knowledge.

References

1. **Levine SB,** *Sex Is Not Simple,* Ohio Psychology Publishing Co., Columbus, 1988, pp 259–260.

2. **Masters WH, Johnson VE,** Sex and the aging process, J Am Geriatrics Soc 29:385, 1981.

3. **Bachmann GA, Leiblum SR, Kemmann E, Colburn DW, Swartzman L, Shelden R,** Sexual expression and its determinants in the post-menopausal woman, Maturitas 6:19, 1984.

4. **Semmens JP, Wagner G,** Estrogen deprivation and vaginal function in postmenopausal women, JAMA 248:445, 1982.

5. **Davidson JM, Chen JJ, Crapo L, Gray GD, Greenleaf WJ, Catania JA,** Hormonal changes and sexual function in aging men, J Clin Endocrinol Metab 57:71, 1983.

6. **Nieschlag E, Lammers U, Freischem CW, Langer K, Wickings EJ,** Reproductive functions in young fathers and grandfathers, J Clin Endocrinol Metab 55:676, 1982.

7. **Traupman J, Eckels E, Hatfield E,** Intimacy in older women's lives, Gerontologist 2:493, 1982.

8. **Pfeiffer E, Verwoerdt A, Davis GC,** Sexual behavior in middle life, Am J Psychiatr 128:1262, 1972.

9. **Martin CE,** Factors affecting sexual functioning in 60–79 year-old married males, Arch Sex Behavior 10:399, 1981.

10. **George LK, Weiler SJ,** Sexuality in middle and late life, Arch Gen Psychiatr 38:919, 1981.

11. **White CB,** Sexual interest, attitudes, knowledge, and sexual history in relation to sexual behavior in the institutionalized aged, Arch Sex Behavior 11:11, 1982.

12. **Renshaw DC,** Sex, intimacy, and the older woman, Women & Health 8:43, 1983.

13. **McCartney JR, Izeman H, Rogers D, Cohen D,** Sexuality and the institutionalized elderly, J Am Geriatrics Soc 35:331, 1987.

14. **Zussman L, Zussman S, Sunley R, Bjornson E,** Sexual reponse after hysterectomy-oophorectomy: Recent studies and reconsideration of psychogenesis, Am J Obstet Gynecol 140:725, 1981.

15. **Andreasson B, Moth I, Jensen SB, Bock JE,** Sexual function and somatopsychic reactions in vulvectomy-operated women and their partners, Acta Obstet Gynecol Scand 65:7, 1986.

16. **Schain WS,** The sexual and intimate consequences of breast cancer treatment, CA 38:154, 1988.

17. **Althof SE, Coffman CB, Levine SB,** The effects of coronary bypass surgery on female sexual, psychological, and vocational adaptation, J Sex Marital Therapy 10:176, 1984.

18. **Papadopoulos C, Beaumont C, Shelley SI, Larrimore P,** Myocardial infarction and sexual activity of the female patient, Arch Intern Med 143:1528, 1983.

19. **Baggs JG, Karch AM,** Sexual counseling of women with coronary heart disease, Heart & Lung 16:154, 1987.

20. **Hellerstein HK, Friedman EH,** Sexual activity and the postcoronary patient, Arch Intern Med 125:987, 1970.

21. **Mallett EC, Badlani GH,** Sexuality in the elderly, Seminars Urology 5:141, 1987.

22. **White CB, Catania JA,** Psychoeducational intervention for sexuality with the aged, family members of the aged, and people who work with the aged, Intl J Aging Human Develop 15:121, 1982.

23. **Steege JF,** Sexual function in the aging woman, Clin Obstet Gynecol 29:462, 1986.

24. **Sherwin BB, Gelfand MM, Brender W,** Androgen enhances sexual motivation in females: A prospective, crossover study of sex steroid administration in the surgical menopause, Psychosom Med 47:339, 1985.

25. **Burger H, Hailes J, Nelson J, Menelaus M,** Effect of combined implants of oestradiol and testosterone on libido in postmenopausal women, Brit Med J 294:936, 1987.

7   Obesity

Because at least 20% of American adults (20–30% of women) over 30 years old are more than 20% overweight, the unrewarding fight against obesity is all too common, not only with our patients, but also with ourselves. Unfortunately, for over 100 years the incidence of obesity has been increasing in the United States, a reflection of an increasingly sedentary life in an affluent society. (1)

The lack of success in treating obesity is not due to an unawareness of the implications of obesity; there is a clear-cut relationship between mortality and weight. The death rate from diabetes mellitus, for example, is approximately 4 times higher among obese diabetics than among those who control their weight. Also higher among obese individuals is the incidence of gallbladder disease, cardiovascular disease, renal disease, and cirrhosis of the liver. The death rate from appendicitis is double, presumably from anesthetic and surgical complications. Even the rate of accidents is higher, perhaps because fat people are awkward or because their view of the ground or floor is obstructed. When the personal and social problems encountered by obese persons are also considered, it is no wonder that a physician without a weight problem cannot comprehend why fat individuals remain overweight.

The frequency with which a practitioner encounters the obese patient whose weight does not decrease despite a sworn adherence to a limited-calorie diet makes one question if there is something physiologically different about this patient. Is the problem due to lack of discipline and cheating on a diet, or does it also involve a pathophysiologic factor? Is the physiology of obese people unusual, or are they simply gluttons?

Definition of Obesity

There is a difference between obesity and overweight. (2) Obesity is an excess of body fat. Overweight is a body weight in excess of some standard or ideal weight. The ideal weight for any adult is believed to correspond to his or her ideal weight from age 20 to 30. The following formulas give ideal weight in pounds:

Women: 100 + [4 × (height in inches minus 60)]
Men: 120 + [4 × (height in inches minus 60)]

At a weight close to ideal weight, individuals may be overweight, but not over fat. This is especially true of individuals engaged in regular exercise. An estimate of body fat, therefore, rather than a measurement of height and weight, is more significant.

121

The most accurate method of determining body fat is to determine the density of the body by underwater measurement. It certainly is not practical to measure density by submerging individuals in water in our offices, therefore skinfold measurements with calipers have become popular as an index of body fat. The skinfold measurement is also not necessary for clinical practice. It is far simpler to utilize the body mass index nomogram, a method that has been found to correspond closely to densitometry measurements. (3)

The body mass index is the ratio of weight divided by the height squared (in metric units). To read the central scale, align a straight edge between the height and body weight scales. A body mass index of about 30 is roughly equivalent to 30% excess body weight, the point at which excess mortality begins. Above 40, the risk from obesity itself is comparable to that associated with major health problems such as hypertension and heavy smoking.

A person is obese when the amount of adipose tissue is sufficiently high (20% or more over ideal weight) to detrimentally alter biochemical and physiologic functions and to shorten life expectancy. Obesity is associated with four major risk factors for atherosclerosis: hypertension, diabetes, hypercholesterolemia, and hypertriglyceridemia. Overweight individuals have a higher prevalence of hypertension at every age, and the risk of developing hypertension is related to the amount of weight gain after age 25. (4) The two in combination (hypertension and obesity) increase the risk of heart disease, cerebrovascular disease, and death.

Unfortunately the basal metabolic rate decreases with age. After age 18, the resting metabolic rate declines about 2% per decade. A 30-year-old individual will inevitably gain weight if there is no change in caloric intake or exercise level over the years. The middle aged spread is both a biological and a psychosociological phenomenon. It is therefore important for both our patients and ourselves to understand adipose tissue and the problem of obesity.

Physiology of Adipose Tissue

Adipose tissue serves three general functions:

1. Adipose tissue is a storehouse of energy.

2. Fat serves as a cushion from trauma.

3. Adipose tissue plays a role in the regulation of body heat.

Each cell of adipose tissue may be regarded as a package of triglyceride, the most concentrated form of stored energy. There are 8 calories per gram of triglyceride as opposed to 1 calorie per gram of glycogen. The total store of tissue and fluid carbohydrate in adults (about 300 calories) is inadequate to meet between-meal demands. The storage of energy in fat tissue allows us to do other things besides eating.

The mechanism for mobilizing energy from fat involves various enzymes and neurohormonal agents. Following ingestion of fat and its breakdown by gastric and pancreatic lipases, absorption of long-chain triglycerides and free fatty acids takes place in the small bowel. Chylomicrons (microscopic particles of fat) transferred through lymph

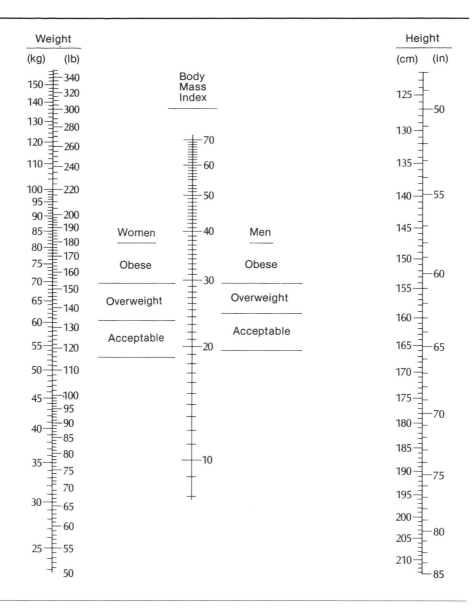

channels into the systemic venous circulation are normally removed by hepatic parenchymal cells where a new lipoprotein is released into the circulation. When this lipoprotein is exposed to adipose tissue, lipolysis takes place through the action of lipoprotein lipase, an enzyme derived from the fat cells themselves. The fatty acids that are released then enter the fat cells where they are reesterified with glycerophosphate into triglycerides.

Glucose serves three important functions:

1. Glucose supplies carbon atoms in the form of acetyl coenzyme A (acetyl CoA).

2. Glucose provides hydrogen for reductive steps.

3. Glucose is the main source of glycerophosphate.

The production and availability of glycerophosphate (required for reesterification of fatty acids and their storage as triglycerides) are considered rate-limiting in lipogenesis, and this process depends on the presence of glucose.

After esterification, subsequent lipolysis results in the release of fatty acids and glycerol. In the cycle of lipolysis and reesterification, energy is freed as heat. A low variable level of lipolysis takes place continuously; its basic function may be to provide body heat.

The chief metabolic products produced from fat are the circulating free fatty acids. Their availability is controlled by adipose tissue cells. When carbohydrate is in short supply, a flood of free fatty acids can be released. The free fatty acids in the peripheral circulation are almost wholly derived from endogenous triglyceride that undergoes rapid hydrolysis to yield free fatty acid and glycerol. The glycerol is returned to the liver for resynthesis of glycogen.

Free fatty acid release from adipose tissue is stimulated by physical exercise, fasting, exposure to cold, nervous tension, and anxiety. The release of fatty acids by lipolysis varies from one anatomic site to another. Omental, mesenteric, and subcutaneous fat are more labile and easily mobilized than fat from other sources. Areas from which energy is not easily mobilized are retrobulbar and perirenal fat where the tissue serves a structural function. Adipose tissue lipase is sensitive to stimulation by both epinephrine and norepinephrine. Other hormones that activate lipase are ACTH, thyroid stimulating hormone (TSH), growth hormone, thyroxine (T_4), 3,5,3'-triiodothyronine (T_3), cortisol, glucagon, as well as vasopressin and human placental lactogen (HPL).

Lipase enzyme activity is inhibited by insulin, which appears to be alone as the major physiologic antagonist to the array of stimulating agents. When both glucose and insulin are abundant, transport of glucose into fat cells is high, and glycerophosphate production increases to esterify fatty acids.

The carbohydrate and fat composition of the fuel supply is constantly changing, depending upon stresses and demands. Since the central nervous system and some other tissues can utilize only glucose for energy, a homeostatic mechanism for conserving carbohydrate is essential. When glucose is abundant and easily available, it is utilized in adipose tissue for producing glycerophosphate to immobilize fatty acids as triglycerides. The circulating level of free fatty acids in muscle will therefore be low, and glucose will be used by all of the tissues.

When carbohydrate is scarce, the amount of glucose reaching the fat cells declines and glycerophosphate production is reduced. The fat cell releases fatty acids, and their circulating levels rise to a point where glycolysis is inhibited. Thus, carbohydrate is spared in those tissues capable of using lipid substrates. If the rise of fatty acids is great enough, the liver is flooded with acetyl CoA. This is converted into ketone bodies, and clinical ketosis results.

In the simplest terms, when a person eats, glucose is available, insulin is secreted, and fat is stored. In starvation, the glucose level falls, insulin secretion decreases, and fat is mobilized.

If only single large meals are consumed, the body learns to convert carbohydrate to fat very quickly. Epidemiologic studies on school children demonstrate a positive correlation between fewer meals and a greater tendency toward obesity. (5) The person who does not eat all day and then stocks up at night is perhaps doing the worst possible thing.

Clinical Obesity

Obesity and the Brain

The hypothalamic location of the appetite center was established in 1940 by the demonstration that bilateral lesions of the ventromedial nucleus produce experimental obesity in rats. Such lesions lead to hyperphagia and decreased physical activity. Interestingly, this pattern is similar to that seen in human beings—the pressure to eat is reinforced by the desire to be physically inactive. The ventromedial nucleus was thought to represent an integrating center for appetite and hunger information. Destruction of the ventromedial nucleus was believed to result in a loss of satiety signals, leading to hyperphagia.

Overeating and obesity, however, may not be due to ventromedial nucleus damage but rather to destruction of the nearby ventral noradrenergic bundle. (6) Hypothalamic noradrenergic terminals are derived from long fibers ascending from hindbrain cell bodies. Lesions of the ventromedial nucleus produced by radiofrequency current fail to cause obesity. These lesions lead to overeating and obesity only when they extend beyond the ventromedial nucleus. Selective destruction of the ventral noradrenergic bundle results in hyperphagia. The lesions that produce hyperphagia also reduce the potency of amphetamine as an appetite suppressant. This noradrenergic bundle may function as a satiety system and be the site of amphetamine action.

Signals arriving at these centers originate in peripheral tissues. Opiates, substance P, and cholecystokinin play a role in mediating taste, the gatekeeper for feeding, while peptides released from the stomach and intestine act as satiety signals. (7)

There may be two kinds of obesity: obesity stemming from a CNS regulatory defect, and obesity due to a metabolic problem occurring despite a normal central mechanism.

Psychologic Factors

Obese and lean people respond differently to their environments. (8) Obese people appear to regulate their desire for food through external signals. Lean people, on the other hand, regulate their intake by endogenous signals of hunger and satiety.

Fear does not inhibit gastrointestinal activity and dull the appetite in obese persons as it does in others. Fat people eat because it is mealtime, and food looks, smells, and tastes good. They also eat because other people are eating, but not necessarily because they themselves are hungry.

Obese people are also less physically active than are people of normal weight. The obese person will drive a car around the block repeatedly until a parking space is available, rather than walk a few blocks. Time-lapse photography studies show that obese people when in a swimming pool spend most of their time floating; lean people move around actively. (9) An obese baby is more willing than is a normal baby to take formula after it has been sweetened, but will take less formula, even though it is sweetened, if the work of eating is increased by a nipple with a smaller hole.

There may be two classes of obesity: one class may include those individuals who clearly eat too much. The other class would be composed of individuals who eat relatively normal diets, but who are extremely inactive.

Fat Cells

Fat cells develop from connective tissue early in fetal life. An important question is whether new fat cells are produced by metaplasia in the adult, or whether an individual achieves a total complement during a certain period of life. In other words, is excess fat stored by increasing the size of the fat cell or by increasing the number of cells? The possibility arises that there is an increase in the total number of fat cells, which just wait to be packed full of storage fat. Furthermore, the total number of fat cells may depend upon an infant's nutritional state during the neonatal period, and perhaps in utero as well.

Studies of fat obtained at surgery indicate that the mean fat cell volume is increased threefold in obese people, but an increase in the number of fat cells is seen only in the grossly obese. (10) When patients diet, the fat cells decrease in size, but not in number. Hypercellular obesity may be a more difficult problem to overcome, since an individual may be saddled with a permanent increase in fat cells.

Some researchers think that, at some period in a person's life, a fixed number of fat cells is obtained. Adolescence, infancy, and intrauterine life seem particularly critical. (11,12) This premise is not solidly established, because there is no certain way to identify an empty fat cell, and potential fat cells cannot be recognized. Nevertheless, a hyperplastic type of obesity (more fat cells) may be associated with childhood and have a poor prognosis; a hypertrophic type (enlarged fat cells) that is responsive to dieting may occur in adults. There certainly appears to be a genetic component. The weights of adopted children in Denmark correlated with the body weights of their biologic parents, but not with their adoptive parents. (13) This would suggest that the genetic influence is even more important in childhood than environmental factors. Other work suggests that the familial occurrence of obesity can be attributed in part to a genetically related reduced rate of energy expenditure. (14)

Some argue that each individual has a setpoint, a level regulated by signals between the fat cells and the brain. According to this argument, previously obese people who have successfully lost weight have to maintain themselves in a state of starvation (at least as far as their fat cells are concerned).

Genetics and biochemistry are against many obese people. It is best to recognize that an obese individual who has suffered with the problem lifelong does have a disorder, a disorder which is not well understood.

Endocrine Changes

The most important endocrine change in obesity is elevation of the basal blood insulin level. Increases in body fat change the body's secretion and sensitivity to insulin. There is a decrease in the number of insulin receptor sites at a cellular level, most significantly in fat, liver, and muscle tissue. The key factors which affect insulin resistance are the amount of fat tissue in the body, the caloric intake per day, the amount of carbohydrates in the diet, and the amount of daily exercise. The mechanism for the increased resistance to insulin observed with increasing weight may be down-regulation of insulin receptors brought about by the increase in insulin secretion. The increase in insulin resistance affects the metabolism of carbohydrate, fat, and protein. Circulating levels of free fatty acids increase as a result of inadequate insulin suppression of the fat cell.

Genetics plays a greater role in the development of maturity onset diabetes than juvenile onset. (15) It is impossible to predict exactly who eventually will develop diabetes, as the tendency is recessive and it will not develop in every generation in a family. But weight is a good tip-off. As weight increases, the frequency of occurrence of diabetes increases. Both gestational diabetes and insulin-dependent diabetes are more common in overweight pregnant patients.

Contrary to popular misconception, hypothyroidism does not cause obesity. Weight gain due to hypothyroidism is confined to the fluid accumulation of myxedema. There is no place, therefore, for thyroid hormone administration in the treatment of obesity when the patient is euthyroid.

Obese people are relatively unable to excrete both salt and water, especially while dieting. During dieting this seems to be mediated by increased output of aldosterone and vasopressin. Since water produced from fat outweighs the fat, people on diets often show little initial weight loss. The early use of a diuretic may encourage a patient to persist with dieting.

The basic question is whether metabolic changes observed in obesity represent adaptive responses to a markedly enlarged fat organ, or whether they are representative of a metabolic or hormonal defect. It appears that the former is true. These changes are secondary responses; they are totally reversible with weight loss. Four-year follow-up in a group of patients who did not regain their weight after dieting revealed persistently normal insulin and glucose responses; patients who regained their weight showed further deterioration in these metabolic factors. (16)

Anatomic Obesity

Gynoid obesity refers to fat distribution in the lower body (femoral and gluteal regions), while android obesity refers to upper body distribution. Gynoid fat is more resistant to catecholamines and more sensitive to insulin than abdominal fat; thus extraction and storage of fatty acids easily occur and fat is accumulated more readily in the thighs and buttocks. This fat is associated with minimal fatty acid flux, and therefore, the negative consequences of fatty acid metabolism are less. Gynoid fat is principally stored fat. The clinical meaning of all this is that women with gynoid obesity are less likely than women with android obesity to develop diabetes mellitus and hypertriglyceridemia.

127

During pregnancy, lipoprotein lipase activity increases in gynoid fat, further promoting fat storage and explaining the tendency for women to gain thigh and hip weight during pregnancy. Also, because this fat is more resistant to mobilization, it is harder to get rid of. This difficulty is related to the adrenergic receptor concentration in the fat cells, the regulation of which remains a mystery.

Android obesity refers to fat located in the abdominal wall and visceral-mesenteric locations. This fat is more sensitive to catecholamines and less sensitive to insulin, and thus more active metabolically. It more easily delivers triglyceride to other tissues to meet energy requirements. This fat distribution is associated with hyperinsulinemia, impaired glucose tolerance, and diabetes mellitus, largely because of decreased hepatic extraction of insulin. (17) It is upper body obesity that is associated with hypertension, and there is reason to believe that the hypertension is directly linked to the hyperinsulinemia. Weight loss in women with lower body obesity is mainly cosmetic, whereas loss of upper body weight is more important for general health.

The waist:hip ratio is a means of estimating the degree of upper to lower body obesity. The ratio is obtained by measuring the body diameters at the levels of the umbilicus and the anterior iliac crests. Interpretation is as follows:

Greater than 1.2 — Android Obesity
From 0.6 to 1.2 — Normal
Less than 0.6 — Gynoid Obesity

Management of Obesity

Aside from not smoking cigarettes, weight reduction is the most important health measure available for reducing the risk of cardiovascular disease. (18) For most patients, after a routine evaluation to rule out pathology such as diabetes mellitus, the physician is left with the frustrating task of prescribing a diet. But it is not enough to just prescribe a diet or prescribe an anorectic drug. An effective weight loss program requires commitment from both patient and physician.

Physician and patient should agree on the goal of a diet program. While the physician may wish the patient to reach ideal weight, the patient may be satisfied with less. Motivation is improved when the goals meet both personal and medical objectives. It is realistic to lose 4–5 pounds in the first month and 20–30 pounds in 4–5 months.

Despite various fads and diet books, the best diet continues to be a limitation of calories to between 900 and 1200 calories per day, the actual amount depending on what the individual patient will accept and pursue.

Ideal Diet: Carbohydrates — 40–45%
Protein — 20%
Fat — 35–40%

The discouraging aspect is that to lose a pound of fat, the equivalent of a 3500 calorie intake must be expended. Dieting has to be slow and steady to be effective. Successful programs include behavior modification, frequent visits to the physician, and involvement of family members. Behavior modification starts with daily recording of activity and behavior related to food intake, followed by the elimination of inappropriate cues (other than hunger) which lead to eating.

Careful studies (performed in hospitalized subjects on metabolic wards) have indicated that the carbohydrate and fat composition of the diet has no effect on the rate of weight loss. (8) Restriction of calories remains the important principle. Substituting one of the liquid formulas for meals has been successful in many individuals. Unbalanced formulations, however, have the same side effects as seen with total starvation (carbohydrate-deprived regimens). Adequate carbohydrate is necessary for utilization of amino acids. In addition, electrolyte problems have been encountered, and there is an initial diuretic phase that can lead to postural hypotension.

The protein-sparing modified fast is a ketogenic regimen providing approximately 800 calories per day. The liquid protein diets have been associated with deaths due to cardiac arrhythmias. The low-calorie diets which utilize protein and carbohydrate supplemented with minerals and vitamins as the sole source of nutrition should be used only for severe obesity and under medical supervision. (19) These diets are still potentially dangerous. The other disadvantage to the semistarvation diet is that short-term success does not guarantee long-term weight maintenance. It is reported that at best only one-fourth to one-third of individuals who lose weight by a semistarvation ketogenic regimen plus behavior modification therapy will have significant long-term weight reduction. (20) On the other hand, for that one-fourth to one-third, this represents a major accomplishment and is worth doing. Unfortunately, repeated dieting and recidivism have a negative impact. With each episode, the body learns to become more efficient, so that with each diet, weight comes off more slowly and is regained more rapidly.

As an index of the general lack of success with diets, a summary of 10 studies (approximately 1200 patients) revealed that only 30% lose 20 pounds or more, and only 4% lose 40 pounds or more. (10) Commercial organizations are no more successful than physician-directed programs or non-profit self-help groups. (21) Thus, it is obvious why gimmicks abound in this area of patient management.

Anorectics are useful as short-term therapy to control hunger, especially at the beginning of a diet and at a plateau or relapse stage. Compared to amphetamines, there is less abuse associated with the amphetamine congeners (diethylpropion, fenfluramine, methamphetamine, and phentermine). Other non-amphetamine anorectics are phendimetrazine and mazindol. All of these agents act on the central nervous system to depress appetite.

Over-the-counter products contain phenylpropanolamine as the active ingredient. This drug is a sympathomimetic derived from ephedrine, and can act synergistically with caffeine to produce amphetamine-like reactions. *It should be noted that phenylpropanolamine taken in combination with bromocriptine or a monoamine oxidase inhibitor can precipitate a hypertensive crisis.*

Surgical treatment and starvation should be reserved for patients who are morbidly obese. Both methods involve many potential problems and require close monitoring.

Controlled studies have not demonstrated the effectiveness of thyroid preparations or human chorionic gonadotropin (HCG). (22) Indeed, adding thyroid hormone increases the loss of lean body mass rather than fat tissue. It is clear that adjunctive drug measures are not successful unless the patient is also motivated either to limit caloric intake or to increase the exercise level in what will be a lifelong battle.

A regular pattern of physical exercise reduces the risk of myocardial infarction in all people. (23) Both weight loss and increased physical activity, through an unknown mechanism, lower the level of low-density lipoprotein (LDL) and increase the level of high-density lipoprotein (HDL). (24) A further benefit of strenuous or prolonged exercise is an inhibition of appetite which lasts many hours, and which is associated with an increase in the resting metabolic rate for 24–48 hours. There is one study, however, that indicates a rebound increase in appetite 1–2 days after exercise. (25) The optimal program includes, therefore, a *daily* period of exercise. The best time for exercise is before meals or about 2 hours after eating. It is probably wise to take a day off at least once a week to give muscles and joints a rest.

Unfortunately one cannot burn up significant calories quickly; it takes 18 minutes of running to compensate for the average hamburger. (26)

Most frustrating is the problem of some patients who limit caloric intake yet do not lose weight. In fact, as the weights of certain patients increase, the number of calories required to remain in equilibrium decreases, probably due to a combination of reduced activity and a change in metabolism. The Vermont study demonstrated that the normal person with induced obesity requires 2700 calories to remain in equilibrium; spontaneously obese patients require only about 1300 calories. (27) Others argue that virtually everyone can lose weight on a diet of 1000 calories per day in that the maintenance requirement for a sedentary adult is about 1.5 times the resting metabolic rate (about 1000–1500 calories per day). (28) The physician must be careful to avoid a condemning or punitive attitude, and understand that it is possible to significantly restrict caloric intake and not lose weight.

Patients appear doomed to frustration and despair unless the physician can motivate them to increase physical activity. In all individuals dieting is more effective when combined with physical exercise, but this is especially true in chronically obese patients. In other words, the lifestyle of an obese person must be changed to overcome the desire to be inactive (walk instead of riding). Only by significantly increasing caloric expenditure will the input-output equilibrium be disturbed.

The obese person feels trapped. Obesity leads to characteristic behavioral manifestations, including passive personality, frequent periods of depression, decreased self-respect, and a sense of being hopelessly overwhelmed by problems. But just as the endocrine and metabolic changes are secondary to obesity, many of the psychosocial attributes surrounding obesity are also secondary. (29)

Motivation to change and emotional support during the change are important. They can be provided by friends, relatives, physicians, or self-help organizations. If the vicious circle of failed diets, resignation to fate, guilt, and shame can be broken, a more effective, happier person will emerge.

References

1. **Van Itallie JB, Hirsch J,** Appraisal of excess calories as a factor in causation of disease, Am J Clin Nutr 32:2648, 1979.

2. **Powers PS,** *Obesity, The Regulation of Weight,* Williams & Wilkins, Baltimore, 1980.

3. **Thomas AE, McKay DA, Cutlip MB,** A nomograph method for assessing body weight, Am J Clin Nutr 29:302, 1976.

4. **Stamler R, Stamler J, Riedlinger WF, Algera G, Roberts RH,** Weight and blood pressure: Findings in hypertension screening of 1 million Americans, JAMA 240:1607, 1978.

5. **Fabry P, Hejda S, Cerny K,** Effects of meal frequency in school children. Changes in weight-height proportion and skinfold thickness, Am J Clin Nutr 18:358, 1966.

6. **Gold RM,** Hypothalamic obesity: The myth of the ventromedial nucleus, Science 182:488, 1973.

7. **Morley JE,** Neuropeptide regulation of appetite and weight, Endocrin Rev 8:256, 1987.

8. **Gordon ES,** Metabolic aspects of obesity, Adv Metab Disord 4:229, 1970.

9. **Mayer J,** Inactivity as a major factor in adolescent obesity, Ann NY Acad Sci 131:502, 1965.

10. **Bray GA, Davidson MB, Drenick EJ,** Obesity: A serious symptom, Ann Intern Med 77:787, 1972.

11. **Ravelli G, Stein ZA, Susser MW,** Obesity in young men after famine exposure in utero and early infancy, New Engl J Med 295:349, 1976.

12. **Charney E, Goodman HC, McBride M, Lyon B, Pratt R,** Childhood antecedents of adult obesity, New Engl J Med 295:6, 1976.

13. **Stunkard AJ, Sorensen TIA, Teasdale TW, Chakraborty R, Schull WJ, Schulsinger F,** An adoptive study of human obesity, New Engl J Med 314:193, 1986.

14. **Ravussin E, Lillioja S, Knowler WC, Christin L, Freymond D, Abbott WGH, Boyce V, Howard BV, Bogardus C,** Reduced rate of energy expenditure as a risk factor for body-weight gain, New Engl J Med 318:467, 1988.

15. **Fanda OP, Soeldner SS,** Genetic, acquired, and related factors in the etiology of diabetes mellitus, Arch Intern Med 137:461, 1977.

16. **Hewing R, Liebermeister H, Daweke H, Gries FA, Gruneklee D,** Weight regain after low calorie diet: Long term pattern of blood sugar, serum lipids, ketone bodies, and serum insulin levels, Diabetologia 9:197, 1973.

131

17. **Stern MP, Haffner SM,** Body fat distribution and hyperinsulinemia as risk factors for diabetes and cardiovascular disease, Arteriosclerosis 6:123, 1986.

18. **Gordon T, Kannel WB,** Obesity and cardiovascular disease: The Framingham study, Clin Endocrinol Metab 5:367, 1976.

19. **Bistrian BR,** The medical treatment of obesity. Arch Intern Med 141:429, 1981.

20. **Bistrian BR, Sherman M,** Results of the treatment of obesity with a protein-sparing modified fast, Int J Obes 2:143, 1978.

21. **Volkmar FR, Stunkard AJ, Woolston J, Bailey RA,** High attrition rates in commercial weight reduction programs, Arch Intern Med 141:426, 1981.

22. **Rivlin RS,** Drug therapy: Therapy of obesity with hormones, New Engl J Med 292:26, 1975.

23. **Paffenbarger RS Jr, Wing AL, Hyde RT,** Physical activity as an index of heart attack risk in college alumni, Am J Epidemiol 108:161, 1978.

24. **Weisweiler P,** Plasma lipoproteins and lipase and lecithin: Cholesterol acyl-transferase activities in obese subjects before and after weight reduction, J Clin Endocrinol Metab 65:969, 1987.

25. **Edholm OG, Fletcher JG, Widdowson EM, McCance RA,** The energy expenditure and food intake of individual men, Brit J Nutr 9:286, 1955.

26. **Konishi F,** Food energy equivalents of various activities, J Am Diet Assoc 46:186, 1965.

27. **Sims EAH, Danforth E Jr, Horton ES, Bray GA, Glennon JA, Salans LB,** Endocrine and metabolic effects of experimental obesity in man, Recent Prog Horm Res 29:457, 1973.

28. **Welle SL, Amatruda JM, Forbes GB, Lockwood DH,** Resting metabolic rates of obese women after rapid weight loss, J Clin Endocrinol Metab 59:41, 1984.

29. **Solow C, Siberfarb PM, Swift K,** Psychosocial effects of intestinal bypass surgery for severe obesity, New Engl J Med 290:300, 1974.

8

The Breast

One of every 10 American women will develop breast cancer during her lifetime. The incidence has been increasing over the past 2 decades and mortality rates have remained disappointingly constant. The breast is the leading site of cancer in women (28% of all cancers), and is now unfortunately (because smoking is obviously the reason) exceeded by lung cancer as the the leading cause of death from cancer in women. (1) Over the years breast cancer has continued this deadly impact despite advances in surgical and diagnostic techniques.

Cancer Site Incidence in U.S. Women

Breast	— 28%
Colorectum	— 15%
Lung	— 11%
Uterus	— 9%
Ovary	— 4%

Cancer Deaths in U.S. Women

Lung	— 21%
Breast	— 18%
Colorectum	— 13%
Ovary	— 5%
Uterus	— 4%

Breast cancer has an increasing frequency with age, although the risk increases less steeply after menopause. A woman at age 70 has almost 10 times the risk as a 40-year-old woman. Over two-thirds of women who develop breast cancer are over the age of 50.

Classically, the single most useful prognostic information in women with operable breast cancer has been the histologic status of the axillary lymph nodes. (2) At 10 years only 25% of patients with positive nodes are free of disease compared to 75% of patients with negative nodes. If more than 3 nodes are involved, the 10 year survival rate drops to 13%. Because of this recognition for the importance of the axillary nodes, the traditional approach to breast cancer (the Halsted surgical approach) was based on the concept that breast cancer is a disease of stepwise progression. *There is an important change in concept. Breast cancer is now viewed as a sys-*

temic disease, with spread to local and distant sites at the same time. Breast cancer is best viewed as occultly metastatic at the time of presentation. Therefore, dissemination of tumor cells has occurred by the time of surgery in many patients, and it is not surprising that radical mastectomy and local irradiation do not prevent metastatic disease.

Because we have been dealing with a disease which has already reached the point of dissemination in most patients, we must move the diagnosis forward several years in order to have an impact on breast cancer mortality. Earlier diagnosis requires that we be aware of what it is that makes a high risk patient.

Risk Factors for Breast Cancer

A constellation of factors influence the risk for breast cancer. (3) These include reproductive experience, ovarian activity, benign breast disease, familial tendency, genetic differences, dietary considerations, and specific endocrine factors. And in addition, another reason not to smoke, an increased risk of breast cancer can be identified in smokers, especially in premenopausal women. (4)

Reproductive Experience.   The risk of breast cancer increases with the increase in age at which a woman bears her first full-term child. A woman pregnant before the age of 18 has about one-third the risk of one who first delivers after the age of 35. To be protective, pregnancy must occur before the age of 30. In fact, women over the age of 30 years at the time of their first birth have a greater risk than women who never become pregnant. There is, however, a significant protective effect with increasing parity, present even when adjusted for age at first birth and other risk factors. (5)

The fact that pregnancy early in life is associated with reduced breast cancer implies that etiologic factors are operating during that period of life. The protection afforded only by the first pregnancy suggests that the first full-term pregnancy has a trigger effect which either produces a permanent change in the factors responsible for breast cancer, or changes the breast tissue and makes it less susceptible to malignant transformation. There is evidence for a lasting impact of a first pregnancy on a woman's hormonal milieu. A small but significant elevation of estriol, a decrease in dehydroepiandrosterone (DHA) and dehydroepiandrosterone sulfate (DHAS), and lower prolactin levels all persist for many years after delivery. (6,7) These changes take on great significance when viewed in terms of the endocrine factors considered below.

Lactation offers a weak to moderate protective effect (20–50% reduced risk) which is stronger for premenopausal breast cancer. (8–10) There is a unique and helpful study of the Chinese Tanka, who are boat people living on the coast of southern China. (11) The women of the Chinese Tanka wear clothing with an opening only on the right side, and they breast-feed only with the right breast. All breast cancers were in postmenopausal women, and the cancers were equally distributed between the two sides, indicating the stronger protection for premenopausal breast cancer. Another significant Chinese study has indicated increasing protection against breast cancer with increasing duration of lactation. (12)

134

Ovarian Activity. Women who have an oophorectomy have a lower risk, and the reduction in risk is greater the younger a woman is when ovariectomized. There is a 70% risk reduction in women who have surgery before age 35. There is a small increase in risk with early menarche and with late natural menopause, indicating that ovarian activity plays a continuing role throughout reproductive life. Obese women have earlier menarche and later menopause, higher estrone production rates and free estradiol levels (lower sex hormone binding globulin [SHBG]), and greater risk for breast cancer. (13)

Benign Breast Disease. With obstruction of ducts (probably by stromal fibrosis), ductule-alveolar secretion persists, the secretory material is retained, and cysts form from the dilatation of terminal ducts (duct ectasia) and alveoli. Women with cystic mastitis have about 4 times the breast cancer rate of comparable normal women. Despite their risk, women with prior benign breast disease form only a small proportion of breast cancer patients—approximately 5%, and fortunately, as the cyclic stimulus of the menstrual cycle is left behind after menopause, symptomatic fibrocystic breasts become less of a problem.

There is strong support to eliminate the phrase fibrocystic disease of the breast. In a review of over 10,000 breast biopsies in Nashville, Tennessee, 70% of the women were found not to have a lesion associated with an increased risk for cancer. (14) The most important variable on biopsies is the degree and character of the epithelial proliferation. Women with atypical hyperplasia had a relative risk of 5.3, while women with atypia and a family history of breast cancer had a relative risk of 11. The point is that we needlessly frighten patients with the use of the phrase fibrocystic disease. For most women, this is not a disease, but a physiologic change brought about by cyclic hormonal activity. *Let's call this problem FIBROCYSTIC CHANGE OR CONDITION.*

The College of American Pathologists supports this position and has offered this classification: (15)

Classification of Breast Biopsy Tissue According to Risk for Breast Cancer:

No increased risk: Adenosis
                       Duct ectasia
                       Fibroadenoma
                       Fibrosis
                       Mild hyperplasia (3–4 cells deep)
                       Mastitis
                       Periductal mastitis
                       Squamous metaplasia

Slightly increased risk (1.5–2.0 times):
                       Moderate or florid hyperplasia
                       Papilloma

Risk increased 5 times:
                       Atypical hyperplasia

Familial Tendency. Female relatives of women with breast cancer have 2–3 times the rate of the general population. There is an excess of bilateral disease among patients with a family history of breast cancer. Relatives of women with bilateral disease have about a 45% lifetime chance of developing breast cancer. In data from the CDC, these relative risks were observed: (16)

Affected aunt or grandmother — 1.5 relative risk.
Affected mother or sister — 2.3 relative risk.
Affected mother *and* sister — 14.0 relative risk.

Hereditary breast cancer (about 8% of all breast cancers) should be suspected when multiple female relatives have developed breast cancer at a relatively young age. Women from such a family have a 50% risk of developing breast cancer and should begin having annual mammography about 5 years earlier than the age at which the earliest breast cancer has been detected in a family member.

Fat in the Diet. The geographical variation in incidence rates of breast cancer is considerable (The United States has the highest rates and Japan the lowest), and it has been correlated with the amount of animal fat in the diet. Lean women, however, have been found to have an increased incidence of breast cancer, although this increase is limited to small, localized, and well-differentiated tumors. (17) Furthermore, studies have failed to find evidence for a positive relationship between breast cancer and dietary total or saturated fat or cholesterol intake. (18) Thus the epidemiologic literature provides little support for the hypothesis that dietary fat intake is related to the risk of breast cancer. This hypothesis was derived from international correlations between per capita fat intake and mortality rates for breast cancer, and has not withstood epidemiologic testing.

Alcohol in the Diet. There is a 60% increase in the risk for breast cancer with the consumption of one or more alcoholic drinks per day. (19) Almost all of many studies conclude that even moderate drinking increases the risk by 40–60%.

Specific Endocrine Factors

1. *Adrenal Steroids*. Subnormal levels of etiocholanolone (a urinary excretion product of androstenedione) have been found from 5 months to 9 years before the diagnosis of breast cancer in women living on the island of Guernsey, off the English coast. (20) A subnormal excretion of this 17-ketosteroid was also found in sisters of patients with breast cancer. A 6-fold increase in the incidence of breast cancer was found between women excreting less than 0.4 mg of etiocholanolone and those excreting over 1 mg/24 hours. Measurement of this 17-ketosteroid might be a useful screening procedure to detect a high risk group of patients because approximately 25% of the population excretes less than 1 mg/24 hours.

2. *Endogenous Estrogen*. Estriol generally has failed to produce breast cancer in rodents, and in fact, estriol protects the rat against breast tumors induced by various chemical carcinogens. The hypothesis is that a higher estriol level protects against the more potent effects of estrone and estradiol. This might explain the protective effect of early pregnancies. Women having had an early pregnancy continue to excrete more estriol than nulliparous women. Premenopausal healthy Asiatic women have a lower breast cancer risk than Caucasians, and also have a higher rate of urinary estriol excretion. (21) When Asiatic women migrate to the United States, however, the risk of breast cancer increases, and their urinary excretion of estriol decreases.

The notion that normal estrogen stimulation unopposed by adequate progesterone secretion is a factor in the pathogenesis of breast cancer was first stated by Sherman and Korenman. (22) Although theoretically appealing on the basis of presumed correlation with epidemiologic risks (infertility, late menopause) clinical research has not always confirmed the thesis. Young women at high genetic risk for breast cancer had normal luteal phases, and a group of premenopausal women with breast cancer also had normal luteal phases. (23) On the other hand, a long-term follow-up study of infertile women with a history of progesterone deficiency indicated a 5.4 times increase in risk of premenopausal breast cancer, while surveys of anovulatory women detected a 3–4 times increase in the risk of cancer which appeared after the age of 50. (24–26)

The logic and epidemiologic support for an estrogen link are impressive arguments. Whether the important factor is the total amount of estrogen, the amount of estrogen unopposed by progesterone, or some other combination is not known. More modern studies implicate biologically available estrogen as a factor. Women who develop breast cancer have higher levels of nonbound estradiol and lower levels of sex hormone binding globulin (SHBG). (27) Perhaps SHBG measurements should be added to our screening efforts.

3. *Exogenous Estrogen.* Epidemiologic and other information continue to suggest some estrogen-related promoter function. These include: a) the condition is 100 times more common in women than in men, b) breast cancer invariably occurs after puberty, c) untreated gonadal dysgenesis and breast cancer are mutually exclusive, d) a 65% excess rate of breast cancer has been observed among women who have had an endometrial cancer, and e) breast tumors contain estrogen receptors which are biologically active as indicated by the presence of progesterone receptors in tumor tissue. Taken together, these data suggest an element of estrogen dependence, if not provocation, in many breast cancers. What is the evidence that exogenous estrogen therapy can provide the same stimulus in vulnerable recipients?

Early studies had in general found little overall effect, but higher risks were suggested for special sub-categories: high parity, nulliparous women, and women with benign breast disease. In several studies, the risk was higher with natural menopause; in one study the risk was highest for menopause due to oophorectomy.

The divergent results are probably due to study size, with positive results based on small numbers. We now have available 3 large studies with comforting results. Data from the Boston Drug Surveillance Program, the CDC Cancer and Sex Hormone Study, and the Nurses' Health Study indicate that postmenopausal use of estrogens does not increase the risk for breast cancer.(28–30) Even better, the studies were large enough to provide data in the various subcategories. The absence of an effect was evident among all of the groups of women for which we have concern. Specifically, there was no evidence for an effect regardless of age at menarche, age at menopause, age of first pregnancy, menopause by surgery, family history of breast cancer, history of benign breast disease, use of estrogen for many years, or use of high doses. Furthermore, the data from the Nurses' Health Study provided strong evidence that estrogen treatment does not substantially accelerate the final subclinical growth phase of breast cancer. (30)

In addition, a recent case-control study from Australia which attempted to control for secular trends in estrogen use, type of menopause, and duration of estrogen use concluded that that there was no evidence for an association between estrogen use and the risk of breast cancer in postmenopausal women. (31) An Australian meta-analysis of 23 studies of estrogen use and breast cancer concluded that estrogen use did not alter the risk of breast cancer. (32)

In a retrospective cohort study of women who underwent biopsy for benign breast disease, the use of exogenous estrogen appeared to lower the risk of developing breast cancer. (33) In women with atypical hyperplasia on biopsy, the risk of developing breast cancer in women not taking estrogen was increased 4.5 times, but in women on estrogen the risk was increased only 3-fold. The importance of this observation is that this evidence indicates that benign breast disease does not represent a contraindication to estrogen replacement treatment.

There are two recent studies on breast cancer and hormone replacement treatment which deserve some discussion. Bergkvist and colleagues from Uppsala, Sweden in a case-cohort study concluded that estrogen use was associated with a slight increase (10%) in the risk of breast cancer, that there was a relationship with duration of use, and that the risk was increased among those women who took a combination of estradiol and progestin. (34) Besides method problems which introduced the possibility of selection bias and surveillance bias, there is reason to be skeptical regarding the significance of the data. The authors correctly indicate that there was a trend toward increasing relative risk with duration of use (in other words, it was not statistically significant), and that the indication of increased risk was based on small numbers of women with breast cancer. A case-control study from Denmark which utilized questionnaires to obtain information from both the cases and controls also indicated a slightly increased risk of breast cancer associated with hormonal replacement therapy. (35) This study contains limitations similar to the Uppsala study (e.g. the relative risk associated with sequential estrogen-progestin use was 1.36 but the confidence interval did not cross 1.0). Indeed, daily use of a combination estrogen-progestin was associated with a reduced risk, RR = 0.63.

As time goes on, more studies and greater duration of use should provide us with more definitive answers to these questions. Until then, it is appropriate to conclude that the bulk of evidence fails to indicate a link between postmenopausal estrogen use and the risk of breast cancer.

4. *Thyroid, Prolactin, Various Nonestrogen Drugs.* Despite isolated suggestions of increased risk, hypothyroidism, reserpine, or prolactin excess, whether spontaneous or drug induced, are not related to an enhanced risk of breast cancer.

5. *Birth Control Pills and Breast Cancer.* The large number of women taking or having taken oral contraceptive steroids, combined with the belief that steroids provoke or promote abnormal breast growth and possibly cancer, has provided a source of major concern for years. The major prospective studies (The Royal College of General Practitioners' Study, The Oxford Family Planning Association Study, and The American Walnut Creek Study) have indicated no significant differences in overall breast cancer rates between users and nonusers. (36–38) However, patients were enrolled in these studies at a time when oral contraceptives were used primarily by married couples spacing out their children. Because this population may not reflect use by younger women delaying their first pregnancy, several case-control studies focused on the use of oral contraceptives before the age of 25. (39–41) All reported an increased risk of breast cancer in early users of oral contraceptives. Another case-control study suggested that the risk of premenopausal breast cancer is increased by long-term use (12 or more years) in young women. (42) In addition, the Royal College of General Practitioners' Study has indicated an increased risk of breast cancer limited to oral contraceptive users who developed breast cancer before the age of 35, while a national United Kingdom case-control study also indicated an increased risk of early breast cancer related to duration of use. (43,44)

These reports prompted the Centers for Disease Control in Atlanta to review information from its on going case control study on steroid use and cancer. No increased risk of breast cancer was found in women using oral contraceptives before the age of 20 with a duration of use greater than 4 years, or before the age of 25 with a duration of use greater than 6 years, or with greater than 4 years use before a first pregnancy. (45) In addition, no increased risk of breast cancer was found among any subgroups of users including women with benign breast disease or a family history of breast cancer.

In a further analysis of the CDC study, the largest on the subject, there was no increased risk associated with any specific type of oral contraceptive, progestin only pills, or the use of 2 or more types. (46) In addition, there was no increased risk associated with any specific progestin or estrogen component, and most importantly, it was demonstrated that long-term use (15 or more years) was not associated with an increased risk of breast cancer. The reliability of the CDC study is reinforced by the fact that the data confirmed the already well-known risk factors, such as nulliparity, late age at first birth, history of benign breast disease, and a family history of breast cancer. Finally, the CDC conclusions are supported by a significant national study from New Zealand. (47)

An updated review of the CDC study confirmed that there was no overall increased risk of breast cancer associated with oral contraceptive use, but an increased risk was identified in women who experienced menarche before age 13, had no children, and used oral contraception for 8 or more years. (48) However, this conclusion

139

was based on only 39 women (1.3% of the cases), and could represent artifactual statistical stratification. Keep in mind that all data on this question are derived from relatively high dose formulations used in the 1960s and early 1970s.

The results of the CDC study, because of its large size, are very reassuring. However, because the population at risk for breast cancer is the age group over 45 years old, and because of the long latent phase for breast cancer, data in the 1990's and 2000's will be required to answer one last very important question: the possibility of very late effects of use. Thus far, the CDC Cancer and Steroid Hormone Study has found no evidence for a latent effect on breast cancer risk through age 54. (49)

A recent case-control study of 407 patients with breast cancer and 424 control women indicated an overall two-fold increased risk of breast cancer before age 45 associated with the use of oral contraception. (50) The authors further indicated (on the basis of a logistic regression model) a four-fold increased risk with oral contraceptive use for 10 or more years. The results of this most recent study by Miller, et al, are directly contrary to previous reports by the same authors which found no increased risk with use at an early age and no overall increased risk. (51,52) The previous studies and the present study involved women of the same age group and used identical methods. The authors address the different results in their discussion and rightly point out that recall of use (the studies depended upon patient recall of oral contraceptive use) could be greater in the cases because of the publicity surrounding this issue. This concern was supported by finding an increased risk in women who used the pills for less than 3 months (an unlikely biological event). Selection bias is also possible due to more attention to the breasts by both physicians and patients in users of oral contraceptives. A similar relative risk across all durations of use also suggests an over-representation of never-users. The four-fold elevated risk with long-term use was an estimate based on a mathematical model. Actually there was no statistical dose-response with duration of use, a finding which argues against a causal relationship.

Thus either there is no increased risk and the different studies reflect methodological biases, or the risk is limited to such specific groups (in terms of age, duration of use, onset of use) that unequal representation can influence a specific study result. An appropriate clinical response is to give greater weight to the larger studies (which would minimize biases and the effects of specific groups). The larger studies (CASH and the study from New Zealand) find no association between oral contraceptive use and breast cancer. The CASH study included nearly 10,000 cases and controls, with 4711 cases of breast cancer in women 20–54 years old and 2088 cases in women under 45 years of age. The New Zealand study consisted of 1330 women. Finally, it is also important to be aware that there is no evidence of an impact of oral contraceptive use (as predicted by the positive reports) on national breast cancer incidence rates in the United Kingdom, Western Germany, and the United States. It is appropriate to tell patients of the conflicting results, pointing out the lack of evidence for an overall increased risk, and to emphasize the probable relative safety of the current lower dose oral contraceptives.

140

Worth emphasizing is a protective effect on benign disease of the breast associated with the progestin component of the pill, an effect which becomes apparent after 2 years of continuous usage. After this time there is a progressive reduction in the incidence of fibrocystic changes in the breast with increasing duration of use. Women who take the pill are one-fourth as likely to develop benign breast disease as nonusers.

6. *Breast Cancer in Diethylstilbestrol (DES)-exposed Women.* Exposure to DES occurred in association with 2 million live births; therefore, the risk for induction of breast cancer during a period of breast differentiation could be significant if DES were a true breast carcinogen. The major study on this subject reported on the follow-up of women who participated in a controlled trial of DES in pregnancy between 1950 and 1952 at the University of Chicago. In this study, no significant association between breast cancer and DES exposure was found. (53) Reinterpretation post hoc in the public press led to a review of the original data and additional information from the national DESAD (DES plus adenosis) Project at the Mayo Clinic. (54) In this new study, among 408 women given DES, there were 8 confirmed cases of breast cancer, in comparison with an expected number of 8.1 based upon breast cancer incidence rates among parous women in the local population. The original Chicago report of no association was confirmed. However, a large collaborative study, involving approximately 6000 women, concluded that there is a small but significant increase in the risk of breast cancer many years later in life in women exposed to DES during pregnancy. (55) Certainly it would be wise to recommend to DES-exposed women that they adhere religiously to screening for breast cancer, including mammography as discussed below.

The Estrogen Window Hypothesis for the Etiology of Breast Cancer

Stanley G. Korenman has promulgated a most interesting thesis concerning the endocrinology of breast cancer. (56,57) Recognizing that the endocrine changes thought to be related to the promotion or provocation of breast cancer were small, inconsistent, did not persist in crossculture or single culture studies, and could hardly account for the 5-fold differential risk of breast cancer among populations, Korenman concluded that *endocrine status is related to breast cancer by influencing the patient's susceptibility to environmental carcinogens.* Recall the dimethylbenzanthracene inducer-promoter model of rodents in which a favorable endocrine environment both increased susceptibility to a single exposure to a known carcinogen and thereafter provided favorable conditions for maintenance and growth of the tumor. Similarly the estrogen window hypothesis in humans has the following components:

1. Human breast cancer is induced by environmental carcinogens in a susceptible mammary gland.

2. Unopposed estrogen stimulation is the most favorable state for tumor induction (the ''open'' window).

3. The duration of exposure to estrogens determines risk (how long the window is ''open'').

4. There is a long latent period between tumor induction and clinical expression.

141

5. Susceptibility to induction ("inducibility") declines with the establishment of normal luteal phase progesterone secretion and becomes very low during pregnancy. (The "open" window is closed, but if tumor has been induced during a previous "open" window period, the hormones which reduce susceptibility nevertheless may promote maintenance and growth.)

The two main induction "open window" periods are the pubertal years prior to the establishment of regular ovulatory menstrual cycles and the perimenopausal period of waning follicle maturation and ovulation. The prolongation of these open windows by obesity, infertility, delayed pregnancy, earlier menarche, and later menopause would be associated with increased susceptibility to an environmental carcinogen. Opposed estrogen (as in birth control pill users and DES exposure during pregnancy) would not increase susceptibility.

Korenman has cited independent support for the estrogen window hypothesis—breast cancer incidence studies of populations exposed to a single carcinogen superimposed on the normal environmental risks. Such data are reported in the extended life span study of atomic bomb survivors from Hiroshima and Nagasaki, and women with tuberculosis receiving repeated fluoroscopies. Inducibility, the presence of windows, and a latency period between induction and clinical expression were demonstrated in each. In the A-bomb survivors, no breast cancer was seen in children irradiated under the age of 10; increased differences in risk occurred if exposure occurred between age 10 and 29 with an especially marked risk exposure period between 10 and 14 years—the period just before ovulation. (58) Excess risk due to irradiation decreased rapidly so that, if exposure occurred between 30 and 49 years of age, there was no significant breast cancer increase over nonirradiated controls. After age 50, increased inducibility seemed to reappear.

In the repeatedly fluoroscoped women with tuberculosis, the greatest incremental risk of breast cancer over un-x-rayed controls occurred in those exposed in the 15–20 year age group with no increase after age 30. (59) The greatest risk appeared 15 years after exposure and persisted at least 40 years.

While the estrogen window hypothesis is not proven it has appealing clarity as well as partial supportive data. It explains many, but not all, the elements of risk in breast cancer. It reminds us of duration as well as the intensity of inducer and promoter substances. It explains the lack of consistent hormonal findings in patients with established breast cancer even though a hormonal factor appears obvious in the pathogenesis of the disorder. It suggests that growth factors regulated by the endocrine environment may be determinants of breast cancer growth. This hypothesis has been stated from a slightly different perspective, emphasizing the importance of progestational resistance to irreversible precancerous proliferation. (60)

Progestational Protection

There is a growing story that exposure to progestational agents is prophylactic against breast cancer. This is consistent with the open window hypothesis. It is progesterone which closes the window, and for that reason, the risk of breast cancer is increased with those factors associated with long-term exposure to unopposed estrogen. On the other hand, progestational agents have been implicated as causal factors for breast cancer. The situation is a very special one, however, being limited only to experiments with beagle dogs. Mammary tumors in the beagle dog are increased as a result of prolonged stimulation with large doses (up to 25 times human luteal phase levels) of progesterone or 17-hydroxyprogesterone derivatives (such as medroxyprogesterone acetate). This has not been reported in any other species, and there is no clinical evidence for a relationship between progestin use and breast cancer in women. Indeed, World Health Organization follow-up of women using Depo-Provera for contraception indicates that exposure to Depo-Provera protects women against breast cancer. (61)

Estrogen normally promotes mitotic growth of the endometrium. Abnormal progression of growth through cystic hyperplasia, adenomatous hyperplasia, atypia, and early carcinoma has been associated with unopposed estrogen activity. Some 10% of women with adenomatous hyperplasia progress to frank cancer, and adenomatous hyperplasia is observed to antedate adenocarcinoma in 25–30% of cases. Retrospective studies have estimated that the risk of endometrial cancer in women on estrogen replacement therapy (unopposed by a progestational agent) is increased by a factor of 4 to 8 times the normal incidence of 1 per 1,000 postmenopausal women per year. It is now apparent, however, that this risk can be reduced by the addition of a progestational agent to the program. Whereas estrogen promotes the growth of endometrium, progestins inhibit that growth. This counter effect is accomplished by progestin reduction in cellular receptors for estrogen, and by induction of target cell enzymes that convert estradiol to an excreted metabolite, estrone sulfate. As a result, the number of estrogen receptor complexes that are retained in the endometrial nuclei is decreased, as is the overall intracellular availability of the powerful estradiol.

One would expect the same mechanism of estrogen receptor depletion to operate in both the endometrium and the breast, and that protection against abnormal mitotic activity should exist in both target tissues. In one long-term follow-up study and one prospective, controlled study, there is an indication that the addition of monthly progestational exposure to an estrogen replacement program lowers the incidence of breast cancer in postmenopausal women. (62,63) There are legitimate criticisms of these studies, and by no means should the conclusions be accepted as definitive. Nevertheless, there is logic to this contention. For example, progestational agents inhibit the in vitro multiplication of human breast cancer cells (64,65), although high doses have been reported to stimulate the growth of cultured malignant cells. (66)

Receptors and Prognosis

There is an excellent correlation between the presence of estrogen receptors and certain clinical characteristics of breast cancer. Premenopausal and younger patients are more frequently receptor negative. Patients with receptor positive tumors survive longer and have longer disease-free intervals after mastectomy than those with receptor negative tumors. The presence of an estrogen receptor correlates with increased disease-free interval regardless of the presence of positive axillary nodes, or the size and location of the tumors. Similarly, patients without axillary lymph node metastases, but with an estradiol receptor negative tumor, have the same high rate of recurrence as do patients with axillary lymph node metastases.

143

It appears that patients with estrogen receptors are those with the more slowly growing tumors. Several reports indicate that estrogen receptor status correlates with the degree of differentiation of the primary tumor. A large proportion of highly differentiated Grade I carcinomas are receptor positive while the reverse is true of Grade III tumors.

It takes estrogen to make progesterone receptors. Therefore the presence of progesterone receptors proves that the estrogen receptor in the tumor is biologically active. Thus, it is not surprising that the presence of progesterone receptors has a correlation with disease-free survival of patients only second to the number of positive nodes. (67) The best prognosis is seen in patients with positive progesterone receptors, even with subsequent disease, if the recurrent disease is still progesterone receptor positive. The loss of progesterone receptors is an ominous sign.

Treatment Selection

The receptor assay is a valuable prognostic indicator which, combined with lymph node status and tumor histologic grade, can be used in management of patients with breast cancer.

The correlation between the presence of estrogen and progesterone receptors and the clinical response to all types of endocrine therapy has been established. Between 50 and 60% of receptor positive postmenopausal patients responded to ablation of hormones, which is almost double the response rate in unselected patients with breast cancer. Less than 10% of receptor negative tumors showed a response (scored as tumor size regression of 50% for a period exceeding a month). Receptor negative patients can be spared unnecessary surgery and months of fruitless trials of hormone therapy by the prompt initiation of chemotherapy.

Current guidelines from the U. S. National Cancer Institute are as follows:

Premenopausal Women:.

Positive Nodes — Treatment with chemotherapy regardless of receptor status.

Negative Nodes — Adjuvant therapy considered only in high risk situations.

Postmenopausal Women:

Positive Nodes — Positive receptor status: treat with tamoxifen. Negative receptor status: consider chemotherapy.

Negative Nodes — Adjuvant therapy considered only in high risk situations.

Some disagree with these recommendations (which they label as conservative), arguing that it makes sense because of the high chance (30%) of recurrence to use aggressive adjuvant therapy for node-negative patients. Older patients have more widespread disease than their younger counterparts at presentation, but the tumors tend to be better differentiated and slower growing with a greater percentage of receptor positive tumors. Thus postmenopausal breast cancers are more relatively resistant to chemotherapy, but susceptible to tamoxifen. (68) Therefore it seems appropriate to advocate a more aggressive use of tamoxifen.

The problem remains that at the time of diagnosis we are usually dealing with a disease which has reached the point of dissemination. Effective treatment requires earlier diagnosis.

Tamoxifen and Endometrial Cancer. A study from Stockholm of 1,846 postmenopausal women who were being treated in a randomized trial of tamoxifen (40 mg daily) following surgery for early breast cancer discovered an increased incidence of endometrial cancer. (69) By the 5th year of tamoxifen treatment, the relative risk of endometrial cancer was increased 6.4 times, although there were 45% fewer cases of recurrent breast cancer. Tamoxifen has both agonistic and antagonistic estrogenic properties. The antagonistic property is the principal feature of its use as therapy for breast cancer. Whether a target tissue responds to the antagonistic action or the agonistic action is dependent upon the individual sensitivity of the tissue. It is apparent that the endometrium is more sensitive to the agonistic action, therefore while the breast is protected against estrogenic effects, the endometrium responds to the weak estrogenic activity of tamoxifen. This has very important clinical application. A woman who is on tamoxifen treatment for longer than 2 years should be treated with either daily or periodic (at least 10 days per month) progestational administration. This should provide effective protection against endometrial cancer. The daily regimen would also offer some protection against osteoporosis.

Needle Aspiration

Needle aspiration of breast lumps should be part of the practice of everyone who cares for women. The technique is easy. A small infiltrate of xylocaine is placed in the skin. Holding the lesion between thumb and index finger with one hand, the other hand passes a 20 or 21 gauge needle attached to a 10 ml syringe several times through the lesion with continuous suction on the syringe. Air is forcibly ejected through the needle on to a cytology slide for smearing and fixing. The usual Pap smear fixative can be used.

The procedure is very cost effective. (70) When aspiration yields clear fluid, no matter what the color, and the mass disappears, the procedure is both diagnostic and therapeutic. Fluid of any other nature (cloudy, opaque, bloody) requires cytologic assessment and/or biopsy. Failure to obtain material for histologic evaluation or the persistence of a mass requires biopsy. Locally recurrent cysts should be surgically removed.

The method used for solid tumor fine needle aspiration is similar to that used for simple cyst aspiration. After the tumor is fixed using the forefinger and thumb of one hand, the needle is inserted into the mass with the other hand. Two ml of air is first drawn into the syringe to later help express the contents onto a slide. Approximately 6 passes are made to different areas of the mass, using short strokes while aspirating. The idea is to secure material within the needle, therefore the negative pressure must be released prior to withdrawing the needle so that the specimen does not become drawn into the syringe. The specimen is then smeared thinly on the slide and fixed.

145

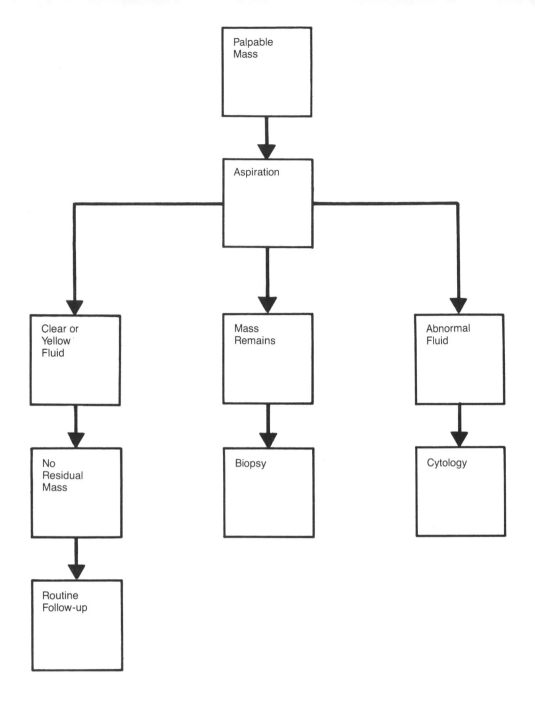

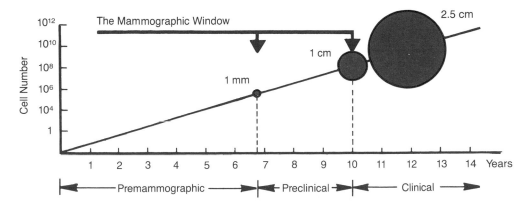

after Wertheimer, et al.

Mammography

Mammography is a means of detecting nonpalpable cancer. In the past few years technical advancements have significantly improved the mammographic image. (71) The doubling time of breast cancer is very variable, but in general, a tumor doubles in size every 100 days. Thus it takes a single malignant cell approximately 10 years to grow to a clinically detectable 1 cm mass, but by this time a tumor of 1 cm has already progressed through 30 of the 40 doublings in size which is estimated to be fatal. (72) Furthermore, the average size at which a tumor is detected (70–75% of tumors are found by patients themselves) is 2.5 cm, a size which has a 50% incidence of lymph node involvement. To decrease the mortality from breast cancer, we must utilize a technique to find the tumors when they are smaller. Mammography is the answer.

In the 1970s, xeromammography significantly reduced the amount of radiation delivered with x-ray mammography. In the 1980s, the film screen system (using special film against a fluorescent screen) was developed, delivering approximately 0.1 rad per examination. With this amount of irradiation, there is no longer a concern for the radiation dose. From a diagnostic point of view, there is no difference between the film screen technique and xeromammography; however, xeromammography delivers more radiation (although the slight increase with the very latest xeromammographic technique is probably insignificant).

Mammography is the technique of choice. Thermography has a high rate of false positive findings. Ultrasound can rarely reveal malignant lesions under 1 cm in size. It is useful, however, to guide the aspiration of lesions. CT scanning has 2 serious limitations. The x-ray dose is large, and the slices are too thick to detect early lesions. Finally, magnetic resonance imaging is not practical because of the long scan times that are necessary.

Mammography is the only method that detects clustered microcalcifications. These calcifications are less than 1 mm in diameter and are frequently associated with malignant lesions. More than 5 calcifications in a cluster are associated with cancer 25% of the time and require biopsy.

147

Mammography has a false negative rate of 8 to 10%. This means that masses are palpable but not visible. Mammography cannot and should not replace examination by patient and physician. Cancer commonly presents as a solitary, solid, painless, hard, unilateral, irregular, nonmobile mass. A decrease in size makes cancer unlikely; however, cancers can stay the same size for many months. A mass requires biopsy regardless of the mammographic picture. A bloody nipple discharge requires cytologic evaluation; about 25% will have breast cancer.

A pattern of dysplasia on the mammogram carries with it an increased risk (2.0–3.5 times normal) of breast cancer. The risk is similar to that seen with the other known risk factors. (73)

The Effectiveness of Mammography. It is now apparent that mammography is effective in reducing the mortality of breast cancer. The Health Insurance Plan of New York screening program demonstrated a 30% decrease in mortality in the screened group over 50 years old. (74) There are currently large scale trials ongoing, but preliminary results are very impressive. In Nijmegan, Netherlands, the breast cancer mortality rate in women of 35 and over was reduced by 50% by annual mammographic screening. (75) In Utrecht, Netherlands, the relative risk of dying from breast cancer among screened women was reduced by 70%. (76)

The first randomized, controlled trial of mammography was begun in Sweden in 1977. Results to the end of 1984 demonstrated a 31% reduction in mortality and a 25% reduction in more advanced breast disease, with a further acceleration of this reduction by the end of 1985. (77,78) Most impressively, these results were obtained with a screening only every 2–3 years and with only a single mediolateral oblique view.

Until recently, it was questioned whether mammography screening was effective for women under 50. The American Breast Cancer Detection Demonstration Project has now demonstrated that screening is just as effective for women in their 40s as in women over 50. (79) This program, which was organized by the American Cancer Society and the National Cancer Institute, began operating in 1973 in 27 locations throughout the United States, enrolling more than 280,000 women. Despite the fact that this is not an organized research study with a control group, the massive database permits many valuable conclusions. From 1977 to 1982, similar high survival rates (87%) for women in their 40s compared with women in their 50s verify that screening was just as effective in the younger women. An important point made by this project is the very significant role played by the women participating in the study.

For an effective breast screening progam, women must be very active in their interaction with the process (including both the medical profession and the detection technology). Cooperation and alertness of the women are key ingredients for achieving success. One obstacle to patient compliance can be traced to shared stories of physical discomfort during mammography (due to the compression of the breast, which is absolutely necessary for films of high quality). A large study assessing this problem concluded that only 10% of women experience severe or moderate discomfort and another 1% complain of moderate pain. (80) This study utilized 7 different centers, and in no center did more than 22% of the women experience moderate or worse discomfort. Not surprisingly, women who harbored an expectation of discomfort, obtained from media, friends, or relatives, were more likely to experience some pain. Most importantly, 88% of the women experienced no or only mild discomfort.

There are problems to be anticipated with extensive mammography screening. Overall, only about 20–30% of biopsy specimens contain carcinoma. That means there will be a large number of biopsies and mammograms performed (including the treatment of clinically ir-relevant lesions), which involves costs to the health care system and cost to the individual in terms of stress and anxiety. The decision to biopsy a slightly suspicious mammographic finding is not made eas-ily. It involves the patient's psychological makeup and experience as well as physician experience, confidence, and medicolegal con-siderations.

One analysis of risks and benefits concluded that because breast cancer is relatively infrequent under the age of 50, it is not cost effective to screen all asymptomatic women aged 40–49. (81) How-ever, mammography is the most potent weapon we possess in the battle against breast cancer, and we believe aggressive screening is worthwhile as outlined below. Mammography not only lowers mor-tality, but it also decreases morbidity because less radical surgery is necessary for smaller lesions.

Every woman should be regarded as being at risk. Health care profes-sionals who interact with women have the opportunity to initiate an aggressive program of preventive health care. The major deterrent to patient use of mammography is the absence of physician rec-ommendations. We urge you to follow these suggested guidelines:

SCREENING FOR BREAST CANCER

All women should be taught self-breast examination by age 20. Because of the changes which occur routinely in response to the hormonal sequence of a normal menstrual cycle, breast examination is most effective during the follicular phase of the cycle.

All women over the age of 35 should have an annual breast exam-ination.

A baseline mammogram should be obtained by age 40, or earlier if high risk factors are present.

From ages 40 to 50, mammography should be performed every 2 years in low risk women and every year in women with significant risk factors.

Annual breast examination and annual mammography should be per-formed in all women over age 50.

SIGNIFICANT HIGH RISK FACTORS

Family history of breast cancer in mother or sister.

Proliferative disease of the breast by biopsy.

First childbirth after age 30.

Dysplasia on mammography.

Relatively low SHBG levels.

The Management of Mastalgia

The frequency and intensity of breast discomfort decrease with increasing age. Nevertheless, a sufficient number of women experience this problem, especially during the perimenopausal years, to warrant a discussion of its management. The cyclic occurrence of breast discomfort is usually associated with dysplastic, benign histologic changes in the breast. Medical treatment of mastalgia has historically included a bewildering array of options. Several are of questionable value. Diuretics have little impact, and thyroid hormone replacement is indicated only when hypothyroidism is documented. Steroid hormone treatment has been tried in many combinations, mostly unsupported by controlled studies. An old favorite, with many years of clinical experience testifying to its effectiveness, is testosterone. One must be careful, however, to avoid virilizing doses. A good practice is to start with small doses, such as 5 mg methyltestosterone every other day during the time of discomfort. In recent years, however, these methods have been supplanted by several new approaches.

Danazol in a dose of 200 mg/day is effective in relieving discomfort as well as decreasing nodularity of the breast. (82) A daily dose is recommended for a period of 6 months. This treatment may achieve long-term resolution of the histologic changes in addition to the clinical improvement; however, there is no evidence that treatment ameliorates atypical epithelial changes and reduces the risk of cancer. Doses below 400 mg daily do not assure inhibition of ovulation, and a method of effective contraception is necessary in premenopausal women because of possible teratogenic effects of the drug. Significant improvement has been noted with vitamin E, 600 units/day of the synthetic tocopheral acetate. No side effects have been noted, and the mechanism of action is unknown. Bromocriptine (2.5–5.0 mg/day) and antiestrogens such as tamoxifen (20 mg daily) are also effective for treating mammary discomfort and benign disease. (82,83)

Clinical observations had suggested that abstinence from methylxanthines leads to resolution of symptoms. Methylxanthines are present in coffee, tea, chocolate, and cola drinks. In controlled studies, however, a significant placebo response rate (30–40%) has been observed. Careful assessments of this relationship have failed to demonstrate a link between methylxanthine use and mastalgia, mammographic changes, or atypia (premalignant tissue changes).(84–86)

Some women on hormone replacement therapy, particularly a combination of estrogen and progestin, develop enlarged, tender breasts. This is usually due to a relatively high dose of the progestin, and responds to lowering the dose or changing the progestin. We have had notable success in switching from medroxyprogesterone to norethindrone (0.35 mg daily).

References

1. **Silverberg E, Lubera J,** Cancer statistics, 1989, CA 39:3, 1989.

2. **Henderson IC, Cannellos GP,** Cancer of the breast, New Engl J Med 302:17,78, 1980.

3. **Bland KI,** Risk factors as an indicator for breast cancer screening in asymptomatic patients, Maturitas 9:135, 1987.

4. **Brownson RC, Blackwell CW, Pearson DK, Reynolds RD, Richens JW Jr, Papermaster BW,** Risk of breast cancer in relation to cigarette smoking, Arch Intern Med 148:140, 1988.

5. **Pathak DR, Speizer FE, Willett WC, Rosner B, Lipnick RJ,** Parity and breast cancer risk: Possible effect on age at diagnosis, Int J Cancer 37:21, 1986.

6. **Musey VC, Collins DC, Brogan DR, Santos VR, Musey PI, Martino-Saltzman D, Preedy JRK,** Long term effects of a first pregnancy on the hormonal environment: Estrogens and androgens, J Clin Endocrinol Metab 64:111, 1987.

7. **Musey VC, Collins DC, Musey PI, Martino-Saltzman D, Preedy JRK,** Long-term effects of a first pregnancy on the secretion of prolactin, New Engl J Med 316:229, 1987.

8. **Byers T, Graham S, Rzepka T, Marshall J,** Lactation and breast cancer: Evidence for a negative association in premenopausal women, Am J Epidemiol 121:664, 1985.

9. **Kvale G, Heuch I,** Lactation and cancer risk: Is there a relation specific to breast cancer? J Epidemiol Comm Health 42:30, 1987.

10. **McTiernan A, Thomas DB,** Evidence for a protective effect of lactation on risk of breast cancer in young women, Am J Epidemiol 124:353, 1986.

11. **Ing R, Ho JHC, Petrakis NL,** Unilateral breast-feeding and breast cancer, Lancet ii:124, 1977.

12. **Yuan J-M, Yu MC, Ross RK, Gao Y-T, Henderson BE,** Risk factors for breast cancer in Chinese women in Shanghai, Cancer Res 48:1949, 1988.

13. **Sherman B, Wallace R, Beam J, Schlabaugh L,** Relationship of body weight to menarchial and menopausal age: Implication for breast cancer risk, J Clin Endocrinol Metab 52:488, 1981.

14. **Dupont WD, Page DL,** Risk factors for breast cancer in women with proliferative breast disease, New Engl J Med 312:146, 1985.

15. **Cancer Committee, College of American Pathologists,** Is 'fibrocystic disease' of the breast precancerous? Arch Path Lab Med 110:171, 1986.

16. **Sattin RW, Rubin GL, Webster LA, Huezo CM, Wingo PA, Ory HW, Layde PM,** Family history and the risk of breast cancer, JAMA 253:1908, 1985.

17. **Willett WC, Browne ML, Bain C, Lipnick RJ, Stampfer MJ, Rosner B, Colditz GA, Hennekens CH, Speizer FE,** Relative weight and risk of breast cancer among premenopausal women, Am J Epidemiol 122:731, 1985.

18. **Willett WC, Stampfer MJ, Colditz GA, Rosner BA, Hennekens CH, Speizer FE,** Dietary fat and the risk of breast cancer, New Engl J Med 316:22, 1987.

19. **Willett WC, Stampfer MJ, Colditz GA, Rosner BA, Hennekens CH, Speizer FE,** Moderate alcohol consumption and the risk of breast cancer, New Engl J Med 316:1174, 1987.

20. **Bulbrook RD,** Urinary androgen excretion and the etiology of breast cancer, JNCI 48:1039, 1972.

21. **Dickinson LE, MacMahon B, Cole P, Brown JB,** Estrogen profiles of Oriental and Caucasian women in Hawaii, New Engl J Med 291:1211, 1974.

22. **Sherman BM, Korenman SG,** Inadequate corpus luteum function: A pathophysiologic interpretation of human breast cancer epidemiology, Cancer 33:1306, 1974.

23. **McFayden IJ, Forrest APM, Prescott RJ, Golder MP, Groom GV, Fahmy DR,** Circulating hormone concentrations in women with breast cancer, Lancet i:1000, 1976.

24. **Cowan LD, Gordis L, Tonascia JA, Jones GS,** Breast cancer incidence in women with a history of progesterone deficiency, Am J Epidemiol, 114:209, 1981.

25. **Coulam CB, Annegars JF,** Chronic anovulation may increase postmenopausal breast cancer risk, JAMA 249:445, 1983.

26. **Ron E, Lunenfeld B, Menczer M, et al,** Cancer incidence in a cohort of infertile women, Am J Epidemiol 125:780, 1987.

27. **Cuzick J, Wang DY, Bulbrook RD,** The prevention of breast cancer, Lancet i:83, 1986.

28. **Kaufman DW, Miller DR, Rosenberg L, Helmrich SP, Stolley P, Schottenfeld D, Shapiro S,** Noncontraceptive estrogen use and the risk of breast cancer, JAMA 252:63, 1984.

29. **Wingo PA Layde PM, Lee NC, Rubin G, Ory HW,** The risk of breast cancer in postmenopausal women who have used estrogen replacment therapy, JAMA 257:209, 1987.

30. **Buring JE, Hennekens CH, Lipnick RJ, Willett W, Stampfer MJ, Rosner B, Peto R, Speizer FE,** A prospective cohort study of postmenopausal hormone use and risk of breast cancer in US women, Am J Epidemiol 125:939, 1987.

31. **Rohan TE, McMichael AJ,** Non-contraceptive exogenous oestrogen therapy and breast cancer, Med J Aust 148:217, 1988.

32. **Armstrong BK,** Oestrogen therapy after the menopause—boon or bane? Med J Aust 148:213, 1988.

33. **Dupont WD, Page DL, Rogers LW, Parl FF,** Influence of exogenous estrogens, proliferative breast disease, and other variables on breast cancer risk, Cancer 63:948, 1989.

34. **Bergkvist L, Hans-Olov A, Persson I, Hoover R, Schairer C,** The risk of breast cancer after estrogen and estrogen-progestin replacement, New Engl J Med 321:293, 1989.

35. **Ewertz M,** Influence of non-contraceptive exogenous and endogenous sex hormones on breast cancer risk in Denmark, Int J Cancer 42:832, 1988.

36. **Royal College of General Practitioners Oral Contraceptive Study,** Further analyses of mortality in oral contraceptive users, Lancet i:541, 1981.

37. **Vessey MP, McPherson K, Yeates D,** Mortality in oral contraceptive users, Lancet i:549, 1981.

38. **Ramcharan S, Pellegrin FA, Ray RM, Hsu J-P,** The Walnut Creek Contraceptive Drug Study. A prospective study of the side effects of oral contraceptives, J Reprod Med 25:366,360, 1980.

39. **Pike MC, Krailo MD, Henderson BE, Duke A, Roy S,** Breast cancer in young women and use of oral contraceptives: possible modifying effect of formulation and age at use, Lancet ii:926, 1983.

40. **McPherson K, Neil A, Vessey MP,** Oral contraceptives and breast cancer, Lancet ii:414, 1983.

41. **Olsson H, Landin-Olsson M, Moller TR, Ranstam J, Holm P,** Oral contraceptive use and breast cancer in young women in Sweden, Lancet i:748, 1985.

42. **Meirik O, Dami H, Christoffersen T, Lund E, Bergstrom R, Bergsjo P,** Oral contraceptive use and breast cancer in young women, Lancet ii:650, 1986.

43. **Kay CR, Hannaford PC,** Breast cancer and the pill—Further report from the Royal College of General Practitioners' oral contraceptive study, Brit J Cancer 58:657, 1988.

44. **UK National Case-Control Study Group,** Oral contraceptive use and breast cancer risk in young women, Lancet i:973, 1989.

45. **Stadel BV, Rubin GL, Webster LA, Schlesselman JJ, Wingo PA,** Oral contraceptives and breast cancer in young women, Lancet ii:970, 1985.

46. **Cancer and Steroid Hormone Study, CDC and NICHD,** Oral contraceptive use and the risk of breast cancer, New Engl J Med 315:405, 1986.

47. **Paul C, Skegg DCG, Spears GFS, Kaldor JM,** Oral contraceptives and breast cancer: A national study, Brit Med J 2923:723, 1986.

48. **Stadel BV, Lai SL,** Oral contraceptives and premenopausal breast cancer in nulliparous women, Contraception 38:287, 1988.

49. **Schlesselman JJ, Stadel BV, Murray P, Lai S,** Breast cancer in relation to early use of oral contraceptives. No evidence of a latent effect, JAMA 259:1828, 1988.

50. **Miller DR, Rosenberg L, Kaufman DW, Stolley P, Warshauer ME, Shapiro S,** Breast cancer before age 45 and oral contraceptive use: New findings, Am J Epidemiol 129:269, 1989.

51. **Miller DR, Rosenberg L, Kaufman DW, Schottenfeld D, Stolley PD, Shapiro S,** Breast cancer risk in relation to early oral contraceptive use, Obstet Gynecol 68:863, 1986.

52. **Rosenberg L, Miller DR, Kaufman DW, Helmrich SP, Stolley PD, Schoffenfeld D, Shapiro S,** Breast cancer and oral contraceptive use, Am J Epidemiol 119:167, 1984.

53. **Bibbo M, Haenszel W, Wied GL, Hubby M, Herbst AL,** A twenty-five year follow-up study of women exposed to DES during pregnancy, New Engl J Med 298:763, 1978.

54. **Brian OD, Tilley BC, LaBarthe DR, O'Fallon WM, Noller KL, Kurland LT,** Breast cancer in DES exposed mothers: Absence of association, Mayo Clin Proc 55:89, 1980.

55. **Greenburg ER, Barnes AB, Resseguie L, Barrett JA, Burnside S, Lanza LL, Neff RK, Stevens M, Young RH, Colton T,** Breast cancer in mothers given diethylstilbestrol in pregnancy, New Engl J Med 311:1393, 1984.

56. **Korenman SG,** The endocrinology of breast cancer, Cancer 46:874, 1980.

57. **Korenman SG,** Estrogen window hypothesis of the etiology of breast cancer, Lancet i:700, 1980.

58. **Tokunaga M, Norman JE, Asano M, Tokuoka S, Ezaki H, Nishimori I, Tsuji Y,** Malignant breast tumors among atomic bomb survivors, JNCI 62:1347, 1979.

59. **Boice JD, Monson RR,** Breast cancer in women after repeated fluoroscopic examinations of the chest, JNCI 59:823, 1977.

60. **De Waard F, Trichopoulos D,** A unifying concept of the aetiology of breast cancer, Int J Cancer 41:666, 1988.

61. **W.H.O. Collaborative Study of Neoplasia and Steroid Contraceptives,** Breast cancer, cervical cancer, and depot medroxyprogesterone acetate, Lancet ii:1207, 1984.

62. **Gambrell RD Jr, Maier RC, Sanders BI,** Decreased incidence of breast cancer in postmenopausal estrogen-progestogen users, Obstet Gynecol 62:435, 1983.

63. **Nachtigall LE, Nachtigall RH, Nachtigall RB, Beckman M,** Estrogen replacement: II. A prospective study in the relationship to carcinoma and cardiovascular and metabolic problems, Obstet Gynecol 54:74, 1979.

64. **Vignon F, Bardon S, Chalbos D, Rochefort H,** Antiestrogenic effect of R5020, a synthetic progestin in human breast cancer cells in culture, J Clin Endocrinol Metab 56:1124, 1983

65. **Mauvais-Jarvis P, Kuttenn F, Gompel A,** Antiestrogen action of progesterone in breast tissue, Breast Cancer Res Treat 8:179, 1986.

66. **Longman SM, Buehring GC,** Oral contraceptives and breast cancer. In vitro effect of contraceptive steroids on human mammary cell growth, Cancer 59:281, 1987.

67. **McGuire WL, Clark LGM,** Role of progesterone receptors in breast cancer, CA 36:302, 1986.

68. **Early Breast Cancer Trialists' Collaborative Group,** Effects of adjuvant Tamoxifen and of cytotoxic therapy on mortality in early breast cancer, New Engl J Med 319:1681, 1988.

69. **Fornander T, Cedermark B, Mattsson A, Skoog L, Theve T, Askergren J, Rutqvist LE, Glas U, Silfversward C, Somell A, Wilking N, Hjalmar M-L,** Adjuvant tamoxifen in early breast cancer: Occurrence of new primary cancers, Lancet i:117, 1989.

70. **Ciatto S, Cariaggi P, Bulgaresi P,** The value of routine cytologic examination of breast cyst fluids, Acta Cytologica 31:301, 1987.

71. **Kopans LDB, Meyer JE, Sadowsky N,** Breast imaging, New Engl J Med 310:960, 1984.

72. **Wertheimer MD, Costanza ME, Dodson TF, D'Orsi C, Pastides H, Zapka JG,** Increasing the effort toward breast cancer detection, JAMA 255:1311, 1986.

73. **Carlile T, Kopecky KJ, Thompson DJ, Whitehead JR, Gilbert FI Jr, Present AJ, Threatt BA, Krook P, Hadaway E,** Breast cancer prediction and the Wolfe classification on mammograms, JAMA 254:1050, 1985.

74. **Shapiro S, Venet W, Strax P, Venet L, Roeser R,** Ten to fourteen year effect of screening on breast cancer mortality, JNCI 69:329, 1982.

75. **Verbeek ALM, Holland R, Sturmans F, Hendriks JHCL, Miravunac M, Day NE,** Reduction of breast cancer mortality through mass screening with modern mammography, Lancet i:1222, 1984.

76. **Collette HJA, Rombach JJ, Day NE, De Waard F,** Evaluation of screening for breast cancer in non-randomized study (the DOM project by means of a case-control study), Lancet i:124, 1984.

77. **Tabar L, Gad A, Holmberg LH, Ljungquist U, Fagerberg CJG, Baldetorp L, Grontoft O, Lundstrom B, Manson JC, Eklund G, Dan NE, Petterson F,** Reduction in mortality from breast cancer after mass screening with mammography, Lancet i:829, 1985.

78. **Tabar L, Faberberg G, Day NE, Holmberg L,** What is the optimum interval between mammographic screening examinations?—An analysis based on the latest results of the Swedish two-county breast cancer screening trial, Brit J Cancer 55:547, 1987.

79. **Seidman H, Gelb SK, Silveraberg E, LaVerda N, Lubera JA,** Survival experience in the breast cancer detection demonstration project, CA 37:258, 1987.

80. **Stomper PC, Kopans DB, Sadowsky NL, Sonnenfeld MR, Swann CA, Gelman RS, Meyer JE, Jochelson MS, Hunt MS, Allen PD,** Is mammography painful? A multicenter patient survey, Arch Intern Med 148:521, 1988.

81. **Eddy DM, Hasselblad V, McGivney W, Hendee W,** The value of mammography screening in women under age 50 years, JAMA 259:1512, 1988.

82. **Pye JK, Mansel RE, Hughes LE,** Clinical experience of drug treatments for mastalgia, Lancet ii:373, 1985.

83. **Fentiman IS, Brame K, Caleffi M, Chaudary MA, Hayward JL,** Double-blind controlled trial of tamoxifen therapy for mastalgia, Lancet i:287, 1986.

84. **Ernster VL, Mason L, Goodson WH III, Sickles EA, Sacks ST, Selvin S, Dupuy ME, Hawkinson J, Hunt TK,** Effects of caffeine-free diet on benign breast disease: A randomized trial, Surgery 91:263, 1982.

155

85. **Lubin F, Ron E, Wax Y, Black M, Funaro M, Shitrit A,** A case-control study of caffeine and methylxanthines in benign breast disease, JAMA 253:2388, 1985.

86. **Schairer C, Brinton LA, Hoover RN,** Methylxanthines and benign breast disease, Am J Epidemiol 124:603, 1986.

Hypertension

Hypertension is the most common chronic disease in older women, contributing significantly to overall morbidity and mortality. (1) There have been substantial advances in understanding the epidemiology, natural history, and treatment of hypertension in both men and women. Because hypertension is the most important, the most frequent, and the most treatable cause for cerebrovascular disease, congestive heart failure, and coronary heart disease in older women, recognition and appropriate management are crucial. Although hypertension in men and women is qualitatively similar, there are meaningful differences.

**Clinical
Definitions**

Cardiovascular risk is related to both systolic and diastolic blood pressures, and the risk increases gradually with each increment in blood pressure. The degree of risk for any increment in blood pressure increases with advancing age. (2) We define a woman as *clinically hypertensive* when the potential benefits of therapy exceed the risks and costs of no treatment. Currently the American diagnosis of hypertension in adults requires a blood pressure greater than 140/90 mm Hg measured on multiple occasions. (3)

The Working Group on Hypertension in the Elderly has provided the following definition for people over age 60: ''An average systolic blood pressure greater than 160 mm Hg and/or an average diastolic greater than or equal to 90 mm Hg on three consecutive visits constitute the diagnosis of hypertension, although the 140–160 mm Hg range represents borderline isolated systolic hypertension when diastolic pressure is less than 90.'' (4)

The following further classification of hypertension applies to older women:

MILD: diastolic pressure = 90–104 mm Hg.

MODERATE: diastolic pressure = 105–114 mm Hg.

SEVERE: diastolic pressure > 115 mm Hg.

Patients with borderline hypertension require close observation, and many will be treated empirically with nonpharmacologic therapy. Those with clinical evidence of cardiovascular disease and borderline or mild hypertension will be treated with drugs. Although the importance of isolated systolic hypertension and its treatment is still under study, women with isolated systolic hypertension are at increased risk of cardiovascular disease and death.

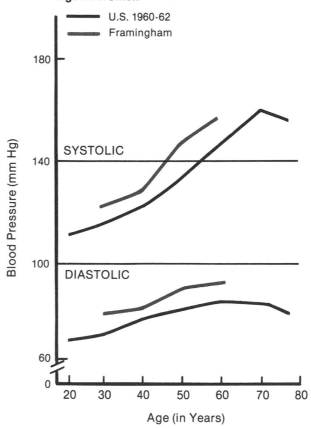

Increasing Blood Pressure with Increasing Age in Women

Epidemiology

The systolic pressure rises progressively with age until age 70 or 80, whereas the diastolic pressure rises to age 50–60, then levels or decreases slightly with advancing age. (5)

Peak blood pressure occurs later in women than in men. However, the systolic blood pressure increase in women between the third and seventh decades is 1–9 mm Hg greater than in men, and the increase in diastolic blood pressure with aging in women is also slightly greater than in men. (6) Women with the lowest blood pressure at younger ages have the smallest rise in blood pressure with increasing age and those with the highest blood pressure when younger have the greatest tendency to increase when older. Increasing blood pressure with increasing age is not inevitable. Many elderly individuals retain normal or low blood pressure throughout life and have lower cardio-vascular mortality and morbidity rates compared to those with higher blood pressures. (2,7)

The figure illustrates the increasing prevalence of hypertension in women with aging. (8) The exact prevalence of hypertension in older women depends upon the selected criteria. Defining hypertension as at least 160/95 mm Hg, about 20% of white women and more than 50% of black women between the ages 45–54 have hypertension. (9) In the 65–74 age group, 48.3% of white women and 72.8% of black women have hypertension.

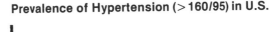

Prevalence of Hypertension (> 160/95) in U.S.

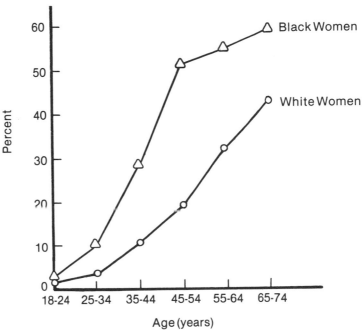

Using a lower limit to define hypertension (140/90 mm Hg), the prevalence in women age 65–74 increases to 66.2% of white women and 82.9% of black women. (9) The prevalence of isolated systolic hypertension in women over age 60 has been estimated to be 12%, increasingly progressive with each decade of advancing age. (10) This remarkable prevalence is a major reason why hypertension in older women is such an important clinical problem.

Risks Associated With Hypertension

Heart disease and stroke rank as the leading causes of death of older women, with the highest cardiovascular mortality found among black women. Twenty-seven percent of all deaths among women are due to coronary heart disease with an additional 25% caused by other forms of cardiovascular disease. (11) Each year, approximately 250,000 women die of coronary heart disease, 100,000 of other forms of heart disease, 100,000 of cerebrovascular disease, and 30,000 of other cardiovascular diseases. Cardiovascular death rates are twice as high among black women compared to white women up to age 75. (12) About 200,000 cardiovascular deaths can be considered to be "premature."

The prognosis for the outcome of hypertension is better for women than for men. After 20 years of comparable hypertension, about twice as many men will die as a result of complications compared to women. Fewer untreated women will go on to develop accelerated or malignant hypertension. The reasons for this better tolerance in women is unknown. Despite this better tolerance, hypertension in older women significantly increases the risk of mortality.

Average Annual Incidence of Cardiovascular Events in Elderly Men and Women
20-Year Follow-up in the Framingham Study (1)
Rate per 1,000 population

Coronary Heart Disease		Cerebro-vascular Disease		Peripheral Arterial Disease		Congestive Heart Failure	
Men	Women	Men	Women	Men	Women	Men	Women
20.4	14.5	8.4	8.6	6.3	3.8	8.2	6.8

Hypertension stands out as the major risk factor for cardiovascular disease and mortality in elderly women. Cardiovascular mortality is increased eight-fold in hypertensive elderly women age 65–74 compared to normotensive elderly women. (1) The risk of hypertension is due to elevation of both systolic and diastolic blood pressures, but with advancing age, the risks of stroke, cardiac enlargement, and congestive heart failure are influenced more by the systolic pressure. (13,14) It is estimated that hypertension in older women accounts for 33% of all cases of cardiac disease and 70% of strokes. (10) Therefore, both combined systolic and diastolic and isolated systolic hypertension are frequent in older women and markedly increase the risk of cardiovascular morbidity and mortality.

Pathophysiology

Hypertension in elderly women is characterized by increased peripheral vascular resistance, a slow heart rate, and reductions in cardiac stroke volume, cardiac output, intravascular volume, renal blood flow, and renin activity. Aortic wall thickness increases and aortic elasticity is reduced, resulting in increased vascular stiffness and rigidity and a decrease in arterial compliance and distensibility which is responsible for the greater rise in systolic pressure compared to diastolic pressure. (15)

A number of hormonal changes characterize hypertension in the elderly. These include a decrease in plasma renin with maintenance of plasma aldosterone, an increase in plasma norepinephrine, and a lack of increase in vasopressin with upright posture. Changes also occur in the autonomic nervous system, including reduced responsiveness for cardiac beta-1 adrenoreceptors, cardiac muscarinic cholinergic receptors, vascular beta adrenoreceptors, and vascular alpha-2 adrenoreceptors. (16) In general, renal blood flow and glomerular filtration decrease with increasing age after 40. The elderly tend to be more inactive physically than younger people, and several studies have demonstrated that physical conditioning in older people can lower the systolic and diastolic blood pressure. (17,18) These observations provide some insights but fail to establish the cause or a leading hypothesis on the etiology of hypertension in older women.

Although the etiology of hypertension in elderly women is unknown, it is provocative that blood pressure increases most after menopause. Another important factor is weight. About 25% of older women are obese, and about half of all hypertensive women are obese. When overweight hypertensive women reduce body weight, blood pressure decreases. A further contributing factor may be the change in reflexes with aging. Older women demonstrate attenuated baroreceptor reflexes in response to sudden increases or decreases in blood pressure. (19) Therefore, mechanisms which increase peripheral resistance may not be countered by appropriate reflex responses to produce vasodilation and changes in heart rate in order to modulate blood pressure.

Diagnosis and Clinical Assessment

Hypertension should not be diagnosed from a single measurement; blood pressure is highly variable. The following techniques are the recommendations derived from a national consensus: (20)

1. There should be no use of cigarettes or caffeine for at least 30 minutes before measurement.

2. The patient should be seated with arm bared, supported, and positioned at heart level.

3. Measurement should begin after 5 minutes of rest.

4. The appropriate cuff size must be used. Use a large cuff if the arm circumference is greater than 32 cm.

5. Measurements should be taken with a mercury sphygmomanometer, a recently calibrated aneroid manometer, or a validated electronic device.

6. The first appearance of sound should be used for the systolic reading, and the disappearance of sound for the diastolic reading.

7. Two or more readings should be averaged. If the first two readings differ by more than 5 mm Hg, additional readings should be obtained and averaged.

8. Initially elevated readings must be confirmed on at least two subsequent visits.

9. An average of 140/90 mm Hg or greater is required for diagnosis. In those over age 60, an average greater than 160/90 mm Hg is required for treatment (with individual exceptions).

10. Patients should be informed of their blood pressure.

161

Three common causes of misdiagnosis are labile (office) hypertension, the auscultatory gap, and pseudohypertension.

Labile Hypertension. Office hypertension (white coat hypertension) is easy to understand and requires repetitive measurements in multiple settings to determine the real blood pressure. Digital readout, electronic devices can be rented or purchased for home measurements, and when used properly are very useful in providing accurate, baseline data. Studies have indicated that patients with blood pressures elevated only in the physician's office have cardiac size and function similar to those of normotensive individuals. (21)

The Auscultatory Gap. This phenomenon occurs when the cuff is deflated; one hears an initial one to three sounds and then a prolonged quiet zone before persistent auscultatory systolic sounds reappear. The systolic pressure is the first systolic sound despite the subsequent quiet zone. If one ignores the first few sounds, the systolic blood pressure will be underestimated.

Pseudohypertension. In pseudohypertension, the sclerotic brachial artery can only be compressed with very high inflation pressures with the cuff. The result is a discrepancy of 10–100 mm Hg between the auscultated systolic pressure and the true intra-arterial pressure, resulting in an overestimation of the blood pressure. To detect pseudohypertension, palpate the radial artery while inflating the cuff to above systolic pressure. When the arterial pulsations are obliterated, with pseudohypertension the artery will remain rigid and palpable (Osler's maneuver). With this condition, the true blood pressure cannot be determined without intra-arterial measurements. (22)

Assessment

The clinical evaluation should answer the following questions:

1. Does the patient have primary or secondary hypertension?

2. Is target organ involvement present?

3. Are cardiovascular risk factors other than high blood pressure present?

Medical History. The following items represent the important historical information:

1. Family history of high blood pressure and cardiovascular disease.

2. Patient history of cardiovascular, cerebrovascular, and renal disease and diabetes mellitus.

3. Known duration and levels of blood pressure.

4. History of weight gain, exercise levels, sodium intake, fat intake, and alcohol use.

5. Symptoms suggesting secondary hypertension.

6. Psychosocial and environmental factors (stress, socioeconomic problems).

7. Other cardiovascular risk factors (obesity, smoking, hyperlipidemia)

8. Over the counter and prescription medications.

9. Results and side effects of previous antihypertensive therapy.

Physical Examination. The following items are especially important:

1. Measurement of height and weight.

2. Funduscopic examination.

3. Carotid pulses, bruits.

4. Thyroid examination.

5. Heart rate, heart size, precordial heave, clicks, murmurs, arrhythmias, S3 or S4 heart sounds.

6. Abdominal bruits, enlarged kidneys, dilatation of the aorta.

7. Peripheral arterial pulsations and bruits, edema.

8. Neurologic assessment.

Secondary Causes of Hypertension. Hypertension may be an important manifestation of a number of clinical disorders, including pheochromocytoma, Cushing's syndrome, primary or secondary hyperaldosteronism, chronic renal disease, acromegaly, hypothyroidism, and renovascular disease. The most common cause of renovascular hypertension is atherosclerosis. The pursuit for a secondary cause of hypertension (in the absence of obvious symptoms or signs of the primary problem) is indicated when any of the following signals are encountered:

1. Difficult to treat or totally refractory hypertension.

2. The onset of a diastolic blood pressure equal to or greater than 105 mm Hg after age 55.

3. Diastolic pressure greater than or equal to 100 mm Hg while on a triple drug regimen.

4. Accelerated hypertension.

5. Spontaneous hypokalemia.

6. A rise in creatinine with or without therapy.

7. Abdominal bruits.

Laboratory Tests. The following minimal evaluation should be performed to detect target organ damage and to aid in treatment:

> Electrocardiogram
> Complete blood count
> Urinalysis
> Creatinine
> Glucose
> Electrolytes
> Uric acid
> Cholesterol
> Calcium

Higher systolic pressure, longer duration hypertension, arrhythmias, or congestive heart failure makes left ventricular hypertrophy more likely. If one chooses drugs (e.g. diuretics) which do not decrease left ventricular hypertrophy during initial therapy, older women should have a diagnostic cardiac ultrasound. The type and frequency of all laboratory tests will be based on the severity of target organ damage, and the effects of the treatment program selected.

Hormone Replacement Therapy and Hypertension

No relationship has been established between hypertension and the doses of estrogen used for replacement therapy. Studies have shown either no effect or a small, but statistically significant, decrease in blood pressure due to estrogen treatment.(23–27) This has been the case in both normotensive and hypertensive women. The very rare cases of increased blood pressure due to estrogen replacement therapy truly represent idiosyncratic reactions. Because of the protective impact of appropriate estrogen replacement on the risk of cardiovascular disease, it can be argued that a woman with controlled hypertension is in need of that specific benefit of estrogen. (see Chapter 5)

The blood pressure impact of the addition of a progestational agent to an estrogen replacement program is yet unknown, although clinical experience and early reports (27) thus far indicate that current low doses have no effect on blood pressure. Until this information is documented long-term, there is no reason to withhold an estrogen-progestin program from women with controlled hypertension; however, close monitoring of the blood pressure makes good clinical sense.

Treatment

Women with diastolic blood pressures greater than 100 mm Hg; women with diastolic blood pressures 90–100 mm Hg and with end organ damage, cardiovascular disease, or other risk factors; and women with high systolic blood pressures or prolonged mild hypertension should be treated. The goal of treatment is to prevent subsequent morbidity and mortality, and to achieve that goal the blood pressure should be maintained below 140/90 mm Hg.

Evidence From Clinical Trials. The Hypertension Detection and Follow-up Study compared rigorous, systematic, antihypertensive therapy in special program centers to existing patterns of care in the community (or more intensive care to less intensive treatment) in mild and moderate hypertensive subjects. The 5 year incidence of fatal and nonfatal cardiovascular end points was reduced by a significant 33% in black women and a nonsignificant 10.7% in white women. (28) Mortality was reduced by 27.8% in black women, while

164

there was no difference in white women. The Australian Therapeutic Trial of Mild Hypertension studied 2,170 men and 1,257 women in a double-blinded, placebo-controlled clinical trial. (29) Trial end-points were significantly lower among actively treated patients compared to placebo-treated patients, but the difference was seen primarily in the male subjects. Women suffered fewer end-points, but no significant difference was observed comparing active to placebo treatment.

The Medical Research Council Study was a 5 year, single-blinded trial of active drug compared to placebo treatment of mild hypertension in patients less than 64 years of age. (30) All cause mortality was decreased in men, but not women. However, there was a significant decrease in stroke in treated women compared to untreated women. In women with diastolic blood pressures greater than 100 mm Hg and 55–64 years of age, there was a significant decrease in events, although there was no decrease in coronary events or mortality. Strokes were decreased in non-smoking women treated with beta blockers or thiazide diuretics, but in smoking women only those treated with a thiazide demonstrated benefit. The European Working Party on High Blood Pressure in the Elderly trial was a randomized, double-blinded, placebo-controlled trial of antihypertensive therapy in patients older than age 60, which demonstrated a significant 44% reduction in all cardiovascular terminating events in older women. (31) There was a decrease (18%, nonsignificant) in cardiovascular mortality in the women. Treatment was not effective in women over age 80.

Overall, the evidence indicates that treatment of hypertension in women decreases the risk of stroke and other cardiovascular morbidity, especially in older women with very high blood pressures, while treatment has less effect on mortality in women than in men. However, most of the studies had relatively few women, and events in women occurred at a lower rate than in men, making it more difficult to demonstrate a treatment effect in the women. In addition, the number of women over age 80 who have been studied is very small, and it is premature to conclude that treatment has no effect in the oldest of women.

When to Treat

Essentially all women in whom the diagnosis of hypertension has been confirmed are candidates for nonpharmacologic therapy. Women less than 80 years old with diastolic blood pressures greater than 100 mm Hg should be treated with drugs if they fail to reach goal blood pressures with nonpharmacologic methods.

Women with diastolic blood pressures 90–100 mm Hg should be treated with drugs if they have any of the following:

1. Systolic blood pressures greater than 160 mm Hg.

2. Black race.

3. Other cardiovascular risk factors (family history of premature cardiovascular disease, elevated LDL-cholesterol, decreased HDL-cholesterol, significantly elevated triglycerides, diabetes mellitus, smoking, evidence of target organ damage: left ventricular hypertrophy, abnormal electrocardiogram, congestive heart failure, cor-

165

onary or cerebrovascular disease, renal disease or proteinuria, or peripheral vascular disease).

4. Some experts believe that drug therapy should be initiated if the diastolic pressure remains elevated in white women for a prolonged period despite nonpharmacologic treatment.

Patients with elevated diastolic blood pressures who are not treated with drugs require close monitoring since 10–20% will progress to higher levels of blood pressure that will require drug treatment. Institution of drug treatment for those over age 80 must be individualized. Those with target organ damage will usually benefit from blood pressure reduction. Those who are biologically "young," vigorous, and without other chronic illnesses may benefit from careful reduction in blood pressure, but data supporting treatment in these very old women are not available.

Nonpharmacologic Therapy

Weight Reduction.   All obese women should participate in weight reduction programs to achieve goal body weight to within at least 15% of desirable weight. One community-based cardiovascular risk reduction program reported that 45% of women ages 65–74 were able to lose weight when appropriately guided and counseled. (32)

Restriction of Alcohol.   Excessive alcohol consumption is associated with hypertension, poor adherence to medication, and refractory hypertension. Hypertensive women should limit alcohol intake to no more than 30 ml (1 oz) per day. This is equivalent to 60 ml of 100 proof whiskey, 240 ml wine, or 720 ml beer.

Restriction of Sodium.   In some patients, hypertension can be controlled with moderate sodium restriction to 70–100 mEq per day (1.5–2.5 g sodium or 4–6 g salt), Therefore, this is a good recommendation for all hypertensive patients. An occasional patient will have an increase in blood pressure with salt restriction, and for that reason careful surveillance of the blood pressure is necessary. This level of salt restriction requires the elimination of table salt and modification of the use of canned, frozen, and processed foods.

Calcium.   Calcium intake is low in many older women, and calcium supplementation has been demonstrated to decrease blood pressure in older patients. (33,34) Because calcium supplementation is advocated to aid in prophylaxis of osteoporosis, the antihypertensive effect can be assessed, and if there is a satisfactory response, drug treatment can be avoided.

Exercise.   Regular aerobic exercise facilitates weight control and lowers blood pressure in some hypertensive patients. However, a conditioning program should be gradual and include careful blood pressure monitoring.

Biofeedback, Relaxation, Stress Management.   Behavioral approaches can produce modest long-term blood pressure reduction in some patients. (35,36) These regimens are most useful in mild hypertension.

Smoking Cessation. Smokers have a higher frequency of malignant hypertension, subarachnoid hemorrhage, coronary artery disease, and sudden death. Furthermore, some drugs, especially beta blockers, do not appear to decrease events in smokers, and risk reduction with treatment of hypertensive smokers is not as great. Certainly the presence of hypertension should give added incentive to both physician and patient to stop smoking.

Modification of Dietary Fats. Reducing saturated fat intake and increasing polyunsaturated fat can decrease arterial blood pressure. (37) Since such dietary changes are recommended to lower blood cholesterol to reduce the risk of developing coronary heart disease, the blood pressure response can be assessed prior to antihypertensive drug treatment.

Pharmacologic
Therapy

Initial Drug Therapy. There are now many drugs in different classes from which to choose for the initial treatment of hypertension. When choosing an initial drug for an older woman, the clinician often finds another clinical condition that could also be treated effectively with a specific antihypertensive drug, or a condition that may be adversely affected. These situations will dictate the drug to be prescribed. Therefore, one should individualize the choice of antihypertensive drug for each patient. This can simplify the regimen for some patients, and improve compliance and avoid adverse effects in many.

As a general rule, it is almost always best to *start low and go slow* with older women (who may have altered metabolism and different responses to drugs). The older the patient, the more this rule applies. The goal blood pressure should be less than 140/90 mm Hg up to age 60, and less than 160/90 mm Hg beyond age 60.

In selecting drugs in older women, other issues are important. The pharmacologic response of the drug may be different in older subjects and the risk of orthostatic hypotension greater. Altered renal and hepatic physiology, coexisting clinical disorders, and concurrent drug therapy will affect the choice of drug. And finally, but not insignificantly, the cost of the drug should be considered.

Few of the many drugs used for treating hypertension produce unique effects or problems in women. In both men and women, drugs like reserpine and alpha methyldopa produce some fatigue and drowsiness. The beta blockers have been associated with decreased exercise tolerance. In women receiving estrogen, reserpine and alpha methyldopa can increase prolactin secretion and cause galactorrhea. However, no antihypertensive drugs are specifically contraindicated in women because of unique side effects or responses.

167

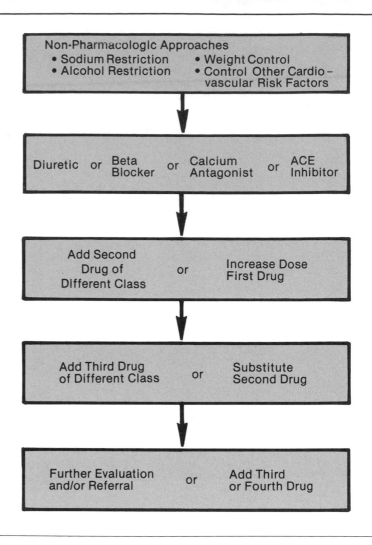

The figure illustrates the 1988 Joint National Committee on Detection, Evaluation, and Treatment of High Blood Pressure recommendation for individualized care therapy. After nonpharmacologic treatment, or with nonpharmacologic treatment as an adjunct, choose a diuretic, beta blocker, calcium antagonist, or angiotensin converting enzyme inhibitor as initial drug therapy.

Diuretic Therapy. The antihypertensive response to thiazide diuretics, alone or in combination with other drugs, is greater in older than in younger patients, and the percent response to this single treatment is 60–70%. (38) In addition, diuretics as first therapy effectively reduced mortality and morbidity in the clinical trials previously cited. The expected decrease in blood pressure will be about 25/10 mm Hg in older women. Initial treatment should be with a drug similar to hydrochlorothiazide 12.5–25 mg/day (often in combination with a potassium sparing diuretic like triamterene or amiloride if there are no contraindications). Salt restriction should be an integral part of the diuretic regimen to enhance response and to minimize potassium loss.

168

Recommended Drugs	Minimal Dose	Maximal Dose
Diuretics		
Hydrochlorothiazide	12.5 mg/day	50 mg/day
Beta Blockers		
Propranolol	40 mg/day	240 mg/day
Atenolol	25	100
Calcium Antagonists		
Diltiazem	90 mg/day	180 mg/day
Nifedipine	30	120
Nitrendipine	10	40
Verapamil	240	480
Verapamil SR (long-acting)	120	480
Angiotensin-Converting Enzyme Inhibitors		
Captopril	12.5–25 mg/day	150 mg/day
Enalapril	2.5–5	40
Lisinopril	5	40

Beta Blockers. Beta blockers effectively lower blood pressure in the elderly, but are considerably less effective than many other drugs. (39) Beta blockers would be a good choice in older women with hypertension who also need treatment for myocardial infarction prevention, arrhythmias, migraine headaches, or senile tremor. These drugs should be avoided in patients with chronic airway disease, brittle insulin-dependent diabetes mellitus, allergic rhinitis, congestive heart failure, AV conduction abnormalities, bradycardia, and depression. Unfortunately, beta blockers often produce fatigue and reduced tolerance for exercise in the elderly, which may decrease functional capacity.

Calcium Channel Blocking Drugs. Calcium channel blockers are an excellent choice for older women with hypertension because they are effective without causing fluid retention, postural hypotension, sedation, depression, or chemical abnormalities. (40,41) Verapamil, nifedipine, diltiazem, nicardipine, and nitrendipine have all demonstrated efficacy in older people. (42,43) Nitrendipine and verapamil are longer acting drugs with fewer side effects related to peak plasma concentration. The others are being evaluated in sustained release formulations. Verapamil and diltiazem depress the sinus node, leading to decreased AV conduction. This can exacerbate sinus node disease or AV conduction abnormalities. Nifedipine and nitrendipine do not demonstrate this effect. All of the drugs depress myocardial function and can worsen congestive heart failure in some patients. The major side effects are dizziness, tachycardia, edema without fluid retention, headache, and gastrointestinal reactions. Verapamil has a high frequency of constipation, especially in older women, and preventive measures to maintain bowel function are necessary when initiating therapy with this drug.

Angiotensin Converting Enzyme Inhibitors. Captopril, enalapril, and lisinopril have demonstrated efficacy in the treatment of older women with hypertension. (44–47) These drugs act as vasodilators and reduce total peripheral resistance without causing a reflex tachycardia. There is a lack of adverse metabolic and central nervous system side effects, and good maintenance of quality of life compared to other drugs. (48) Hyperkalemia is a potential problem with this class of drugs, and they should be used cautiously in patients with renal disease and in combination with nonsteroidal anti-inflammatory agents. They should not be used in combination with potassium salts or potassium retaining diuretics. All of the drugs can cause rash, cough, angioedema, taste disturbances, and in some patients decreased renal function.

Subsequent Steps in Therapy

One to 3 months should be allowed to evaluate the response to initial therapy, unless there are adverse effects or no initial response. There are 3 options for the next step:

1. Increase the dose of the initial drug.

2. Add a drug from a different class.

3. Stop the initial drug; substitute a drug from a different class.

Ordinarily one will add a drug if there is a partial response to the first drug, and substitute if there is no response or if there are side effects. If the first drug was not a diuretic, the second drug will usually be a thiazide diuretic since it will enhance the effect of most other drugs.

Before proceeding to the addition of other drugs, potential reasons for failure should be considered.

CAUSES OF REFRACTORY HYPERTENSION

Nonadherence to therapy.

Drug related:
  Doses too low.
  Inappropriate combinations.
  Rapid inactivation.
  Effects of other drugs.

Associated conditions:
  Increasing body weight.
  Excessive alcohol intake.
  Renal insufficiency.
  Renovascular hypertension.
  Malignant or accelerated hypertension.
  Other causes of hypertension.

Volume overload:
  Inadequate diuretic therapy.
  Excessive sodium intake.
  Fluid retention because of reduced BP.
  Progressive renal damage.

Step-Down Therapy	If a patient had uncomplicated hypertension and is controlled for more than one year, consider a careful slow reduction in dose or number of drugs while emphasizing nonpharmacologic treatment. Many will initially maintain normal blood pressure, but most will eventually require the reinstitution of drug therapy, thus careful monitoring of blood pressure is necessary.
Compliance	Most older women take an active interest in their treatment, and several studies have documented very high compliance and control rates in older hypertensive patients. Older patients have a relatively low 5 year incidence of adverse drug reactions requiring discontinuation of treatment. Adverse drug effects from antihypertensive drugs do not appear to be more frequent in the elderly than in the young.
Systolic Hypertension	There is no doubt that there is increased health risk associated with isolated systolic hypertension (systolic pressure greater than 160 mm Hg and a diastolic pressure less than 90 mm Hg). Data, however, are unavailable to demonstrate a reduction in morbidity and mortality with treatment. A number of trials have documented that systolic blood pressure can be safely reduced with diuretics, methyldopa, clonidine, calcium channel blockers, and others. Therefore, the decision to treat must be individualized, although the same drug regimens will be used as for combined systolic and diastolic hypertension.
Conclusion	Hypertension in older women is frequent and markedly increases the risk of cardiovascular morbidity and mortality, while treatment is safe and effective in decreasing that risk. The selection of specific antihypertensive drugs is empiric, but we have presented a logical initiation and modification strategy. Therapy should be initiated with low doses of drugs and carefully monitored for effectiveness, failure, or adverse effects. A patient's quality of life should remain a paramount concern of the physician, and drug treatment should be modified accordingly.

References

1. **Kannel WB,** Some lessons in cardiovascular epidemiology from Framingham, Am J Cardiol 37:269, 1976.

2. **Kannel WB,** Hypertension and aging, in Finch CE, Schneider EL, editors, *Handbook of the Biology of Aging*, Van Nostrand Reinhold, New York, 1985.

3. **Joint National Committee,** The 1984 report of the Joint National Committee on detection, evaluation, and treatment of high blood pressure, Arch Intern Med 144:1045, 1984.

4. **Working Group on Hypertension in the Elderly,** Statement on hypertension in the elderly, JAMA 256:70, 1986.

5. **Gordon T,** Blood pressure of adults by age and sex, United States 1960–62, National Center for Health Statistics, PHS Pub. 1000, Ser. 11, No. 4, 1964.

6. **Roberts J, Maurer K,** Blood pressure levels of persons 60–74 years, United States, 1971–1974, National Center for Health Statistics 11:1, 1977.

7. **Lowenstein FW,** Blood pressure in relation to age and sex in the tropics and subtropics: A review of the literature and an investigation in two tribes of Brazil Indians, Lancet i:389, 1961.

8. **Shapiro AP, Rutan GH,** Hypertension in women: Differences and implications, in Eaker ED, Packard B, Wenger NK, Clarkson TB, Tyroler HA, editors, *Coronary Heart Disease in Women*, Haymarket Doyma, Inc., New York, 1987, pp 172–176.

9. **Subcommittee on Definition and Prevalence of Hypertension,** Hypertension prevalence and the status of awareness, treatment, and control in the United States, Hypertension 7:457, 1985.

10. **Vogt TM, Ireland CC, Black D, Camel G, Hughes G,** Recruitement of elderly volunteers for a multicenter clinical trial: The SHEP Pilot Study, Controlled Clinical Trials 7:118, 1986.

11. **National Center for Health Statistics,** U.S. mortality data 1968–1983.

12. **Thom TJ,** Cardiovascular disease mortality among U.S. women, in Eaker ED, Packard B, Wenger, NK, Clarkson TB, Tyroler HA, editors, *Coronary Heart Disease in Women*, Haymarket Doyma, Inc., New York, 1987, pp 33–40.

13. **Kannel WB, Dawber TR, McGee, DL,** Perspectives on systolic hypertension—The Framingham Study, Circulation 61:1179, 1980.

14. **Kannel WB, Wolf PA, McGee DL, et al,** Systolic blood pressure, arterial rigidity, and risk of stroke, JAMA 245:1225, 1981.

15. **Messerli FH, Ventura HO, Glade LB, Sundgaard K, Dunn FG, Frohlich ED,** Essential hypertension in the elderly: Hemodynamics, intravascular volume, plasma renin activity, and circulating catecholamine levels, Lancet ii:983, 1983.

16. **Docherty JR,** Aging and the cardiovascular system, J Auton Pharmacol 6:77, 1986.

17. **Barry AJ, Daly JW, Pruett EDR, Steinmatz JR, Page EF, Biskhead NC, Rodahl K,** The effects of physical conditioning on older individuals, J Gerontol 21:182, 1966.

18. **DeVries HA,** Physiologic effects of an exercise training regimen upon men aged 52–58, J Gerontol 25:325, 1970.

19. **Shimada K, Kitazumi T, Sadakane N, Ogura H, Ozawa T,** Age-related changes of baroreflex function, plasma norepinephrine, and blood pressure, Hypertension 7:113, 1985.

20. **Joint National Committee,** The 1988 report on detection, evaluation, and treatment of blood pressure, Arch Intern Med 148:1023, 1988.

21. **White WB, Schulman P, McCabe EJ, Dey HM,** Average daily blood pressure, not office blood pressure, determines cardiac function in patients with hypertension, JAMA 261:873, 1989.

22. **Messerli FH, Ventura HO, Amodeo C,** Osler's maneuver and pseudo-hypertension, New Engl J Med 312:1548, 1985.

23. **Lind T, Cameron EC, Hunter WM, Leon C, Moran PF, Oxley A, Gerrard J, Lind UCG,** A prospective, controlled trial of six forms of hormone replacement therapy given to postmenopausal women, Brit J Obstet Gynaecol (Suppl 3) 86:1, 1979.

24. **Pfeffer RI, Kurosaki TT, Charlton SK,** Estrogen use and blood pressure in later life, Am J Epidemiol 110:469, 1979.

25. **Lutola H,** Blood pressure and hemodynamics in postmenopausal women during estradiol-17β substitution, Ann Clin Res (Suppl 38) 15:9, 1983.

26. **Wren BG, Routledge AD,** The effect of type and dose of oestrogen on the blood pressure of postmenopausal women, Maturitas 5:135, 1983.

27. **Hassager C, Christiansen C,** Blood pressure during oestrogen/ progestogen substitution therapy in healthy post-menopausal women, Maturitas 9:315, 1988.

28. **Langford HG, Stamler J, Wassertheil-Smoller S, Prineas RJ,** All cause mortality in the HDFP Program, Prog in Cardiovasc Dis 29:29, 1986.

29. **Management Committee, The Australian Therapeutic Trial of Mild Hypertension,** Treatment of hypertension in the elderly, Med J Australia 2:309, 1981.

30. **Miall WE, Greedber G,** editors, *Mild Hypertension: An Account of the MRC Trial,* Cambridge University Press, New York, 1987.

31. **Amery A, Birkenhager W, Brixko P, et al,** Mortality and morbidity results from the European Working Party on High Blood Pressure in the Elderly trial, Lancet i:1349, 1985.

32. **Jeffery RW, Folsom AR, Luepker RV, Jacobs DR Jr, Gillum RF, et al,** Prevalence of overweight and weight loss behavior in a metropolitan adult population: The Minnesota Heart Survey experience, Am J Public Health 74:349, 1984.

33. **Tabuchi Y, Ogihara T, Hashizume K, Saito H, Kumahara Y,** Hypotensive effect of long term oral calcium supplementation in elderly patients with essential hypertension, J Clin Hypertension 3:254, 1986.

34. **McCarron DA,** Calcium metabolism and hypertension, Kidney Internat 35:717, 1989.

35. **Health and Public Policy Committee, American College of Physicians,** Biofeedback for hypertension, Ann Intern Med 102:709, 1985.

36. **Patel C, Marmot MG, Terry DJ, et al,** Trials of relaxation in reducing coronary risk: Four year follow-up, Brit Med J 290:1103, 1985.

37. **Iacono JM, Dougherty RM, Puska P,** Reduction of blood pressure associated with dietary polyunsaturated fat, Hypertension 4 (Suppl 3):34, 1982.

38. **Freis ED,** Relationship of age and antihypertensive drug therapy, Cardiology Board Review 10:49, 1988.

39. **Niarchos AP, Laragh JH,** Hypertension in the elderly, Mod Concepts Cardiovasc Dis 59:49, 1980.

40. **Muller FB, Bolli P, Erne P, Kiowski W, Buhler FR,** Use of calcium antagonists as monotherapy in the management of hypertension, Am J Med 77 (Suppl 2B):11, 1984.

41. **Ben-Ishay D, Leibel B, Stessman J,** Calcium channel blockers in the management of hypertension in the elderly, Am J Med 81 (Suppl 6A):30, 1986.

42. **Schnapp P, Hermann H, Cernak P, Kahay J,** Nifedipine monotherapy in the hypertensive elderly, Curr Med Res Opin 10:407, 1987.

43. **Schwartz JB, Abernathy DR,** Responses to intravenous oral diltiazem in elderly and younger patients with systemic hypertension, Am J Cardiol 59:1111, 1987.

44. **Jenkins AC, Knill , Dreslinski GR,** Captopril in the treatment of the elderly hypertensive patient, Arch Intern Med 145:2029, 1985.

45. **Ajayi AA, Hockings N, Reid JL,** Age and the pharmacodynamics of angiotensin converting enzyme inhibitor enalapril and enalapritat, Br J Clin Pharmacol 21:349, 1986.

46. **Woo J, Wook S, Kin T, Vallance-Owen J,** A single-blind randomized crossover study of angiotensin-converting enzyme inhibitor and triamterene and hydrochlorothiazide in the treatment of mild to moderate hypertension in the elderly, Arch Intern Med 147:1386, 1987.

47. **Laher MS, Natin D, Rao SK, Jones RW, Carr P,** Lisinopril in elderly patients with hypertension, J Cardiovasc Pharmacol 9 (Suppl 3):569, 1987.

48. **Croog SH, Leveine S, Tests MA, et al,** The effects of antihypertensive therapy on the quality of life, New Engl J Med 314:1657, 1986.

10 Cardiovascular Disease in Older Women

Heart disease is the leading cause of death in women, accounting for about 28% of all deaths. (1) Premenopausal women have a very low rate of heart disease; however, after menopause, coronary heart disease increases in women, soon approximating the rate found in men 10 years earlier. Because hypertension is such a major contributor to cardiovascular disease risk in older women, it is reviewed in a separate chapter (Chapter 9). Other than hypertension, the most common cardiovascular disorders are coronary artery disease, congestive heart failure, and chronic atrial fibrillation. Syncope and peripheral vascular disease account for additional important cardiovascular disorders in aging women.

Coronary Heart Disease

The most common manifestations of coronary heart disease in women are angina pectoris (56%), myocardial infarction (35%), and sudden cardiac death (9%). (2) Chest pain is obviously a symptom of coronary heart disease, but it is more difficult to interpret in women. Typical angina pectoris is characterized by a pressing substernal chest discomfort which occurs repetitively with exercise, occasionally radiates to the arm or the jaw, may be accompanied by shortness of breath or perspiration, and is usually relieved by rest. In women with apparent typical angina pectoris, coronary heart disease is present in 35–65%, and in women with atypical chest pain, coronary heart disease is present in less than 20%. (3)

Although angina pectoris remains the most common (more than 80%) presenting symptom of coronary heart disease in older women, chest pain may be confused with pain due to arthritis, gastroesophageal reflux, or other chest conditions. In addition, many older women exercise so little that they never reach their limitation, and thus avoid the induction of pain. It should be noted that dyspnea is a more common presenting symptom in older patients, and it is said to be the most common complaint with myocardial infarction and transient myocardial ischemia. Since systolic murmurs and S4 gallops are frequent in healthy older women, the physical findings of coronary heart disease are limited in this age group.

The clinician should keep in mind that even very nonspecific symptoms such as unexplained episodes of weakness, perspiration, neck and shoulder pain, and indigestion can be atypical manifestations of heart disease.

Approximately 50% of people over age 65 have abnormal cardiograms. Many of these reflect age-related anatomic changes. Unequivocal pathologic q waves are an important diagnostic finding for ischemic heart disease.

The most common cause of angina pectoris in older women is atherosclerotic obstruction of the coronary arteries, resulting in a decreased myocardial blood flow with increased left ventricular thickness and stiffness. Coronary artery spasms can also cause angina pectoris in older women. Spasms with or without obstructive coronary arteries explain cold-induced angina, angina at rest, and angina occurring at variable and unpredictable levels of physical exertion. A patient with atherosclerotic obstruction will usually have the onset of chest pain at nearly the same level of work in a repetitive fashion. Patients with either spasms or combined obstruction and spasms can have chest pain with a limited amount of exertion on one occasion, and at another time endure a fairly high exercise load. It is now recognized that in addition to episodes of angina pectoris, most patients who have coronary heart disease that is symptomatic have even more frequent silent myocardial ischemia with daily activity. (4)

Variant angina pectoris (Prinzmetal's angina) is characterized by attacks occurring during rest, a preservation of exercise capacity, and elevated ST segments during attacks. Prinzmetal's angina is a clear manifestation of coronary artery spasms and occurs more commonly in women. (5) In men, the course is more unstable and usually associated with atherosclerotic obstructive changes in the coronary arteries.

Despite the availability of numerous high technologic diagnostic tests, many women with chest pain cannot be given a specific diagnosis. The prognosis for these women is excellent. In one study of women with normal coronary arteries and chest pain followed for 8 years, none had a coronary heart disease event, although more than half continued to have chest pain. (6)

Elderly women with typical angina pectoris should be treated; however, they do not require further non-invasive diagnostic studies unless surgical treatment is contemplated. In patients with less typical chest pain, the exercise electrocardiogram with or without thallium myo-
cardial imaging is the preferred non-invasive test. In addition to the cardiogram changes in the exercise test, it is important to observe the ability of the patient to exercise, the time of onset of signs and symptoms correlated with the work load, the blood pressure response, and the heart rate. If a patient can only exercise to a very modest level, the test may be falsely negative. If a patient has the onset of chest pain at a very low level of exercise, especially with ST-segment changes, this is indicative of a positive test. If a patient develops hypotension at low work levels, this is an ominous sign. Patients who develop symptoms at very low levels of exercise or who develop hypotension should be considered for coronary arteriography and surgery.

Thallium imaging of the myocardium during exercise increases the sensitivity and specificity of the exercise test; however, little diagnostic value is obtained from myocardial imaging if the routine exercise test is entirely normal. (7)

Acute Myocardial Infarction	A higher percentage of clinically unrecognized myocardial infarctions occurs in women (35%) compared to men (26%). On the other hand, women with a new myocardial infarction have a worse prognosis than men because the right coronary arteries are more dominant. In addition, early recurrent myocardial infarction is more common in women than in men.
	A number of studies have indicated a higher mortality rate for women compared to men. Women, particularly black women, more frequently experience congestive heart failure and angina pectoris after myocardial infarction. Whereas substernal chest pain with or without radiation is the most common symptom in younger patients, sudden dyspnea and an exacerbation of previously controlled heart failure are the most common presenting complaints in older individuals. In addition, acute confusion, sudden death, syncope, peripheral artery occlusion, vertigo, and palpitations are common presenting manifestations in older patients.
	Mortality from acute myocardial infarction increases with age, approximating 70% in those over age 70. Older patients are more likely to develop heart failure, pulmonary edema, or cardiogenic shock. Most arrhythmic deaths from acute myocardial infarction occur shortly after the onset of symptoms. In elderly patients, atypical symptoms must prompt a consideration of acute myocardial infarction, and patients must be transported to the hospital early to treat this life-threatening problem. Patients with suspected acute myocardial infarction should be admitted to the hospital and be under the care of a skilled internist or cardiologist.
Treatment of Coronary Heart Disease	Older women with coronary disease with or without angina pectoris should be treated initially with medical therapy (lifestyle changes and drugs). Surgical treatment is reserved for patients with refractory symptoms or severe disease. It is prudent for the clinician to search for treatable contributing factors such as hypertension, congestive heart failure, hyperthyroidism, hypothyroidism, or severe anemia.
Nitroglycerin	The mainstay of treatment of chronic stable angina pectoris remains nitroglycerin. It is important that the nitroglycerin be fresh and that it be utilized under the tongue immediately with the onset of discomfort. Adverse effects include orthostatic hypotension, headache, and syncope. For those patients who have very frequent symptoms, preventive therapy may be required.
Beta Blockers	For those patients who have purely exercise-induced angina pectoris, beta blockers provide the most effective therapy. Beta blockers decrease the heart rate response to exercise and limit the systolic rise in blood pressure. Because myocardial infarction often occurs in the early morning hours, a long acting beta blocker is recommended which can be taken at bedtime and have its maximal effect early in the morning. Side effects of beta blockers include fatigue, depression, heart failure, heart block, symptomatic bradycardia, and bronchospasm. A greater benefit with beta blockers has been demonstrated in women compared to men, and it is especially recommended that women who have had a myocardial infarction be treated with beta blockers to prevent a second infarction. (8)

Calcium Channel Blockers	If a patient has chest pain at rest, with or without exertional angina, many experts recommend a calcium channel blocker because of the probable presence of coronary artery spasm. The major side effects are orthostatic hypotension, flushing, edema, and syncope.
Aspirin	Aspirin-treated women who have survived an acute myocardial infarction demonstrated a 52% reduction in subsequent infarctions. (9) There was also a beneficial trend in the prevention of stroke and transient ischemic attacks, as well as a 58% reduction in the onset of new angina. There is some controversy over aspirin dosage, and consultation is recommended for advice regarding this important prophylactic treatment.
Surgical Treatment	If a patient fails to respond to medical therapy, coronary angiography should be considered to document the anatomic changes and extent of disease. The treatment options at this point are percutaneous transluminal coronary angioplasty or coronary artery bypass surgery. Coronary bypass surgery in patients aged 65–69 is associated with a higher mortality rate (4.6%) compared to younger patients, and in those over age 75, there is a mortality rate of 9.5%. (10) Because coronary angioplasty has a lower morbidity and mortality rate, it is an attractive alternative. Success rates for angioplasty vary with patient selection; however, from 60–89% are considered successful, with a mortality rate of 1.8–2.9%. Complication rates are high (15–20%), including arrhythmias, myocardial infarction, and emergency coronary bypass surgery.

Coronary bypass surgery in the elderly is associated with an overall 6 year survival rate of 79%. There is not much difference in survival comparing those aged 65 to those over age 75, nor is there much difference in those with more than one vessel involved. Those with normal left ventricular function have the highest survival rates. Older patients who are considered to be low risk with mild angina, good left ventricular function, and no left main artery disease have a 6 year survival rate of 88% compared to 62% in those who have severe symptoms, unstable angina, left ventricular dysfunction, severe three vessel disease, or left main coronary disease. Elderly women have a higher mortality rate than their male counterparts, 6.9% vs 4.7%. |
| **Congestive Heart Failure** | The incidence of congestive heart failure rises steeply with age in each decade after age 50. In the Framingham Study, 75% of heart failure was caused by hypertension, 39% by coronary artery disease, and 21% by rheumatic heart disease. (11) Heart failure is equivalent to a malignancy in terms of mortality, an overall 10–20% annual mortality rate, and 50% in those with severe heart failure.

Heart failure is due to an inability to meet the oxygen demands of the body because of decreased cardiac output or pulmonary or systemic venous congestion because of back pressure from a failing heart. The classic view of heart failure attributed the failure to a volume overload of the myocardium resulting in decreased contractility and systolic dysfunction. It is now recognized that stiffer left ventricles and left ventricular hypertrophy in the elderly lead to diastolic dysfunction. (12) |

Four major factors determine cardiac performance: preload, afterload, contractility, and heart rate. An abnormality in each of these factors can result in congestive heart failure. When cardiac output fails there is a simultaneous increase in sympathetic nervous system activity, an increase in renin-angiotensin-aldosterone, and an increase in vasopressin. These compensatory mechanisms result in vasoconstriction and salt and water retention, further worsening the heart failure. During an acute fall in cardiac output, one can understand how these compensatory mechanisms serve to maintain blood pressure and perfusion of vital organs; however, with chronic failure, these mechanisms increase cardiac work and overburden the heart.

Congestive heart failure is diagnosed by the typical signs and symptoms. Common manifestations of low cardiac output are a limitation in exercise, muscle fatigue, confusion, and somnolence. Pulmonary congestion is manifested by dyspnea on exertion, orthopnea, and paroxysmal nocturnal dyspnea. The signs of heart failure are the same in older women as in younger patients. Because many older people have heart murmurs and S4 sounds, these are not as specific as they are in younger patients. A third heart sound is indicative of heart failure in older patients. Chest x-ray is often helpful to document pulmonary venous congestion, redistribution of blood flow, and an increase in cardiac heart size. Newer techniques such as Doppler and radionucleotide studies require expert consultation for performance and interpretation.

It is important to consider precipitating factors for congestive heart failure in older women. Noncompliance with complicated medical regimens or an inability to restrict dietary sodium are preventable precipitating factors. Older women frequently take nonsteroidal anti-inflammatory agents for joint problems. These agents can cause fluid retention. Cardiac arrhythmias, anemia, abnormal thyroid function, and systemic infections can precipitate heart failure.

There are common pitfalls in diagnosis encountered in older women. Dyspnea and fatigue may be due to deconditioning, obesity, or chronic lung disease. Pulmonary rales are a frequent finding in older individuals because of atelectasis and chronic lung disease. Older women frequently develop ankle edema because of venous insufficiency. A palpable liver may not be due to hepatomegaly. Occasionally one can even find jugular venous distention due to an age-related change in the aortic arch.

Treatment of
Heart Failure

Initially one should try to remove precipitating factors, treat underlying medical conditions, and remove drugs such as alcohol or nonsteroidal anti-inflammatory agents. In addition, patients should have dietary sodium restricted, and rest prescribed.

The drug of choice for congestive heart failure is a diuretic. Thiazide diuretics induce a moderate natriuresis, with less volume depletion, although there is more hypokalemia. (13) After a therapeutic trial with a thiazide, one can use one of the newer, more potent diuretics, such as furosemide. Carbohydrate intolerance and lipid disorders can be induced by diuretics, and hyperuricemia can be induced or worsened. Potassium-sparing diuretics are useful in combination with thiazides.

After evaluating the clinical effects of diuresis and discovering an inadequate response or an elevation of BUN and creatinine, the choice is between digitalis and vasodilators. Patients with systolic dysfunction demonstrate the best response to digitalis. Cardiac arrhythmias are the most important manifestation of digoxin toxicity. Other symptoms which suggest toxicity include central nervous system reactions (confusion, hallucinations) and gastrointestinal changes (nausea, anorexia). Mood drugs affect digoxin activity, and this interaction must be kept in mind.

The most important new addition to the treatment of heart failure has been the development of angiotensin converting enzyme inhibitors. (14,15) These drugs have been demonstrated to benefit patients 70 years old. These inhibitors block the conversion of angiotensin-I to angiotensin-II, thereby decreasing vasoconstriction and the secretion of aldosterone. Maximal response requires several weeks, and symptomatic improvement should not be expected immediately. The most worrisome side effect is hypotension. Renal function and electrolytes must be monitored.

Syncope

Syncope in older people is defined as a transient loss of consciousness with a lack of responsiveness and postural tone, followed by spontaneous recovery. It occcurs in about 2% of those 65–69 years old, increasing to 12% in those over age 85. (16–18) Syncope deserves diagnostic analysis because while unexplained syncope is associated with a slight increased mortality rate within one year, when syncope can be linked to a cardiovascular cause, the one year mortality rate is increased to 18%.

Syncope is often due to a failure to maintain blood pressure because of changes in the cardiovascular and neuroendocrine systems. Specific problems include a blunted change in heart rate with postural change, an inability to conserve sodium (reduced renin and aldosterone secretion), and diminished thirst resulting in volume depletion. The risk is further increased when these changes are combined with cardiovascular and neurologic diseases and drugs which induce hypotension. The most common causes of syncope are hypotensive reactions, severe anemia, cardiac disease, and primary cerebral disease.

Asymptomatic orthostatic hypotension occurs in as many as 20% of older people. About half of older individuals who complain of dizziness on standing have demonstrable orthostatic hypotension. In the remainder, the dizziness appears to be a central nervous phenomenon unrelated to a change in blood pressure or heart rate. Symptomatic orthostatic hypotension, however, is usually caused by significant disease or drugs.

A careful history emphasizes precipitating circumstances and the use of drugs. Measure the blood pressure lying and then upright at 1–3 minute intervals. Both the carotid and peripheral pulses are examined for regularity, intensity, and upstroke. In the examination, look for findings of aortic stenosis, evidence of volume depletion, manifestations of bleeding, and an assessment of neurologic condition. Laboratory evaluation includes the blood count, electrolytes, renal function, and glucose levels. An electrocardiogram is essential to identify myocardial ischemia, myocardial infarction, arrhythmias, and heart block. If an arrhythmia is suspected, 24 hour ambulatory cardiac monitoring may be necessary in order to make an accurate diagnosis.

Most experts do not recommend routine neuro-diagnostic studies (such as magnetic resonance imaging or CT scanning of the head, or electroencephalography) unless there are focal neurologic findings.

A cardiovascular cause for syncope is found more often in elderly than in young patients, but less than half of the cases of syncope in older patients yield a diagnosis. In institutionalized elderly, most of the cases have a cardiovascular cause. (18) The most common cardiac causes are conduction problems, including sinus node disease, tachyarrhythmias, and bradyarrhythmias. Occasionally a silent myocardial infarction will present with syncope. This is the easiest diagnosis to make because the electrocardiogram will be abnormal.

From 20–40% of syncope is non-cardiac in origin. Orthostatic hypotension can be secondary to volume loss, drugs (antihypertensives, narcotics, nitrates, sympathetic blockers, phenothiazines, diuretics, antidepressants, alcohol, barbiturates, L-dopa), prolonged immobility, or autonomic insufficiency. Syncope may be associated with meals, defecation, cough, and other situational stresses which cause increased intrathoracic pressure with impaired venous return and bradycardia. Postprandial hypotension is of uncertain etiology, due either to gastrointestinal vasodilator peptides or splenic blood pooling in patients with impaired cardiovascular reflexes.

A true seizure is likely if the patient experiences an aura, tonic chronic motor activity, tongue biting, incontinence, and amnesia. Strokes and transient ischemic episodes can masquerade as syncope. In many cases, the presentation is atypical. The overall problem is so complex that expert consultation is worthwhile.

The goal of treatment is to prevent further episodes of syncope, with an aim to prevent falls, trauma, and fractures. Treatment intervention includes the elimination of unnecessary drugs and teaching patients how to take proper actions if they anticipate a syncopal attack. Patients must be taught ways to cope with situations which can induce hypotension (for example, calf muscle exercise while sitting, prior to getting up). Drug interventions should be limited to the treatment of specific disorders. Arrhythmias should be treated only after clear, symptomatic disturbances are documented. Because of the current difficulty in selecting the proper drug, arrhythmia problems should be referred to an internist or cardiologist.

Cardiac Arrhythmias

The incidence of conduction disturbances increases significantly with age. An arrhythmia should be suspected when a patient describes palpitations, skipped beats, or syncope. Diagnosis frequently requires ambulatory continuous monitoring.

Arrhythmias are frequently present in patients who have other heart disease, especially hypertension, valvular heart disease, or coronary artery disease. Always consider hyperthyroidism as a possible cause for atrial fibrillation; this is extraordinarily important in older patients in whom the symptoms of hyperthyroidism may be masked.

It is difficult to decide whether treatment outweighs toxicity and risks in older patients. There is no evidence that treatment of asymptomatic ventricular premature contractions prevents sudden death. This is one of the clinical situations in which therapeutic nihilism is frequently justifiable. Atrial fibrillation is associated with a greater risk of stroke and a higher mortality rate, and deserves oral anticoagulation. Patients with rheumatic mitral valve diseases combined with atrial fibrillation should definitely receive oral anticoagulation; however, patients who have had atrial fibrillation for a long time and are currently not on anticoagulation probably should not be anticoagulated unless they have clinical symptoms or events of embolization.

Atrial fibrillation of new onset deserves conversion to sinus rhythm with antiarrhythmic drugs, with or without electrical cardioversion. There is a risk of embolization associated with conversion and anticoagulation is indicated prior to the attempt. The goal of treatment is to achieve a heart rate less than 90–100 at rest and a relatively normal heart rate response to exercise. These problems require management by a cardiologist.

Degenerative disease in the sinus node (the sick sinus syndrome) is a common consequence of coronary heart disease. The hallmark of this disease is the sinus beat pause. Pauses of more than 3 seconds in duration can lead to syncope or dizziness. The tachy-brady syndrome is a tachyarrhythmia followed by symptomatic pauses due to delayed sinus conduction. Treatment is usually with a permanent pacemaker to ameliorate symptoms; however, pacemaker placement does not lower mortality, therefore asymptomatic patients are usually not treated. Heart blocks should be evaluated by a cardiologist.

The evaluation of ventricular arrhythmias is very perplexing because ventricular ectopic beats increase in frequency with age. Ventricular ectopic beats in older people with normal cardiovascular systems have no influence on mortality. When ventricular ectopic beats occur in patients with underlying heart disease (especially congestive heart failure), then the risk of sudden death increases dramatically. Currently, symptomatic patients with demonstrable ventricular arrhythmias should be evaluated for treatment by a cardiologist, especially in the presence of heart failure or left ventricular dysfunction. (19)

Valvular Heart Disease

There are two important valvular heart diseases in older women, mitral valve prolapse and aortic stenosis.

Mitral Valve Prolapse.   Mitral valve prolapse is very common, the most common cause of mitral regurgitation. Specific diagnostic criteria have been developed, divided into major and minor categories. (20) Major criteria include a mid-to-late systolic click and late systolic murmur, and positive findings on a two dimensional echocardiogram. Minor criteria include a loud first heart sound with an apical, holosystolic murmur, echocardiographic changes of the posterior mitral valve leaflet, or alterations in both mitral valve leaflets.

Most patients are asymptomatic. (21) The most frequent symptoms are chest pain, dyspnea, fatigue, weakness, dizziness, and syncope. Patients can have premature ventricular beats or ventricular tachycardias. In general, the duration of the systolic murmur is a function

182

of the severity of the mitral regurgitation. The physical findings can be exaggerated by auscultation in the standing position (a decrease in venous return with a decrease in the ventricular volume enhances any prolapse which is present).

The prognosis with mitral valve prolapse is exceptionally good. In some patients, the mitral regurgitation will become progressive, resulting in increased volume overload of the left ventricle, left ventricular hypertrophy, and occasionally left atrial enlargement and congestive heart failure. Some will be candidates for mitral valve replacement. The treatment of asymptomatic patients is limited to antibiotic prophylaxis for endocarditis. It is controversial whether prophylaxis is necessary in the absence of a murmur (the only finding being isolated clicks).

Aortic Stenosis. Systolic murmurs occur in more than half of patients over age 65. Most of these are benign and result from flow changes over the aortic valve because of aortic sclerosis. Differentiation of aortic sclerosis from aortic stenosis is important.

The murmur of aortic stenosis is usually heard loudest in the second right intercostal space and is maximal in the suprasternal notch. (22) Unfortunately, older people do not present many of the typical manifestations of aortic stenosis seen in young patients, including a diminished second sound and limitation of the systolic blood pressure. (23) In addition, symptoms of exercise intolerance, syncope, and angina are frequently manifestations of other diseases. However, if one finds this type of heart murmur in association with left ventricular hypertrophy and cardiac enlargement, especially in the absence of hypertension, then aortic stenosis is a very good possibility.

The definitive non-invasive diagnosis is made by echocardiography. Valve replacement is technically feasible with good results in the elderly.

Peripheral Vascular Disease

The prevalence of peripheral vascular disease increases with age; the major symptom, intermittent claudication, reaches an incidence of 12 per 10,000 women. (23) The rate of new cases is about one quarter the rate of new coronary heart disease each year. Intermittent claudication is an exercise-induced aching or cramping in the calf, thigh, or buttocks, relieved within minutes by rest and reproducibly induced again by exercise. With a very severe decrease in blood flow, significant vascular changes in the extremities cause ulcerations, infections, and osteomyelitis.

Peripheral vascular disease indicates a diffusive atherosclerotic process, and most patients have concomitant coronary artery disease, and often cerebral vascular disease as well. More than 80% of patients will remain stable; less than 10% require surgery.

The most important non-invasive diagnostic maneuver is to compare the systolic blood pressure in the arms to that in the ankle or popliteal space. If the ratio of the ankle to arm systolic pressure is greater than 0.95, significant peripheral vascular disease is not present.

Treatment is directed to smoking cessation, control of cardiovascular disease, and exercise rehabilitation. Patients should be referred for expert evaluation and exercise prescription.

183

References

1. **Thom TJ,** Cardiovascular disease mortality among U.S. women, in Eaker ED, Packard B, Wenger NK, Clarkson TB, Tyroler HA, editors, *Coronary Heart Disease in Women,* Haymarket Doyma, Inc., New York, 1987, pp 35–36.

2. **Beard CM, Foster B, Annegers JF,** Reproductive history in women with coronary heart disease: A case-controlled study, Am J Epidemiol 120:108, 1984.

3. **Detry JR, Kapita BM, Cosyns J, Sottiaux B, et al,** Diagnostic value of history and maximal exercise electrocardiography in men and women suspected of coronary heart disease, Circulation 56:756, 1977.

4. **Deanfield JE, Selwyn AP, Chierchia S, Maseri A, Ribeiro P, Krikler S, Morgan M,** Myocardial ischemia during daily life in patients with stable angina: Its relation to symptoms and heart rate changes, Lancet ii:753, 1983.

5. **Selzer A, Langston M, Ruggeroli C, Cohn K,** Clinical syndrome of variant angina with normal coronary arteriogram, New Engl J Med 295:1343, 1976.

6. **Proudfit WL, Welch CC, Sequeira C, Morcerf FP, Sheldon WC,** Prognosis of 1000 young women studied by coronary angiography, Circulation 64:1185, 1981.

7. **Beller G,** Nuclear cardiology: Current indications and clinical usefulness, in O'Rourkera K, editor, *Current Problems in Cardiology,* Year Book Medical Publishers, Chicago, 1985.

8. **Beta Blocker Heart Attack Trial Research Group,** A randomized trial of propranolol in patients with acute myocardial infarction, JAMA 247:1107, 1982.

9. **Aspirin Myocardial Infarction Study Research Group,** A randomized, controlled trial of aspirin in persons recovered from myocardial infarction, JAMA 243:661, 1980.

10. **Gersh BJ, Kronmal RA, Frye RL, Schaff HV, Ryan TJ, Gosselin AJ, Kaiser GC, Killip T III,** Coronary arteriography and coronary artery bypass surgery: Morbidity and mortality in patients aged 65 years or older, Circulation 67:483, 1983.

11. **McKee PA, Castelli WP, MacNamara PM, Kannel WB,** The natural history of heart failure in the Framingham Study, New Engl J Med 285:1441, 1971.

12. **Topol EJ, Traill TA, Fortuin NJ,** Hypertensive hypertrophic cardiac myopathy of the elderly, New Engl J Med 312:277, 1985.

13. **Flambaum W,** Diuretic use in the elderly: Potential for diuretic-induced hyokalemia, Am J Cardiol 57:38A, 1986.

14. **Cohn JN, Archibald DG, Ziesche S, Franciosa JA, et al,** Effect of vasodilator therapy on mortality and chronic congestive heart failure: Results of a Veteran's Administration Cooperative Study, New Engl J Med 314:1547, 1986.

15. **Consensus Trial Study Group,** Effects of enalipril on mortality and severe congestive heart failure, New Engl J Med 316:1429, 1987.

16. **Lipsitz LA,** Syncope in the elderly, Ann Intern Med 99:92, 1983.

17. **Robbins AS, Rubenstein LZ,** Postural hypotension in the elderly, J Am Geriatrics Soc 32:769, 1984.

184

18. **Kappoor W, Snustad D, Peterson J, Wieland HS, Cha R, Karpf M,** Syncope in the elderly, Am J Med 80:419, 1986.

19. **Dreifus LS,** Clinical arrhythmias in the elderly: Clinical aspects, Cardiol Clinics 4:273, 1986.

20. **Perloff JK, Child JS, Edwards JE,** New guidelines for the clinical diagnosis of mitral valve prolapse, Am J Cardiol 57:1124, 1986.

21. **Hickey AJ, Wilcken DEL,** Age and the clinical profile of idiopathic mitral valve prolapse, Br Heart J 55:582, 1986.

22. **Forssell G, Jonasson R, Orinius E,** Identifying severe aortic valve stenosis by bedside examination, Acta Med Scand 218:397, 1985.

23. **Wei JY, Gersh BJ,** Heart disease in the elderly, Cur Probl Cardiol 12:7, 1987.

24. **Criqui MH, Fronek A, Barrett-Connor E, Klauber MR, Gabriel S, Goodman D,** The prevalence of peripheral arterial disease in a defined population, Circulation 71:510, 1985.

11   Common Pulmonary Problems

Although lung function declines with advancing age, older individuals do not have respiratory complaints unless disease is present. At least part of the decline in lung function occurs because of exposure to pulmonary infections and environmental pollutants, including passive cigarette smoking.

The most important pulmonary problems in older women include chronic bronchitis, chronic obstructive pulmonary disease (COPD), adult-onset asthma, pneumonia, tuberculosis, and carcinoma of the lung. Another disorder which has recently achieved significant recognition is sleep apnea, a sleep disorder which results in nocturnal hypoxia.

Changes with Aging

In older women, the anterior-posterior diameter of the chest tends to increase and kyphosis frequently develops. With significant osteoporosis, kyphosis is progressive, causing the lower ribs to reach the upper portion of the pelvis and resulting in decreased pulmonary function with an increased susceptibility to infection. Calcification of the costal cartilages, decreased respiratory muscle strength, increased chest wall stiffness, and age-related enlargement of the respiratory bronchioles and alveolar ducts all further contribute to decreased lung function and diminished capacity to cope with pulmonary stress and exercise. (1) These changes lead to a decrease in vital capacity with age, although total lung capacity does not decline. Residual volume increases nearly 50% with aging. Other measurements of lung function decline with age, such as spirometric measurements of the forced expiratory volume (FEV), expiratory flow rate, and maximal expiratory flow volume. Forced expiratory volume for one second (FEV_1) declines about 30 ml per year. This age-related decline is markedly accelerated by cigarette smoking.

With increasing age, there is a progressive decline in healthy alveolar capillary surface area, resulting in a decreased diffusing capacity. Arterial oxygen tension declines by about 4 mm Hg per decade. This is believed to be due to an imbalance between ventilation and perfusion caused by the collapse of small airways in the lower lung fields during tidal breathing. (2–4) Older people appear to have decreased central respiratory control with an attenuation of response to hypoxemia and hypercapnia. (5) Disorders of sleep and problems of nocturnal control of breathing with accompanying respiratory ir-

187

regularities causing apneic episodes, hypopnea, and oxygen desaturation are more common and more severe in the elderly. (6)

An important function of the respiratory tract is to purify inspired air in order to maintain infection-free lung tissue. (7) Aging results in decreased cough, ciliary action, clearing of inhaled particles, decreased respiratory secretion of IgA, and alteration in alveolar macrophage phagocyte cell function (and these changes are more marked in smokers). The decrease in these functions contributes to an increased susceptibility in older people to chronic bronchitis and pneumonia.

Manifestations of Disease

Cough associated with sputum production is one of the most common respiratory complaints. An acute change in cough usually signifies an upper respiratory or lower pulmonary infection. Besides acute infections, other common causes of cough include chronic bronchitis, asthma, and post nasal drip. Less frequent causes include esophageal reflux with aspiration, congestive heart failure, lung cancer, interstitial lung disease, and inspiratory irritants such as tobacco smoke. A newly appreciated cause of chronic cough is treatment with the angiotensin converting inhibitors (captopril, enalapril, lisinopril). Shortness of breath, with or without cough, indicates a significant pulmonary illness in 50% of women with this complaint. (8) On the other hand, it is important to recognize that many older women have significant shortness of breath because of inactivity and deconditioning.

Hemoptysis (or blood-streaked sputum) is a manifestation of an upper respiratory infection or lung cancer. After age 45, hemoptysis is most likely to be due to a bronchogenic carcinoma, bronchitis, tuberculosis, or pulmonary embolism. Chest pain is frequently a manifestation of pulmonary disease rather than a cardiac problem.

Normal people breathe 8–16 times per minute, with a tidal volume of 400–800 ml. Variations in the breathing pattern can signify important underlying pulmonary disease. Obstructed breathing is characteristic of chronic obstructive pulmonary disease (COPD), distinguished by a slow respiratory rate with an increased tidal volume and wheezing. Restricted breathing has a small tidal volume and a rapid rate. Gasping respiration, characteristic of severe heart failure or cerebral hypoxia, is distinguished by quick inspirations with long expiratory pauses. Cheyne-Stokes respiration, associated with COPD, cardiac failure, or cerebral vascular disease, is a cyclic pattern of alternating apnea and hypernea. Hypoventilation is characterized by low tidal volume and low rate. The presence of each of these breathing patterns can help identify patients with significant pulmonary pathology.

Chronic Bronchitis

Chronic bronchitis is characterized by mucus hypersecretion with cough and expectoration on most days for at least 3 months of the year with no identifiable cause for 2 consecutive years. Cigarette smoking is the most common cause, but atmospheric pollution and occupational exposures may also be contributory. Clinical examination is usually normal unless there is associated chronic obstructive disease. Chest x-rays are usually normal, except for increased bronchial vascular markings. Pulmonary function tests can reveal airway obstruction with normal lung volumes. Treatment usually involves removal of the irritant, especially cigarette smoking. Acute purulent infections should be treated with antibiotics. Some patients will require bronchodilators and intermittent courses of antibiotics. One should look for chronic sinusitis with post nasal drip or esophageal reflux as causes for the chronic cough.

Chronic Obstructive Pulmonary Disease (COPD)

Chronic obstructive pulmonary diseases are characterized by limitation of *expiratory* flow and include asthma, bronchitis, emphysema, bronchiectasis, and some localized disorders of the upper airway. Emphysema is characterized by disruption of the terminal alveolar septa and loss of the terminal air units. In its presence, pulmonary function studies indicate airway obstruction, increased total lung capacity, diminished elastic recoil, and decreased diffusion capacity. (9) The diagnostic hallmark of both is a decrease in the FEV_1:FEV ratio.

Treatment of COPD. Treatment of COPD involves the control of symptoms and attention to complications. Patients with emphysema and no bronchospasm are difficult to treat, and one should be very conservative in utilizing bronchodilators, corticosteroids, and antibiotics. Those with bronchitis and obstruction to airflow are treated with bronchodilators, theophylline derivatives, intermittent antibiotics, and occasionally corticosteroids.

TREATMENT PROGRAM FOR COPD

1. Smoking cessation.

2. Patient and family education.

3. Relief of bronchospasm:
   —localized anticholinergic drugs,
   —localized beta adrenoreceptor agonists,
   —theophylline derivatives,
   —corticosteroids.

4. Reduce secretions (by avoiding irritants and treating infections with antibiotics).

5. Prevent infections by administering influenza and pneumococcal vaccines (see Chapter 18). In patients who have not been vaccinated for influenza for the current season, or who appear to have an influenza infection despite immunization, amantadine should be administered in a dose of 100 mg bid for 14 days. This medication can also be used prophylactically in the presence of an epidemic. Side effects are uncommon, but include confusion, ataxia, tremor, and convulsions.

6. Chest physical therapy, including postural drainage with chest percussion, breathing retraining, exercise conditioning, and low flow oxygen therapy for those with chronic mild hypoxia.

Anticholinergics. Atropine or ipratropium bromide decreases secretions and relieves bronchospasm. They should be administered with the beta adrenoreceptor agonists. (10)

189

Adrenoreceptor Agonists. Selective beta adrenoreceptor agonists include terbutaline, metaproterenol, bitolterol, and albuterol. These drugs are administered via metered-dose inhalers, 1–2 puffs two or more times a day. Careful instruction in the proper use of these inhalers is important.

Theophylline. Theophylline (sustained release form 100–300 mg bid) is a bronchodilator which stimulates respiration, improves diaphragmatic function, and results in diuresis. Theophylline clearance is influenced by drugs such as cimetidine and erythromycin and other factors such as diet, illness, smoking, heart failure, and liver disease. Toxicity is characterized by restlessness, insomnia, tremor, nausea, and vomiting. The therapeutic blood level of theophylline is 8–20 μg/ml. Very high levels can result in cardiac arrhythmias or seizures. This is one of the drugs for which monitoring of blood levels is important. (11)

Corticosteroids. Corticosteroids should be reserved for patients who fail simple pharmacologic treatment and who have proven significant reversible bronchospasm documented by pulmonary function tests. The following characteristics indicate possible good response to steroid treatment: eosinophilia in the sputum or blood, a 30% increase in the FEV_1 from baseline in response to beta adrenoreceptor agonist administration, and improvement in exercise tolerance after administration of a beta adrenoreceptor agonist. The most frequently used steroid regimen is 40 mg prednisone daily or its equivalent for 2–3 weeks. The dose should then be tapered to the lowest dose which will maintain improved function, preferably an alternate day schedule. Keep in mind that steroid side effects can be devastating, and older women are especially susceptible to osteoporosis.

Antibiotics. Acute bronchitis can exacerbate COPD. In fact, respiratory infections are one of the major causes of increased morbidity and mortality in COPD. Most respiratory infections begin with viral infections; however, these patients frequently develop secondary bacterial infections with the following organisms: *Haemophilus influenzae*, *Streptococcus pneumoniae*, and occasionally *Staphylococcus aureus*. Sputum cultures rarely are helpful in directing treatment. All of the following antibiotics can be used effectively: ampicillin, amoxacillin, tetracycline, erythromycin, trimethoprim/sulfamethoxazole, ampicillin/clavulinic acid. The duration of treatment is 7–14 days. It is reasonable to provide thoughtful patients with prescriptions for the self-administration of antibiotics early in the course of an infection.

Bronchial Asthma

Bronchial reactivity causes episodic shortness of breath, wheezing, and cough. Bronchial smooth muscle spasm, mucosal inflammation and edema, and mucus hypersecretion with narrowing and plugging of the bronchial tree result in airflow obstruction. Most asthmatics have the onset of their illness before age 40. Only 3% present from 40–60 years of age, and less than 1% develop new asthma after age 70. (12) Because of this infrequent new occurrence later in life, older patients are often incorrectly diagnosed as having chronic bronchitis. Asthmatic episodes usually develop after exercise, viral respiratory infections, or exposure to cold air or environmental irritants. It should be remembered that some drugs, such as aspirin, will precipitate bronchospasm in susceptible individuals. When asthma develops after the age of 60, it often requires continuous bronchodilator therapy, including corticosteroids. Treatment is similar to that of COPD; however, in contrast to COPD, corticosteroid inhalers are useful, especially if utilized as a preventive measure when the patient is symptom free. Another preventive approach is to provide a nasal preparation such as cromolyn (which decreases histamine release from mast cells) for use after exercise or exposure to cold.

Pneumonia

Pneumonia occurs frequently in older women. In the oldest patients, symptoms are often atypical (non-specific deterioration, rapid heart rate, and increased respiratory rate), although most patients still have the classic symptoms of cough, chest pain, sputum, and fever. Physical findings are very useful when present, but again, they may be absent in older women. The appropriate diagnostic test is the chest x-ray. The most common causes of an acute pulmonary infiltrate are nonbacterial. The most common bacteria causing pulmonary infection are *Streptococcus pneumoniae* and *Haemophilus influenzae*. Legionella pneumonia is more common in men. Treatment requires early antibiotic administration. Penicillin is the drug of choice for patchy bronchopneumonia or lobar pneumonia with Gram-positive diplococci in the sputum smear. For *Haemophilus influenzae*, ticarcillin/clavulinic acid, cefamandole, ceferozine, or trimethoprim/sulfamethoxazole is effective. If one suspects mycoplasma pneumonia or legionella pneumonia, erythromycin is the drug of choice. If the pneumonia is hospital-acquired or nursing home-acquired, an aminoglycoside should be administered. Supportive therapy is an important component in the treatment of pneumonia in older women. Adequate hydration must be maintained; deep breathing, good coughing, and sputum production improve prognosis.

Tuberculosis

Tuberculosis still represents an important clinical problem in older people, often presenting with nonspecific complaints. (13) Chest x-rays usually performed because of the classic symptoms of fever, night sweats, weight loss, anorexia, and hemoptysis demonstrate upper lung field infiltrates with or without cavitation. Occasionally chest x-ray reveals single or multiple nodules, miliary spread, or infiltrates in other locations. (14) Remember that up to 20% of patients with active tuberculosis have negative skin tests.

It is imperative to consider pulmonary tuberculosis in elderly women with a variety of symptoms when a diagnosis is not apparent. A skin test should be performed immediately. A positive test (10 mm induration or more) indicates prior infection, while a negative reaction requires a repeat test a week later. Early morning sputum specimens should be collected and examined on 3 consecutive days. Induced sputums should be obtained if necessary. If these methods are ineffective and tuberculosis is still suspected, bronchoscopic examination or gastric aspiration may be necessary to obtain specimens for culture. Treatment is highly effective with isoniazid and rifampin but requires referral for expert guidance and supervision.

Lung Cancer

The most important comment to be made in regard to lung cancer in a book devoted to preventive care is to lament the increasing incidence which can be directly attributed to smoking. Lung cancer is now the the leading cause of death from cancer in U.S. women. (15)

Cancer Site Incidence in U.S. Women

Breast	28%
Colorectum	15%
Lung	11%
Uterus	9%
Ovary	4%

Cancer Deaths in U.S. Women

Lung	21%
Breast	18%
Colorectum	13%
Ovary	5%
Uterus	4%

Because of this new prominence for lung cancer in older women, liberal use of chest x-rays for any respiratory complaint is recommended. Treatment is complicated and requires specialist consultation.

Interstitial Lung Diseases

Interstitial lung diseases represent a heterogeneous group of disorders characterized by an interstitial and interlobular inflammatory process, with fibrosis in the distal lung architecture. There are a number of causes for lung fibrosis, including toxicity from drugs or poisons, autoimmune disorders, chronic infections, and idiopathic injury. Typical symptoms are shortness of breath with exercise and a nonproductive cough.

Occasionally patients will have systemic symptoms with fever, weight loss, fatigue, myalgia, and arthralgia. Physical findings may be absent or rales will be present in the lower lung fields. Clubbing also may be present. Diagnosis requires a chest x-ray, demonstrating interstitial infiltrates in the lower lungs.

Sleep Disorders

Sleep apnea is an important cause of serious psychologic and physiologic disruption in older people. Sleep apnea is characterized by a cessation of breathing for 10 seconds or longer, underventilation, and oxygen desaturation.

Normal sleep is quite variable. Nonrapid eye movement sleep (or quiet sleep) is associated with slow waves with increased amplitude on EEG. This quiet sleep has 4 progressively deeper stages. Stages 1 and 2 are characterized by irregular breathing, even periods of Cheyne-Stokes breathing. The sleep becomes established in the deeper stages 3 and 4; breathing stabilizes and becomes more regular. During sleep, intercostal muscle activity decreases, and there is paradoxical movement of the rib cage with a decrease in residual lung capacity. These are of no consequence in a normal, healthy individual.

In the sleep apnea syndrome, both sleep and respirations are disturbed. The patient usually reports very restless sleep with tossing and turning. Patients are not rested upon awakening, and are sleepy throughout the day. The etiology of sleep apnea is not always clear. It can be due to a central nervous system problem or associated with obstructed upper airways. In the past this syndrome has typically been associated with massive obesity or with COPD. However, sleep apnea is increasingly being recognized in women of normal body weight with no underlying pulmonary disease.

The diagnosis of sleep apnea requires a sleep study in a laboratory, during which ventilatory status and oxygen saturation are monitored. Management includes weight reduction in overweight individuals and the administration of drugs to enhance respiration. The drug of choice is protriptyline, 20 mg at bedtime. Occasionally patients will require nocturnal oxygen administration.

References

1. **Krumpe PE, Knudson RJ, Parson G, Reiser K,** The aging respiratory system, Clin Geriatr Med 1:143, 1985.

2. **Knudson RJ, Lebowitz MD, Holberg CL, Burrows B,** Changes in the normal maximal expiratory flow-volume curve with growth and aging, Am Rev Respir Dis 127:725, 1983.

3. **Muiesan G, Sorbini CA, Grassi V,** Respiratory function in the aged, Bull Physiopath Resp 7:973, 1971.

4. **Holland J, Milic-Emili J, Macklem PT, Battes BV,** Regional distribution of pulmonary ventilation and perfusion in elderly subjects, J Clin Invest 47:81, 1968.

5. **Kronenberg RS, Adrage CW,** Attenuation of the ventilatory and heart rate responses to hypoxia and hypercapnia with aging in normal men, J Clin Invest 52:1818, 1973.

6. **Naifeh KH, Smith PL, Bleecker K,** Ventilatory control during sleep in the elderly, Geriatr Clin No Am 2:227, 1986.

7. **Reynolds HY,** Lung host defenses, Chest 75:239, 1979.

8. **Lfandahl S, Sten B, Svanborg A,** Dyspnea in 70 year old people, Acta Med Scand 107:225, 1983.

9. **Petty TL, Silvers GW, Stanford RE,** Mild emphysema is associated with reduced elastic recoil and increased lung size, but not with air-flow limitation, Am Rev Respir Dis 136:867, 1987.

10. **Mann JS, George CF,** Anticholinergic drugs in the treatment of airway disease, Br J Dis Chest 79:209, 1985.

11. **Staiv AH, Bodem G, Wiesbock D,** Theophylline pharmacokinetics in the aged: Results of a dose finding study in 12 geriatric patients, Clin Pharmacol 9:199, 1987.

12. **Derrick EH,** The significance of the age of onset of asthma, Med J Aust 1:1317, 1971.

13. **Fullerton JM, Dyer L,** Unsuspected tuberculosis in the aged, Tubercle 46:193, 1965.

14. **Chang S-C, Lee PY, Perng RP,** Lower lung field tuberculosis, Chest 91:320, 1987.

15. **Silverberg E, Lubera J,** Cancer statistics, 1989, CA 39:3, 1989.

12 Gastrointestinal Function and Diseases

Increasing age is associated with alterations in major functions in the gastrointestinal tract; however, older women's abdominal symptoms should not be attributed to age alone. Serious GI disease (cancer) is a prevalent problem in older life. For example, it would be unusual for irritable bowel to present for the first time in an elderly woman, and a recent change in bowel habits would be unlikely to be "functional." Even though we prefer not to attribute symptoms to functional causes, functional gastrointestinal complaints continue to be a major problem in elderly women. However, gastrointestinal tumors and cancers increase with aging, and there is greater concern when an older person presents with a new or changing GI symptom.

Physical findings often do not assist in establishing a diagnosis. An accurate and detailed history is paramount. Diagnostic evaluations of the GI tract have improved dramatically in the past decade, but are generally more difficult to perform in older people and are associated with higher complication rates. In addition, purgatives frequently used to prepare for diagnostic studies can result in significant dehydration in very old people.

Changes with Aging

Two major changes occur in the aging gut which contribute to anatomic and physiologic alterations. (1) The mucosa of many gut surfaces tends to atrophy, and submucosal nerve plexuses degenerate. These changes in the jejunum result in changes in absorption. Lactase deficiency occurs commonly. Fat malabsorption results from a combination of the GI changes and decreased pancreatic secretion. Decreased acid secretion in the stomach leads to a decrease in iron absorption in the duodenum. Vitamin absorption is decreased but usually does not result in true vitamin deficiencies. Nevertheless, many recommend vitamin supplementation in later years. Vitamin D and calcium absorption decreases with age, due to a combination of decreases in sun exposure, renal conversion of vitamin D to its active metabolite, and intestinal absorption. Colonic transit time decreases in older people, producing more constipation. (2) Liver weight decreases with age, associated with decreasing numbers of hepatocytes. This results in a decreased hepatic metabolism for many drugs. Liver function tests, however, change little with age. Basal and stimulated gastric acid secretion declines with age, yet many older women still secrete excessive amounts of acid and suffer from peptic ulcer disease.

195

**Esophageal
Disease**

Difficulty or pain on swallowing, a lump in the throat, heartburn, nasopharyngeal regurgitation, coughing, wheezing, morning hoarseness, sore throat, pulmonary infection, and substernal chest pain can all be associated with esophageal disorders. Because normal swallowing requires coordination between the mouth and the pharynx and is mediated by muscular mechanisms, many muscular diseases result in impaired swallowing. Cerebral vascular disease which involves the nuclei in the brain stem commonly causes dysphagia with uncoordinated oropharyngeal swallowing. Some demyelinating diseases, for example Parkinson's disease, can cause dysphagia. Uncommon causes include mechanical obstruction by tumors or abscesses. Upper esophageal dysphagia usually results in symptoms with swallowing liquids. Lower esophageal dysphagia causes a problem in handling solids.

Diagnostic evaluation includes careful examination of the oral pharynx, a neurologic examination, barium x-ray studies, esophageal manometric studies, and laryngoscopy. These patients deserve referral to a specialist.

Presbyesophagus. Presbyesophagus is characterized by abnormal frequency of tertiary or non-peristaltic contractions and inadequate relaxation of the lower esophageal sphincter. (3,4) These changes can be the result of aging or vascular, metabolic, or neurologic events. Although presbyesophagus can cause dysphagia, dysphagia should not be attributed to presbyesophagus until intrinsic or extrinsic compression has been excluded.

Cricopharyngeal Achalasia. Cricopharyngeal achalasia usually presents with a lump in the throat or a sensation of food getting stuck high in the chest or throat, and occasionally in association with nasopharyngeal regurgitation with swallowing. Paradoxical contractions of the cricopharyngeal muscle or failure of the muscle to relax normally during the pharyngeal phase of swallowing causes the symptoms. Regardless of the etiology, treatment is surgical, myotomy.

Hiatus Hernia and Esophageal Reflux. Hiatal hernias increase in frequency in older women until approximately 70% of women after age 70 have this problem. (5) The hiatal hernia itself rarely causes symptoms unless there is associated reflux esophagitis from an incompetence of the lower esophageal sphincter. The symptoms of reflux are usually substernal burning and regurgitation with acid regurgitation into the throat. Acidic foods such as citrus fruits can cause burning and discomfort. Overeating, obesity, and cigarette smoking contribute to the severity and frequency of esophageal reflux. Reflux can also cause symptoms of dysphagia secondary to inflammatory stricture in the distal esophagus. This problem can even cause respiratory symptoms, including coughing, wheezing, morning hoarseness, and sore throat. Recurrent pulmonary infections can result from aspiration of gastric contents during the night. Frequently patients and clinicians misinterpret substernal chest discomfort from esophageal reflux and inflammation for cardiac pain. (6)

Usually pain from esophageal reflux worsens with drinking coffee, tea, and fruit juices. The pain is frequently relieved by antacids, assuming upright posture, or exercising (of course, pain due to ischemic heart disease does not display these characteristics).

Evaluation includes an esophageal barium study or endoscopy. At times the diagnosis can be difficult if there is no inflammation or stricture. Occasionally a provocative challenge with ergonovine or another cholinergic drug during esophageal manometry will be needed to diagnose this condition. These agents can induce coronary vasospasm and probably should not be used in older people.

Esophageal injury due to medications should be considered. Antibiotics, potassium chloride, iron tablets, clonidine, and non-steroidal anti-inflammatory drugs can cause ulcerations in the lower esophagus. Patients should be instructed to take medications upright with adequate amounts of fluid. Immobilized older women are more likely to develop esophageal disease secondary to medications.

Patients with typical symptoms and an uncomplicated history can be treated symptomatically for 2–4 weeks without diagnostic studies. If there is a more complicated history or a less than optimal response to the therapeutic trial, prompt evaluation is indicated.

TREATMENT OF ESOPHAGEAL REFLUX

1. Eat 3 small meals a day.

2. Avoid foods that decrease lower esophageal sphincter pressure: alcohol, fats, chocolates, peppermint.

3. Take nothing by mouth for 3–4 hours before bedtime.

4. Elevate the head of the bed 6 or more inches.

5. Avoid stooping and straining, especially after a meal.

6. Overweight patients should lose weight.

7. Limit the use of drugs such as nicotine, theophylline, anticholinergics, caffeine, beta adrenergic blockers, and calcium channel blockers.

8. Take liquid antacids 1 and again 3 hours after meals, and at bedtime.

9. Consider ranitidine, 150 mg bid.

10. For persistent symptoms, consider bethanecol, 10 or 25 mg tid and at bedtime, or metaclopramide, 10 mg tid and at bedtime.

11. Treatment may require bougienage or surgery.

Achalasia. Achalasia in women over 50 is uncommon. If evaluation of dysphagia demonstrates the typical narrowed bird-beak distal esophagus on a barium swallow, then endoscopy is required to exclude a tumor of the cardia of the stomach which may cause secondary achalasia. Achalasia can also be caused by tumors of the lung and pancreas.

Esophageal Infection. Esophageal infections with *Candida* occur in association with malignancy, diabetes mellitus, malnutrition, antibiotic treatment, or immunosuppression. In older, debilitated patients, esophageal candidiasis can occur in the absence of other contributing conditions. Diagnosis usually requires endoscopic biopsy, although barium esophageal studies can be diagnostic. (7)

Peptic Ulcer

Gastric ulcers reach their peak frequency at approximately ages 55–65. In older individuals, gastric and duodenal ulcers occur with about equal frequency. Symptoms, as is often the case in older people, are often atypical or nonspecific. Peptic ulcers may present without antecedent symptoms as an acute hemorrhage, perforation, or obstruction. Because gastric ulcers require biopsy and brushing for cytologic examination, fiberoptic endoscopy is now utilized for initial evaluation. Although duodenal ulcers can be easily diagnosed radiographically, fiberoptic endoscopy is superior, especially for small ulcers. Because symptoms are not always specific for duodenal versus gastric ulcers, endoscopy is preferred no matter what the presentation.

Treatment of Peptic Ulcers. Initial treatment utilizes one of the H_2-receptor antagonists: cimetidine, ranitidine, or famotidine. All of these drugs demonstrate 89% efficacy in healing uncomplicated duodenal ulcers within 6 weeks, and have high cure rates for gastric ulcers. Sucralfate can be used for patients who have problems tolerating the H_2-receptor antagonists.

Antacids, 1 and 3 hours after meals and at bedtime, are effective, but poor compliance and GI symptoms make this less attractive. Gastric secretagogues, including alcohol, coffee, salicylates, nonsteroidal anti-inflammatory drugs, and cigarette smoking should be avoided.

Most ulcers heal within 6–8 weeks, and therefore treatment should be discontinued after 8 weeks. Exceptions to this rule include very large ulcers. Ulcers tend to recur. A bedtime dose of cimetidine (400 mg), ranitidine (150 mg), or famotidine (20 mg), or sucralfate 1 gr bid is about 80% effective in preventing duodenal ulcer recurrences. This treatment is also effective in decreasing the risk of ulcers due to ulcerogenic drugs.

Diseases of the Colon

Lower bowel disease typically presents with abdominal pain, gastrointestinal bleeding and weight loss, or changes in bowel movements. About one-third of women over the age of 60 have colonic diverticula. Diverticular disease is predominantly an affliction of Western culture, and the high frequency has been attributed to the low fiber content of our diet. Many symptoms attributed to diverticular disease may be due to other causes. About 80% of people with diverticula remain asymptomatic throughout life. The one symptom reliably associated with diverticula is colicky or gripping pain in the left lower quadrant, which is worse after meals. Frequently a cord-like loop of colon can be palpable in the left lower quadrant.

The diagnosis is best made by barium enema. Treatment utilizes a high fiber diet with psyllium or other soluble and insoluble fibers. Bran in the diet controls symptoms in most patients. Surgery is reserved for only the most severe cases to alleviate serious sequelae.

Diverticulitis is usually a single episode of acute left lower quadrant pain with associated signs of abdominal infection (fever, leukocytosis, peritonitis). Typical findings may be absent in older patients. Diagnostic studies include plain x-rays of the abdomen, and sigmoidoscopy; barium enemas should not be performed during an acute episode of inflammation. Broad spectrum antibiotics for 7–10 days are used for treatment, as well as nasogastric suction and bowel rest with careful food management. Bleeding from a diverticulum usually is located in the right colon and can be massive and unabated. These serious problems require consultation with a gastroenterologist.

Ulcerative colitis and Crohn's disease, inflammatory bowel diseases, have a second peak in incidence in older life. These conditions also deserve referral for management.

Colorectal Neoplasms.   Cancers of the colon and rectum increase rapidly after age 40, doubling every 10 years to a peak at age 75. They rank third in cancer deaths in women, after lung cancer and breast cancer. Colorectal cancer is a preventable disease. The majority of carcinomas begin as an adenomatous polyp. Removal of premalignant polyps dramatically reduces the frequency of this cancer. An intensive surveillance program with removal of any visualized polyps demonstrated an 85% reduction in subsequent development of rectal and sigmoid carcinoma. (8)

Adenomatous polyps can be diagnosed by flexible sigmoidoscopy, barium enema, or colonoscopy. Most polyps can be easily removed through a scope. The malignancy rate in polyps less than 1 cm in diameter is about 1%. In contrast, those more than 2 cm in size have a 50% likelihood of being cancer. (9) The time for progression from early adenoma formation to the development of carcinoma is believed to be 5–15 years.

Screening for Colonic Neoplasia.   Hemoccult II, a guaiac impregnated paper, is the most widely used test for fecal occult blood. Only 3–4% of asymptomatic patients over age 40 have a positive test, and the predictive value for adenoma or carcinoma is about 45%. The positive predictive value increases to about 80% for people over age 70 because of the increased incidence of colonic carcinoma. Foods such as turnips, horseradish, broccoli, and caulifower can cause a false positive test. Vitamin C inhibits oxidation and can cause a false negative test. Patients are instructed to collect at least 6 fecal smears, and the tests must be developed within 4 days. A single positive test is regarded as significant. The test is relatively insensitive, and this has resulted in advocacy for routine flexible colonoscopy at 3 to 5 year intervals in people over age 50. Once an individual is discovered to have an adenomatous polyp, frequent colonic examinations must be performed.

Functional Bowel Disease.   Frequently no organic disease can be identified after a thorough diagnostic evaluation in a patient with gastrointestinal symptoms. Indeed, functional bowel disease may be twice as common as any other GI diagnosis. (10) The symptoms mimic other serious pathology. Symptoms are exacerbated by dietary indiscretions or life stresses. Depression frequently accompanies irritable bowel symptoms.

Treatment includes careful evaluation for serious underlying GI disorders, adequate psychological support, dietary manipulations including a high fiber diet, and occasional antispasmodics such as Donnatal or tincture of belladonna. Stress management improves symptoms in many patients. Antidepressant treatment is useful, using drugs which combine antidepressant action with anticholinergic properties.

Constipation. Constipation is difficult to define, and it is best to accept the patient's definition. An acute change, associated with pain or bleeding, requires GI evaluation. Constipation can occur due to spasticity associated with an irritable colon. Atonic constipation is more common in older women, due to decreased motility. Constipation is frequently multifactorial, a manifestation of neurological disorders, hypothyroidism, depression, dehydration, and medications.

Treatment requires fiber supplementation with increased food intake. An exercise program may increase bowel transit time, and a review of medications is imperative. Chronic laxative abuse can cause constipation and be very refractory to treatment. Laxatives, therefore, should be avoided. If they are necessary, lactulose is preferred.

Diarrhea. Acute diarrhea is a serious problem in very old women because of the increased susceptibility to dehydration. A frequent cause of diarrhea is lactose intolerance, which progresses with aging. A therapeutic trial of elimination of lactose is worthwhile. Chronic diarrhea requires evaluation for malabsorption and colonic lesions.

Hemorrhoids and Anal Fissures. Rectal bleeding should not be attributed to hemorrhoids in older women without an examination to exclude inflammatory and other causes of GI bleeding. Nonthrombosed hemorrhoids are not painful and present either with rectal bleeding or as an anal mass that appears during defecation. Anal fissures cause burning or sharp pain initiated and relieved by defecation. A failure to respond to the usual treatments (Sitz baths, stool softeners, bran and psyllium, topical anesthetics, and emollient suppositories) requires further evaluation by a gastroenterologist or proctologist.

Diseases of the Liver

Although liver diseases decrease in frequency with aging, some diseases are more severe in the elderly.

Viral Hepatitis. In older people, hepatitis A decreases in frequency while the others increase. (11) Typical symptoms of viral hepatitis include malaise, anorexia, nausea and vomiting, and abdominal discomfort. Other symptoms include urticarial rash, arthralgias, arthritis, jaundice, dark urine, altered mental status, and depression. Physical examination usually reveals a large tender liver with mild jaundice. Aminotransferase enzymes are more than 10 times normal. Older women have more severe symptoms and a more prolonged course of biochemical abnormalities compared to younger women. Chronic hepatitis and cirrhosis occur in about 3–5% of patients with hepatitis B, and up to 55% in patients with the non A and non B hepatitis secondary to transfusions. There is no curative treatment for acute viral hepatitis.

Hepatotoxicity from Medication. Medication as the cause for liver disease or abnormal liver function tests should be considered in any older individual. When liver function abnormalities are identified, only urgently required medications should be continued. Hepatocellular disease due to drugs usually resolves in a short period of time.

Cirrhosis. Alcohol is not the only cause of cirrhosis. Cirrhosis can be due to drugs or toxins, hepatitis, metabolic derangements, and vascular disease, including heart failure. Primary biliary cirrhosis can first present in elderly women. (12) An elevation in alkaline phosphatase in an asymptomatic individual suggests this possibility.

Cholelithiasis

Biliary tract disease in older women presents in various ways. Chronic cholecystitis can cause unexplained fevers and weight loss. Acute cholecystitis presents typically with right upper quadrant pain, nausea, vomiting, fever, chills, right upper quadrant tenderness, leukocytosis, and abnormal liver tests (especially alkaline phosphatase and bilirubin). The transaminase may initially be high, but within a few hours it decreases to near normal levels.

Cholelithiasis increases in frequency with increasing age, and is twice as common in women at all ages. Between the ages of 80–89, 38% of women have cholelithiasis. Only 5% of acute cholecystitis is not due to stones.

The diagnostic procedure of choice is real time ultrasonography, 90–95% sensitive and 95% specific. Cholecystography can still be performed when ultrasonography yields poor results. Both tests are insensitive for common duct stones. Persistent symptoms with biliary type pain or abnormal liver function tests without an abnormal ultrasound may require endoscopic retrograde cholangiography.

Most gall stones are asymptomatic. The natural history of asymptomatic gall stones indicates that only 18% of patients will develop symptoms of pain during a 15 year follow-up. (13) There is no advantage for prophylactic cholecystectomy over conservative management. Prophylactic cholecystectomy is indicated in patients with diabetes mellitus or chronic hemolytic anemias, and in patients who travel to remote countries where medical care is suboptimal.

Acute cholecystitis in older women is associated with greater morbidity and mortality. (14) If the presence of stones is confirmed by ultrasonography, surgery should be performed with minimal delay. The therapeutic choice for chronic cholecystitis is also surgery.

References

1. **Holt P,** Aging in the gut, Geriatric Med Today 4:44, 1985.

2. **Brandt LJ,** *Gastrointestinal Disorders of the Elderly*, Raven Press, New York, 1984.

3. **Hollis JB, Castell DO,** Esophageal function in elderly men: A new look at presbyesophagus, Ann Intern Med 80:371, 1974.

4. **Soergel KH, Zboralski FE, Amberg JR,** Presbyesophagus: Esophageal mortality in nonagenarians, J Clin Invest 43:1472, 1964.

5. **Pridie RB,** Incidence and co-incidence of hiatus hernia, Gut 7:188, 1966.

6. **Benjamin SB, Castell DO,** Chest pain of esophageal origin, Arch Intern Med 143:772, 1983.

7. **Levine MF, Macones AJ, Laufer I,** *Candida* esophagitis: Accuracy of radiographic diagnosis, Radiology 154:581, 1985.

8. **Sherlock P, Lipkin M, Winawer SJ,** Prevention of colon cancer, Am J Med 68:917, 1980.

9. **Enterline HT,** Polyps and cancer of the large bowel, Curr Top Path 63:65, 1976.

10. **Sklar M,** Gastrointestinal diseases in the aged, in Reichel W, editor, *Clinical Aspects of Aging,* Williams & Wilkins, Baltimore, 2nd edition, 1983, p 205.

11. **Dupinski K,** Hepatitis in the aged, Digestion 8:254, 1973.

12. **Lehan NNA, Bassendine MF, James OFW,** Primary biliary sclerosis: A disease increasingly recognized in the elderly, Geriatric Med Today 3:64, 1984.

13. **Gracie WA, et al,** Natural history of silent gall stones, Gastroenterology 80:1161, 1981.

14. **Glen F,** Surgical management of cholecystitis in patients 65 years of age and older, Ann Surg 193:56, 1981.

13 The Urinary Tract and Pelvic Floor

Problems of the lower urinary tract are common in elderly women. Symptoms include urinary incontinence, dribbling, frequency, and urgency. To a significant degree, these problems reflect changes with aging in the genitourinary system, including relaxation of the pelvic floor. From an individual and a social point of view, incontinence is the most prevalent and the most disturbing problem.

Incontinence in the elderly is often neglected. On the contrary, urinary incontinence should not be underrated. It has a profound effect on the quality of life for elderly women and their families. It is one of the most difficult problems for a family to manage. The physician must aggressively seek its presence. It cannot be assumed that women will voluntarily discuss their symptoms. Most importantly, incontinence should not be dismissed as a natural consequence of aging. There is a rational and simple approach to the problem, which yields effective management, usually without invasive tests or surgery. (1)

In this chapter, we will consider the changes that occur with aging in the urinary tract as well as in the pelvic floor. We will offer a program of evaluation and management for the clinical consequences of these changes.

Renal Function with Aging

Despite renal senescence manifested by marked decreases in renal blood flow, glomerular filtration rate, and tubular function, the aging kidney effectively maintains body fluid volumes and electrolyte concentrations. Therefore, despite the loss of both renal mass and function, the majority of elderly people exhibit no signs or symptoms of renal disease. (2) Although not well studied, the following are probably all reduced in elderly women: bladder capacity, ability to postpone voiding, urethral closure pressure, and urinary flow rate; while the following are increased: residual volume and detrusor instability (uninhibited bladder contractions). All of these changes predispose to incontinence.

Aging Renal Anatomy. Renal mass (primarily cortical), the number and surface area of glomeruli, and the proximal tubule length and volume all decrease with age. These changes (about 20% of kidney weight) can be largely, if not totally, attributed to vascular changes (medial hypertrophy, intimal proliferation, and hyalinization of the renal arteries). The anatomical changes (about 50% of all glomeruli are lost) are consistent with a decrease in outer cortical blood flow, while inner cortical and medullary perfusion is relatively unchanged with age.

Aging Renal Physiology

Renal Blood Flow. A marked decrease in renal blood flow occurs after age 50 (about 10% per decade), consistent with an increase in renal vascular resistance. Studies indicate that decreased blood flow is the primary event, inducing parenchymal atrophy.

Glomerular Filtration Rate. A progressive reduction in glomerular filtration rate (GFR) occurs with age (markedly after age 50), consonant with the decrease in blood flow and renal mass. Creatinine clearance falls to less than 100 ml per minute. This reduction in renal function has important clinical implications, especially regarding the use of drugs. Muscle mass, creatinine production, creatinine release, and creatinine excretion are all reduced, and therefore serum creatinine is unchanged despite the decrease in creatinine clearance. The BUN rises only a few mg/dl with aging.

Tubular Function. A decrease in renal tubular function parallels the progressive decline in GFR. This suggests that nephrons are lost as entire functional units. Distal tubular function is reduced to a greater degree than GFR, manifested by defects in concentrating and diluting capacity (not explained by central defects in vasopressin secretion). Studies are consistent with an abnormal response to adequate circulating levels of vasopressin. Independent of the decrease in GFR, elderly tubules demonstrate a diminished ability to acidify the urine (usually a clinical problem only with diabetic ketoacidosis or shock). Responses to sodium loading and sodium restriction are slower with old kidneys, which can lead to volume problems. The aging tubules do not leak red or white blood cells, glucose, or protein into the urine.

Endocrine Function. In normotensive people, renin activity and blood aldosterone levels progressively decline with age. The response of the renin-angiotensin-aldosterone system to sodium changes is sluggish and contributes to impaired sodium conservation. The prostaglandin and kallikrein systems have been inadequately studied in the elderly.

Clinical Importance of Renal Aging

Because of the decrease in renal function with age, estimation or measurement of the creatinine clearance is necessary to avoid renal damage with nephrotoxic drugs and to prevent overdosage (e.g. with digoxin). When the creatinine clearance is known, drug dosage can be selected from tables. Creatinine clearance in elderly women can be estimated by the following formula utilizing age, serum creatinine, and body weight: (3)

$$CC \ (ml/min) = \frac{(140 \ - \ age) \times (weight \ in \ kg)}{72 \times Cr} \times 0.85$$

Decreased renal function predisposes elderly patients to dangerous volume depletion when exposed to the combination of bowel preparation, overnight dehydration, and the use of x-ray contrast media. An IVP is associated with a high incidence of renal injury in the elderly. The consequence can be acute renal failure. Sensorium problems (and a reduced intake of water) combined with the defect in renal concentrating ability can lead to a problem of hypernatremia in the elderly. Hyponatremia is also encountered, but it is a less serious problem, and usually is due to drug or illness-stimulated vasopressin secretion.

The decreased activity of the renin-angiotensin-aldosterone system can induce hypoaldosteronism secondary to insufficient stimulation of the adrenal gland. Unexplained and persistent hyperkalemia with only a mild decrease in renal function is the usual clue.

External Atrophic Changes

Due to low estrogen production, atrophy of mucosal surfaces takes place during the postmenopausal years. This genitourinary atrophy leads to the symptoms of vaginitis, pruritus, dyspareunia, and stenosis, which affect the ease and quality of living. Urethritis with dysuria, urgency, incontinence, and urinary frequency is a further result of mucosal thinning, in this instance of the urethra and bladder. Pelvic relaxation with cystocele, rectocele, enterocele, and uterine prolapse, as well as vulvar dystrophies, are not a consequence of estrogen deprivation.

The Urethral Caruncle. The urethral caruncle is a polyp of urethral mucosa, protruding from the urethral meatus, the result of chronic inflammation or irritation in atrophic tissue. It is usually asymptomatic, although it can bleed and cause dysuria, frequency, and urgency. This condition is best treated with estrogen replacement therapy, although, if asymptomatic, it can be ignored except for one proviso. Persistent or recurrent caruncles should be biopsied. About 2% are malignant (usually ca-in-situ).

Urethral Prolapse. This condition is an eversion of mucosa through the external urethral meatus, usually due to estrogen deficiency. It can be secondary to trauma or repeated coughing and straining. Excision may be necessary, but estrogen treatment should be tried first. The diagnosis is easy: this is the only condition in which a red mass of tissue completely surrounds the meatus.

Relaxation of the Pelvic Floor

Aging and parturition alter the integrity of the pelvic floor musculature. Intact levator muscles are capable of strong contraction which closes the opening through which the genital organs can pass. This sphincter-like action is weakened by childbirth and by the postmenopausal involution of muscle mass. Prolapse due to pelvic relaxation results in the following clinically recognized anatomical conditions: cystocele, rectocele, enterocele, and uterine prolapse.

Physical examination requires observation both at rest and while straining. With coughing or straining, the order and extent of the pelvic structures can be noted. It is not appropriate to assess the degree of relaxation by applying traction to the cervix.

Classification of Pelvic Relaxation

Descent of cervix, bladder, or rectum *to* introitus *only* with straining.	First degree—Slight
Descent of cervix, bladder, or rectum *beyond* the introitus *only* with straining.	Second degree—Moderate
Descent of cervix, bladder, or rectum *beyond* the introitus *at rest*.	Third degree—Severe
Complete prolapse: entire cervix and uterus protrude beyond the introitus and the vagina is inverted.	Procidentia

The main symptoms of prolapse are a sense of something falling out or sitting on a mass, and backache. Symptoms are also due to the usual association with cystocele, rectocele, and enterocele. A bulge in the anterior vaginal wall is usually a downward displacement of the bladder: a cystocele. Symptoms include a fullness or bulging sensation in the vagina, and in extreme cases, discomfort and difficulty with walking and sitting. Stress incontinence is a symptom of urethral and bladder neck defects, not of a pure cystocele, but urinary incontinence is the most common symptom with a cystocele because the vesicourethral angle is usually also relaxed. Relaxation of this area allows the proximal urethra to fall from its intraabdominal location. The change in anatomical relationships in this area is the key to incontinence.

A small cystocele causes no symptoms, and often a large cystocele can be asymptomatic. The pressure of a protruding mass can be significantly uncomfortable and is aggravated by activity, standing, or straining. Anterior vaginal colporrhaphy is the most effective treatment for cystocele, usually combined with vaginal hysterectomy and posterior colporrhaphy, because the cystocele is usually associated with general pelvic floor relaxation.

A bulge of the posterior vaginal wall is due to downward movement of the rectum: a rectocele. The most common complaints are constipation or the need to apply digital pressure in the vagina in order to defecate.

An enterocele is a herniation of the pouch of Douglas into the rectovaginal septum, essentially a cul-de-sac hernia. Usually asymptomatic, vaginal pressure and aching discomfort may be present. Incarceration of bowel does not occur. This is almost always a component of uterine prolapse. Obliteration of the enterocele sac should accompany all surgical procedures. Recurrent cases require suspension of the vaginal apex (usually to the sacrospinous ligaments) with nonabsorbable material. (4)

A retroverted uterus is more subject to prolapse because the corpus is aligned with the axis of the vagina. Most women with uterovaginal prolapse have a composite problem, including cystocele, rectocele, enterocele, and stress incontinence. The best management consists of a composite surgical procedure: vaginal hysterectomy, anterior colporrhaphy, and posterior colporrhaphy. Proper technique requires evaluation of the cul-de-sac, with elimination of redundant peritoneum and plication of the cul-de-sac to correct and prevent an enterocele. For massive eversion of the vagina or for a failed enterocele repair, sacrospinous ligament fixation is recommended.

There are some simple things which can be done to relieve the symptoms of prolapse. Anything which reduces intraabdominal pressure helps. Therefore, the patient and physician should pay attention to smoking, excessive body weight, heavy lifting, and constipation. The use of a vaginal pessary should be considered.

The Vaginal Pessary

The vaginal pessary is a very old treatment. The ancient Greeks used half a pomegranate soaked in wine to hold a prolapsed uterus in place. The vaginal pessary can support prolapsing pelvic tissues or hold a symptomatic retroverted uterus in the anteroversion position. In some cases, urinary stress incontinence can be improved by pessary support of the vesicourethral junction. Another important benefit of pessary use is relief of chronic backache due to pelvic relaxation. Note that this type of backache characteristically is absent in the morning, worsens through the day, and is relieved by lying down. A pessary is useful for women who are poor risks for surgery or to assess whether symptoms might be alleviated by corrective surgery.

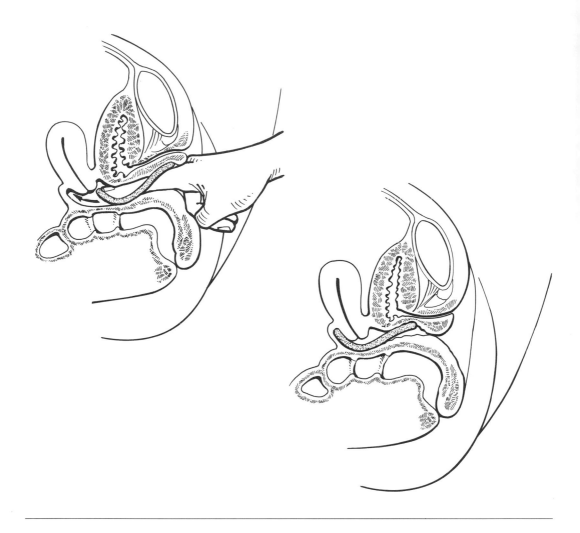

Fitting a pessary is exactly the same as fitting a diaphragm. To determine the proper length of a pessary, pass any instrument (e.g. a uterine sound) to the top of the posterior vaginal vault. Mark the instrument at the introitus; this length minus 1 cm is the appropriate length for the pessary. The posterior portion sits behind the cervix in the posterior vaginal fornix. The midportion supports the vesicourethral junction, and the anterior portion is supported by the posterior, inferior surface of the pubis. *The pessary should fit the vagina loosely enough so that a finger can be placed between the pessary and the vaginal walls.* After a pessary is fitted, the patient should stand and walk. If pain occurs or the pessary is displaced, the size or shape is not appropriate. If a pessary is uncomfortable or interferes with bowel or bladder function, it is not fitted properly.

A pessary must be removed periodically for cleaning, and the vagina inspected for infection or ulceration. For most pessaries, examination in 1–2 weeks and then every 2–3 months is adequate. Prolonged pessary use inevitably leads to pressure necrosis and ulceration of the vagina. It is almost a requirement that women wearing pessaries receive estrogen treatment to minimize vaginal wall ulceration. If vaginal reaction is present, the pessary should not be re-inserted for 1–2 weeks. Take care not to abandon a vaginal pessary; serious complications can ensue. These patients should be followed closely.

Most, if not all, of these pessaries are available from Milex Products, Inc., Chicago, Illinois 60631.

The Smith Pessary. The rounded top is better suited where there is excellent and well-defined support by the pubis.

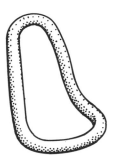

The Hodge Pessary. The squared top is appropriate when there is limited pubic support. The Smith and Hodge pessaries are primarily for converting a retroverted uterus to the anterior position, with no more than a mild cystocele present.

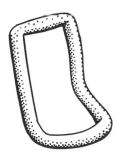

The Gehrung Pessary. This pessary is recommended for prolapse associated with cystocele and rectocele.

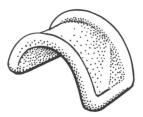

The Gellhorn Pessary. This pessary, shaped like a collar button, rests the stem on the perineum and provides a platform for the cervix. It is intended to support a prolapsed uterus.

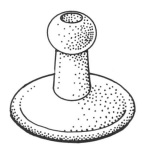

The Ring and Donut Pessaries. These pessaries are recommended for prolapse of the uterus and are effective in reducing cystocele and rectocele. The ring pessary is most suitable for old women. It is especially useful for prolapse and should be asymptomatic if properly fitted.

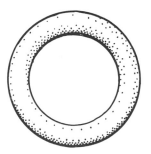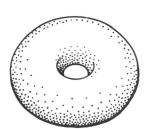

The Cube Pessary. This is the pessary of last resort for prolapse, especially for severe cases with cystocele and rectocele in very old women. Support is due to the suction action of the six concave surfaces against the vaginal walls. The cube pessary can be compressed for greater ease of insertion well up into the vagina. Removal may require insertion of finger tips between the vaginal mucosa and the pessary to break the suction. The attached cord is only for the purpose of locating the pessary; *it is not meant to be pulled for removal*. The pessary should be removed every night for washing and reinsertion in the morning (this is necessary to avoid vaginal ulceration). Vaginal drainage can be achieved by burning small holes in the center of the concavities.

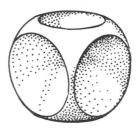

Urinary Incontinence

The Physiology of Micturition. The urinary bladder is a hollow organ containing a muscular layer called the detrusor muscle. The detrusor muscle is an intricate meshwork of circularly arranged smooth muscle fibers sandwiched between longitudinal bundles. This arrangement allows the bladder to expand and contract in all directions.

Urination has two requirements: the storage of urine and the expulsion of urine. The bladder and urethra function as a single unit. When the bladder fills, the detrusor remains quiet and relaxed under sympathomimetic control. When bladder capacity is reached, urgency is experienced until voiding is accomplished. During micturition the parasympathetic tone is activated via acetylcholine receptors and the detrusor contracts voluntarily, the only smooth muscle organ in our bodies under volitional control. Thus the bladder sphincter tightens under alpha-adrenergic influence, and the detrusor relaxes under beta-adrenergic influence.

The sphincter of the bladder is the entire length of the urethra (a functional sphincter rather than a true anatomic sphincter). During emptying, the detrusor contracts and the urethra actively relaxes. During voiding, the pelvic floor musculature relaxes and the vesicourethral angle changes to permit full drainage. Conversely, continence (storage of urine) requires pelvic floor tautness. Thus stress incontinence is usually associated with pelvic floor relaxation.

The urethra is about 4 cm long in women. The smooth muscle layers of the urethra form a functional internal sphincter. The striated muscle external sphincter allows voluntary interruption of voiding and provides a mechanism to empty the urethra after the internal sphincter has closed.

The process of voiding begins with activation of a reflex arc between the detrusor and the brain indicating a sensation of bladder fullness. The brain then amplifies bladder contraction by parasympathetic stimulation. The net effect of vesicourethral innervation is to communicate bladder volume to the brain. When a critical degree of bladder distension is reached, the detrusor muscle contracts, unless inhibited by higher brain centers.

Urinary Incontinence

Classification	Treatment
Urge Incontinence (Detrusor Instability) —inability to inhibit reflex bladder contractions in response to filling	Focus on cause: infection, mucosal atrophy, CNS disease, irradiation. Behavioral bladder retraining, drug therapy includes estrogen, anticholinergics.
Stress Incontinence —sphincter insufficiency	Kegel exercises, surgical treatment, pessary
Overflow Incontinence —obstruction or impaired sensation	Catheter, alpha-adrenergic antagonists
Functional Incontinence —inability to reach the toilet	Improve mobility or cognition which prevent normal voiding, avoid drugs.

Urge Incontinence (Detrusor Instability). Urge incontinence occurs when a woman senses the need (the urge) to urinate but cannot inhibit leakage before reaching the bathroom. This is the most common type (70%) of incontinence in elderly women. Detrusor instability is associated with reduced bladder capacity because of excessive, inappropriate detrusor contraction. In elderly women, a significant contribution to this problem is loss of cortical inhibition of detrusor contraction, hence this type of incontinence is seen with CNS conditions such as stroke, Alzheimer's disease, tumors, and Parkinson's disease. Peripheral causes include hypoestrogenic atrophy, obstruction, bladder irritation due to infection or irradiation, fecal impaction, diabetic neuropathy, and spinal cord lesions secondary to degenerative joint disease or herniation of a disc. Symptoms include frequent episodes of urgency, nocturnal wetting, and normal volumes of urine (residual volume is small). This is the most common problem associated with estrogen-deficient atrophy of genitourinary mucosa.

Genuine Stress Incontinence. Genuine stress incontinence (loss of urine with coughing or physical activity) is the result of increased bladder pressure and decreased urethral resistance. The most common cause of urinary incontinence in women is pelvic floor relaxation. But any condition which alters the usual pressure differential between bladder and urethra can cause stress incontinence, e.g. abdominal tumors or chronic pulmonary disease. Women are especially sensitive to intraabdominal pressure changes because one-half to two-thirds of the urethra is intraabdominal. Symptoms include loss of urine with straining, normal volumes, no nocturnal wetting, and small residual volumes.

Overflow Incontinence.   Overflow incontinence is due to obstruction (mainly in men due to prostatic hypertrophy) or impaired sensation. The bladder is hypotonic and distended. Detrusor insufficiency can occur due to neurogenic injuries or peripheral neuropathy. This is a condition commonly encountered with medications (anticholinergics and antidepressants). The patient reports incomplete emptying, slow flow, and a need to strain, and there is a large residual volume (over 100 ml). Leakage of small amounts of urine is frequent through the day and night without the sensation of need to void or the sense of fullness. *The bladder is usually palpable after voiding.*

History and
Examination

Urinary incontinence is an important problem in older women. It can contribute to decubitus ulcers, psychosocial isolation and depression, and frequent urinary tract infections. An accurate history is usually sufficient to distinguish genuine stress incontinence from urge incontinence. Inspection and palpation of the anterior vaginal wall and urethra should be performed at rest and during the Valsalva maneuver. A quick neurologic assessment of the sacral nerves can be accomplished by tapping the clitoral glans or labia minora. This should elicit reflex contraction of the anal sphincter. Failure to do so warrants full neurologic evaluation.

Important Historical Information:

1. Type of incontinence: urge, stress, overflow, functional.

2. Frequency, severity, duration.

3. Symptoms (dysuria, dribbling).

4. Medications.

5. Other illnesses, mental state.

Incontinence with coughing is a reliable test confirming the presence of genuine stress incontinence due to sphincter weakness. Genuine stress incontinence is associated with normal cystometry, normal residual volumes, normal bladder capacity, and the absence of involuntary bladder contractions. Most women with stress incontinence have a cystocele. In the past, the Bonney test was utilized to predict a favorable response to surgery. In the Bonney test, two fingers are placed along the urethra, pressing upwards to stop the incontinence. The Bonney test is no longer considered reliable, as urodynamic testing has revealed that urethral mechanical obstruction is produced, obviously yielding a good effect.

Important Parts of the Examination:

1. Examine with straining.

2. Palpate bladder after voiding.

3. Pelvic examination (atrophy, prolapse).

4. Rectal examination (fecal impaction).

5. Neurologic examination (perineal sensation, anal sphincter tone).

213

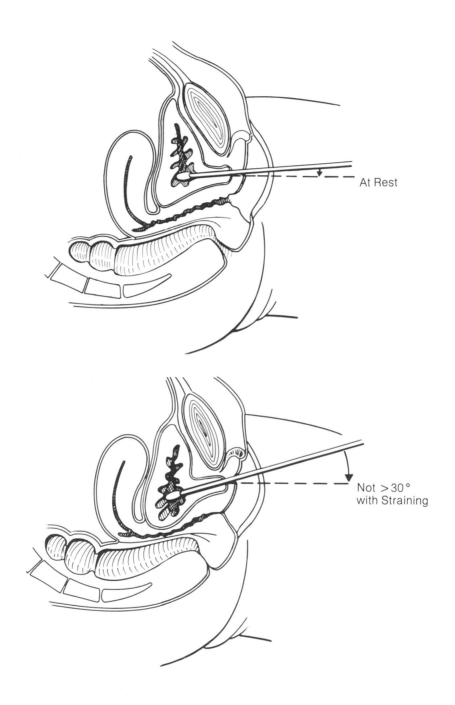

At Rest

Not > 30°
with Straining

214

Since control of the anal sphincter is similar to that of the bladder, the autonomic reflex arc can be tested by assessing anal tone on examination, including voluntary sphincter contraction.

Perineal Sensation	Autonomic Reflex Tone	Problem
Present	Absent	Motor neuron lesion
Absent	Present	Reflex incontinence: diabetes mellitus, multiple sclerosis, cord injury
Absent	Absent	Overflow incontinence: neurologic injuries
Present	Present	Urge incontinence, genuine stress incontinence, overflow incontinence

The Q-Tip Test. The Q-tip test assesses the degree of urethral mobility. A lubricated cotton-tipped applicator is introduced into the urethra. At rest, the angle of the applicator with the floor is about 10°. With straining, the angle should not exceed 30°. This test has been claimed to be abnormal in 95% of patients with genuine stress incontinence. (5) It is significantly correlated with the presence of a cystocele. Excessive movement is due to urethral mobility secondary to relaxation of the vesicourethral angle.

Laboratory Tests

Only a few office tests and procedures are necessary for the vast majority of women with urinary incontinence. Urinalysis and culture are indicated to screen for the presence of infection. Women with overflow incontinence should be tested for syphilis. The residual volume is a helpful discriminator for the various diagnostic categories. Pelvic ultrasound can be used if straight catheterization is unacceptable. The normal residual volume is less than 50 ml.

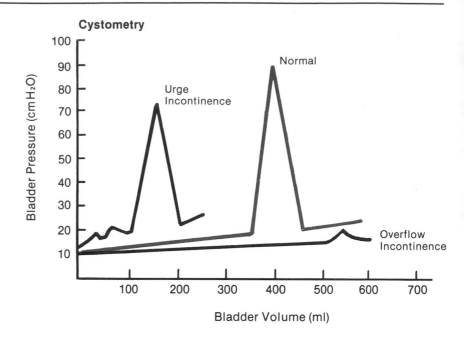

Cystometry

Bladder Pressure (cm H₂O) — y-axis labeled: $Bladder\ Pressure\ (cm\ H_2O)$

Bladder Volume (ml)

Office cystometry is easy to perform and provides important information. After voiding, insert a 16 F Foley catheter; measure the residual volume. Use a recording cystometer or a central venous pressure monitor zeroed at the level of the bladder to record pressures. Fill the system with sterile saline, then begin a continuous flow of the saline into the bladder. The patient is asked to report the sensation of fullness and the urge to void. The following responses are normal and can be compared with abnormal responses in the figure:

NORMAL CYSTOMETRY

Normal sense of bladder filling: 100–200 ml.
Desire to void: 250–300 ml.
Detrusor contraction: 400–600 ml (functional capacity).

Urge incontinence is the commonest type in the elderly, and detrusor motor instability is the commonest finding on cystometry. The bladder with detrusor instability contracts spontaneously, although provocation (coughing, bladder tapping) may be necessary in that simple filling is often insufficient to stimulate contractions. Despite the patient's attempts, the contractions cannot be inhibited. With full urodynamic studies, abnormalities in urethral pressure profiles consistent with genuine stress incontinence are found in 30–40% of ambulatory incontinent elderly women. (1) In institutionalized elderly, the same variety of causes for incontinence is found, including patients with dementia and/or immobility. (6) Appropriate treatment, therefore, requires accurate diagnosis.

Incontinence is common immediately after a stroke. Incontinence persisting 3–12 months after a stroke is usually due to detrusor hyperreflexia (urge incontinence). The same finding occurs in 75% of cases of urinary incontinence in women with Parkinson's disease.

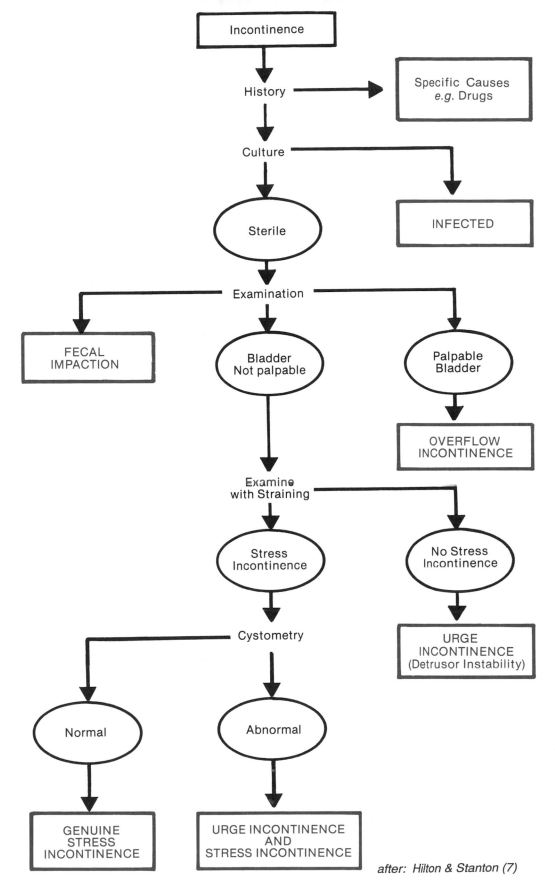

after: Hilton & Stanton (7)

The value and cost-effectiveness of urodynamic testing in the elderly have been questioned. (7,8) Furthermore, urodynamic studies are not absolutely accurate. Many elderly continent women have abnormal studies, and some incontinent patients have normal urodynamics. Straight-forward clinical evaluation according to the algorithm is sufficient. The accuracy of the Q-tip test has also been questioned. It is not necessary for diagnosis, and in the algorithm, it is not included.

The purpose of the algorithm is to identify the small number of incontinent women who truly need urodynamic tests. The simple flow plan readily separates those patients who can be treated medically and those who need referral to surgical colleagues. There are several useful key points.

KEY POINTS IN THE INCONTINENCE ALGORITHM

1. A palpable bladder identifies essentially all patients with overflow incontinence. These patients should have urodynamic studies to rule out obstruction.

2. Only 40% of patients require cystometry. The remainder can be managed by history and examination.

3. Urodynamic studies are indicated for treatment failures.

Approximately one-third of elderly incontinent patients have an acute problem. Recovery can be achieved within a few weeks when attention is directed to the elimination of reversible causes such as infection, drug overdosage, acute illnesses, hyperglycemia, fecal impaction, and mucosal atrophy. In the remainder of patients, over one half can be cured or substantially improved. (1,9,10)

Estrogen replacement therapy is very successful in reversing mucosal atrophy. Both patient and physician should be aware that a significant response can be expected in one month, but it takes up to 6–12 months to fully restore the genitourinary mucosa. Do not be discouraged by an apparent lack of immediate response.

Treatment of Urge Incontinence. Often no specific cause of urge incontinence is found and detrusor instability is best treated empirically with antispasmodic drugs (after first making sure the problem is not due to mucosal atrophy, which is easily reversed with estrogen). Anticholinergic agents decrease detrusor contractions, increase bladder capacity, decrease urgency, and improve incontinence. Unfortunately the severity of side effects is a problem in older women. Side effects include confusion, agitation, orthostatic hypotension, dry mouth, and delayed gastric emptying. The dosage must be titrated carefully. One can produce increased residual volumes at high doses (which would aggravate the condition). Imipramine and bladder retraining should be the first approach. If one drug fails, try another. Results are unpredictable and can be dramatic. Combining low doses of two agents with complementary actions, such as oxybutynin and imipramine, will maximize the benefit and minimize side effects. Propantheline is best avoided in patients with dementia or in patients on other anticholinergic agents.

Bladder Training. The basic principle underlying bladder training protocols is improvement of central nervous system control of micturition, although changes in bladder capacity could also be a contributing factor. Cure rates for urge incontinence (detrusor instability) range from 44% to 97%. (10) Training protocols appear to be better than drug therapy when conscientious and dedicated participants are involved. Indeed, under such circumstances, the addition of drug therapy does not improve results. Studies indicate that behavioral training is very effective when combined with biofeedback and verbal feedback.

Bladder Retraining Protocols:

1. Bladder Training—progressive extension of the interval between voiding, aiming for 3–4 hours.

2. Habit Retraining—a schedule of toilet use adjusted to timed episodes of incontinence and desire to void.

3. Timed Voiding—voiding is always at a fixed time.

4. Prompted Voiding—usually for institutionalized patients; assistance is offered when patient perceives need to void.

   There is no evidence that training approaches are useful for overflow incontinence, and the impact on genuine stress incontinence is a minor one (probably due to strengthening of the pelvic floor muscles). However, a significant number of older incontinent women have detrusor instability with urge symptoms, and therefore, there is a real place for training protocols. Those incontinent women with detrusor instability without urge symptoms have a lower success rate with bladder training.

Treatment of Overflow Incontinence. Treatment is usually directed to surgical correction of a lesion causing obstruction. If there is no obstruction problem, drug therapy is utilized in an empiric fashion.

Treatment of Genuine Stress Incontinence. The long-term surgical correction rate for genuine stress incontinence is approximately 70% for the primary procedure. (11) However, if a cystocele is not greater than first degree, a good response can be anticipated with Kegel exercises. (12) Kegel exercises are isometric exercises which strengthen the levator ani and pubococcygeal muscles. The exercise is simple: contraction of the pelvic floor muscles consists of closing the anal sphincter and shutting off the flow of urine in midstream. Once learned, *use the 5–10 rule:* the contraction should be maintained for 5–10 seconds, and repeated a minimum of 5–10 times per day. Kegel exercises have classically been considered to be less effective in postmenopausal women. However, Kegel exercises combined with estrogen replacement therapy may prove to be effective, and it is worth trying.

Relief of incontinence can be obtained by support of pelvic relaxation with a vaginal pessary. Urodynamic studies indicate that a pessary stabilizes the urethra and the vesicourethral junction, and increases urethral functional length. (13) A pessary does not block or obstruct the flow of urine, but restores continence by supporting the urethra and the base of the bladder.

Alpha-adrenergic agonists have been shown to improve stress incontinence in a significant number of older women. This is worth trying in women who are not candidates for surgery. Most clinicians report that imipramine is the single most effective bladder relaxant in elderly women. Imipramine has the unique combination of alpha-adrenergic stimulation and anticholinergic activity. This is especially useful in combined detrusor instability and stress incontinence. Pure stress or urge incontinence is unusual in the very old. More often it is a mixed picture. It makes sense to first try a pharmacologic approach, an approach reported to be successful in the majority of cases, thus avoiding surgery. (14) Combining the alpha-adrenergic agent with estrogen replacement therapy may be even more effective, although it is argued that genuine stress incontinence is not affected by treatment with estrogen. (15) On the other hand, others argue that estrogen improves or cures genuine stress incontinence in over 50% of patients due to a direct effect on the urethral mucosa. (16) Bladder capacities under 300 ml or over 800 ml contraindicate the surgical approach.

Drug Therapy for Incontinence

Drugs	Dose	Action
Urge Incontinence:		
Imipramine (Tofranil)	10–25 mg qhs to qid	Decreases detrusor tone, increases sphincter tone
Oxybutynin (Ditropan)	2.5–5.0 mg qhs to qid	Decreases detrusor tone
Flavoxate (Urispas)	100–200 mg bid to qid	Decreases detrusor tone
Propantheline (Norpanth, Pro-Banthine)	7.5–15.0 mg bid to qid	Decreases detrusor tone
Estrogen	See Chapter 5	Removes atrophy as irritant
Overflow Incontinence:		
Bethanechol (Urecholine)	5–25 mg bid to qid	Increases detrusor tone
Prazosin	1–5 mg bid to qid	Decreases sphincter tone
Phenoxybenzamine	10 mg qhs	Decreases sphincter tone
Stress Incontinence:		
Imipramine (Tofranil)	10–25 mg qhs to qid	Decreases detrusor tone, increases sphincter tone
Phenylpropanolamine	25 mg daily to qid	Increases sphincter tone

Long-Term Catheterization. As a last resort, an indwelling catheter may be necessary to solve the problem of urinary incontinence in very old patients. (17) Because of the potential for complications, this is not a trivial decision. Even with a closed collecting system, bacteriuria is the major complication, although it may take 30 or more days for its development. Other complications of chronic use include stones, vesicoureteral reflux, cystitis, and nephritis.

Once inserted, the catheter should be replaced only for leakage or obstruction that cannot be corrected by flushing the catheter. Obstruction can occur due to precipitated crystals associated with urinary tract infections. Long-term catheterization leads to polymicrobial bacteriuria with both familiar and less common pathogens. Because of its inevitability and prevalence, bacteriuria need be assessed by urine cultures only in the presence of signs of illness, such as fever or deterioration.

Not every episode of fever requires treatment. Women with long-term, indwelling catheters have occasional febrile episodes that are low-grade and self-limited. High temperatures are more serious and are associated with a significant risk of death. Mild fever should be treated if it persists beyond 24 hours, and temperatures $\geq 102°$ should be treated immediately.

Careful maintenance of the closed system is necessary to prevent bacterial entry. There is no advantage to putting antibacterial substances in the collection bag or along the catheter. Nor is there any reduction in bacteriuria utilizing irrigations of the catheter, either continuous or intermittent. Prophylactic antibiotics only yield resistant organisms.

Urinary Tract Infections

Clinical studies have generally supported empiric treatment for acute, uncomplicated urinary tract infections. From a cost-effective point of view, it is acceptable to omit a culture in this circumstance. The drugs of choice are trimethoprim, trimethoprim/sulfamethoxazole, nitrofurantoin, and sulfa. Ampicillin is not recommended for first-line therapy.

It is important to identify patients with recurrent infections because of the significant risk of renal impairment. Urinary tract infections are usually secondary to stepwise colonization of the vaginal introitus and urethral mucosa by uropathogenic organisms from the rectal flora. Bacterial adherence to epithelial receptors is an important part of the mechanism. Although not documented, it is likely that estrogen replacement therapy will reduce the frequency of urine infections in the postmenopausal years because of its support of a normal vaginal flora.

Women with recurrent infections should have urologic evaluation, including urography and cystoscopy, to identify correctable causes for reinfection, e.g. a urethral diverticulum. The urethral diverticulum is probably an acquired problem following trauma, catheterization, labor and delivery, or infections. The classic symptoms are dysuria, post-voiding dribbling, and a purulent exudate expressible from the urethra. Surgical repair is necessary.

A midstream clean catch specimen which yields a positive result should be confirmed by a urine sample obtained by catheterization. (Single catheterization for diagnostic purposes should be followed by single dose prophylaxis of an antimicrobial agent). The traditional requirement for a colony count of 100,000 or more per ml is no longer acceptable. Lower counts (as low as 100/ml) can be associated with significant infections.

Recurrent reinfection should be given a course of low-dose prophylaxis (maintained for at least 6 months). (18) An agent must be used that has no risk of causing resistance in the fecal flora.

Agents for Low-Dose Prophylaxis

1. Nitrofurantoin 100 mg qhs.

2. Cephalexin 250 mg qhs.

3. Trimethoprim-sulfamethoxazole (Bactrim, Cotrim, Septra) 40–200 mg qhs or trimethoprim 50 mg qhs.

4. Cinoxacin 250–500 mg qhs.

For difficult, recalcitrant cases, the patient can be educated to utilize self-start therapy. Treatment follows the demonstration of infection with one of the home testing kits. A 3 day full dose, empirical broad spectrum antimicrobial agent is used. Full doses of nitrofurantoin, cinoxacin, or norfloxacin are recommended. Ampicillin, tetracycline, sulfisoxazole, and cephalexin all should be avoided because of the propensity for resistant bacteria. Bacteriuria persistent 10 days after treatment requires follow-up evaluation.

Asymptomatic Bacteriuria. Asymptomatic bacteriuria (a colony count greater than 100,000/ml in asymptomatic patients) is more common in older women. A lack of estrogen lowers the vaginal pH, promoting colonization of the vagina by uropathogens. Pelvic floor relaxation can lead to urinary tract obstruction and incomplete voiding. It is not cost-effective to routinely culture all older women. However, if asymptomatic bacteriuria is identified, single-dose antibiotic therapy is worthwhile: 3 tablets of double-strength trimethoprim sulfamethoxazole (Bactrim DS, Septra DS) or 3 gm of amoxicillin.

References

1. **Ouslander JG, Hepps K, Raz S, Su H-L,** Genitourinary dysfunction in a geriatric outpatient population, J Am Geriatrics Soc 34:507, 1986.

2. **Bichet DG, Schrier RW,** Renal function and diseases in the aged, in Schrier RW, editor, *Clinical Internal Medicine in the Aged*, W.B. Saunders Co., Philadelphia, 1982, pp 211–221.

3. **Cocroft DW, Gault MH,** Prediction of creatinine clearance from serum creatinine, Nephron 16:31, 1976.

4. **Morley GW, DeLancey JOL,** Sacrospinous ligament fixation for eversion of the vagina, Am J Obstet Gynecol 158:872, 1988.

5. **Karram MM, Bhatia NN,** The Q-tip test: Standardization of the technique and its interpretation in women with urinary incontinence, Obstet Gynecol 71:807, 1988.

6. **Resnick NM, Yalla SV, Laurino E,** The pathophysiology of urinary incontinence among institutionalized elderly persons, New Engl J Med 320:1, 1989.

7. **Hilton P, Stanton SL,** Algorithmic method for assessing urinary incontinence in elderly women, Brit Med J 282:940, 1981.

8. **Williams ME, Pannill FC III,** Urinary incontinence in the elderly, Ann Intern Med 97:895, 1982.

9. **Resnick NM, Yalla SV,** Management of urinary incontinence in the elderly, New Engl J Med 313:800, 1985.

10. **Hadley EC,** Bladder training and related therapies for urinary incontinence in older people, JAMA 256:372, 1986.

11. **Park GS, Miller EJ Jr,** Surgical treatment of stress urinary incontinence: A comparison of the Kelly plication, Marshall-Marchetti-Krantz, and Pereyra procedures, Obstet Gynecol 71:575, 1988.

12. **Burgio KL, Robinson FJC, Engel BT,** The role of biofeedback in Kegel exercise training for stress urinary incontinence, Am J Obstet Gynecol 154:58, 1986.

13. **Bhatia NN, Bergman A, Gunning JE,** Urodynamic effects of a vaginal pessary in women with stress urinary incontinence, Am J Obstet Gynecol 147:876, 1983.

14. **Karram MM, Bhatia NN,** Management of coexistent stress and urge urinary incontinence, Obstet Gynecol 73:4, 1989.

15. **Wilson PD, Faragher B, Butler B, Bullock D, Robinson EL, Brown ADG,** Treatment with oral piperazine oestrone sulphate for genuine stress incontinence in postmenopausal women, Brit J Obstet Gynaecol 94:568, 1987.

16. **Bhatia NN, Bergman A, Karram MM,** Effects of estrogen on urethral function in women with urinary incontinence, Obstet Gynecol 160:176, 1989.

17. **Muncie HL Jr, Warren JW,** Long-term urethral catheters in older women, Am Fam Physician 37:103, 1988.

18. **Schaeffer AJ,** Recurrent urinary tract infections in women, Postgrad Med 81:51, 1987.

14

The External Genitalia

Vulvovaginal problems in postmenopausal women are to a significant degree influenced by the absence of estrogen. But not all problems should be attributed to a lack of estrogen. Infections and specific lesions do occur in older women, and every effort must be made to obtain a specific diagnosis in order to prescribe specific treatment. Almost all of the vulvovaginal problems which bring a postmenopausal woman to a physician can be easily diagnosed in the office and promptly and effectively managed.

For a detailed description of vulvar lesions (along with excellent pictures), the textbook by E.G. Friedrich Jr, *Vulvar Disease*, is highly recommended. (1) This is a book beautifully written for the clinician, a classic in its own time which endures because of its timeless lessons and practical value.

We will first consider the vaginal and vulvar changes which occur with aging, then review the clinical problems of vulvovaginitis, vulvar disorders, and vulvodynia.

Changes with Aging

In the absence of estrogen, the vaginal epithelium is thin, undifferentiated into the well-recognized layers (basal, intermediate, and superficial) characteristic of the reproductive years. Estrogen is also responsible for the deposition of glycogen in the vaginal epithelium, mainly in the superficial cells. The superficial cells are a direct reflection of estrogen stimulation and provide a protective function for the vagina.

The absence of glycogen-containing superficial cells results in a decreased production of lactic and acetic acids. During the reproductive years, the vaginal flora utilize glycogen and its metabolic products in a dynamic equilibrium which must be maintained to prevent symptomatic problems. The normal flora consist largely of lactobacilli and acidogenic corynebacteria in large numbers which overwhelm and hold in check the small numbers of fungi present. The normal low vaginal pH (3.8–4.2) is the result of the acids produced by the vaginal flora, thus maintaining a milieu which favors the continued growth of the normal flora.

In the absence of estrogen, the superficial layer becomes thinner and fails to differentiate into mature glycogen-producing forms. Consequently the vagina is not acidic (pH 6.5–7.5). The vagina assumes a characteristic pale, atrophic appearance (thin, dry, and shiny), and

225

the discharge is scanty and yellowish. The most common cause of postmenopausal bleeding due to benign conditions is atrophic vaginitis (followed by cervical polyps). Other symptoms include dyspareunia, pruritus, and urinary complaints (urgency, frequency, dysuria). A commonly voiced complaint by menopausal and postmenopausal women is vaginal dryness.

Vaginal dryness due to the loss of estrogen-supported lubrication directly leads to the symptoms of vaginitis, vaginismus, and dyspareunia. Vaginal fluid production is estrogen-dependent and significantly mediated by maintenance of vaginal blood flow. (2) It is important for both physicians and patients to know that restoration to a normal estrogen state requires 6–12 months of therapy. Also of practical note, the assessment of vaginal cytology is not useful. Variations in interpretation, as well as the exquisite sensitivity of the mucosal pattern to estrogen, make it impossible to judge estrogen need or dosage by vaginal cytology (known as the maturation index).

Vulvovaginitis

The Ecosystem

The vaginal environment is a dynamic system influenced by the secretions of the epithelial cells, the pH, the hormonal milieu, trauma, coitus, and the microbial flora. (3) In an estrogen-supported vagina, the superficial epithelial cells have a high glycogen content. The normal flora of the vagina utilize this rich supply of glycogen, and as a result of the organic acids produced, the normal pH of the vagina is acidic (pH 3.8–4.2). This acidic pH inhibits the overgrowth of pathogens. After menopause, without estrogenic support, the epithelium becomes atrophic, leading to a decrease in the acid production and an increase in pH to 7.0. Such a vagina is subject to increased colonization with anaerobic organisms. Maintenance of an acidic pH is an important benefit of estrogen replacement therapy. As with restoration of lubrication, maximal acidic pH normalization can require a year of treatment.

Vaginal lubrication and an acidic pH are also maintained to some degree by sexual activity. This is probably due to maintenance of vaginal vascularity.

The cervical mucus and the menstrual flow are alkaline, providing better growth media for pathogens. Coitus and sexual excitement also raise the vaginal pH and can predispose to vaginitis.

Candidiasis

Candida organisms grow well in the normal acidic pH of the vagina. Control of their growth depends heavily upon the presence of the other organisms in the normal vaginal flora. The disruption of the normal pH or the normal flora (e.g with the use of broad-spectrum antibiotics or immunosuppressive agents) allows the growth of a foreign bacteria or the overgrowth of *Candida*. *Candida* species are opportunists; their growth to the point of vaginitis follows escape from inhibition by the normal flora. *Candida albicans* is the most common fungus, with *Candida glabrata* a distal second. *C. glabrata*, as with other *Candida* species, is more resistant to the usual treatment, but more sensitive to gentian violet. *Candida* species other than *C. albicans* are probably associated with chronicity and recurrence.

Symptoms. The major complaint is almost always pruritus, followed by burning and dysuria, and a vaginal discharge. Burning after intercourse is a characteristic symptom.

Discharge. The discharge, classically thick, white or yellow and curdlike, is not always prominent. It usually has a noticeable odor.

Diagnosis. In most postmenopausal women, vaginal candidiasis is due to antibiotic treatment, diabetes mellitus, or the recent initiation of hormone replacement. An erythematous (sometimes shiny) appearance of the vagina and vulva is the usual finding. When found on the vulva, *Candida* are always present in the vagina and require intravaginal treatment. The vaginal pH is 4.0 to 4.5. *Note: If the pH is 4.5 or less, the patient either has Candida or a normal discharge. If symptoms are present, an infection with Candida is inevitably present.* The standard diagnostic tool consists of the vaginal smear, both the saline smear (to detect other pathogens) and the KOH smear (to lyse cellular material and allow *Candida* to stand out). The microscopic examination reveals budding filaments and spores with *C. albicans*, while only spores will be seen with *C. glabrata*.

The smears are often unrewarding and in obvious contrast to the presenting complaints. Empiric treatment is worthwhile, but it is helpful to have tubes of Nickerson's media in the office. Inoculation and culture at room temperature will yield a definitive answer within a day or two. However, a sufficient number of organisms can be present to yield a recurrent infection but at the same time this number can be insufficient to produce a colony on culture. Furthermore, significant infection can be present with minimal discharge and a normal-appearing vagina.

Treatment. The first line of treatment consists of one of the imidazole drugs or terconazole, used as vaginal creams or suppositories. While 3-day courses of treatment (2 suppositories qhs) have become popular and their effectiveness has been supported by clinical trials, clinical experience still indicates that longer treatment schedules (administration bid for 7–14 days) are more effective with lower recurrence rates.

As a last resort, an old tried and true treatment is recommended for resistant and recurrent *Candida* infections: gentian violet applied topically. The cervix, vagina, introitus, and inner vulva are painted with a 1% aqueous solution of gentian violet; residual liquid should be removed. Gentian violet impregnated in tampons or as a vaginal suppository is not as effective. Repeat treatment need not be more frequent than weekly, and usually no more than once or twice. It is equally effective against *C. albicans* and *C. glabrata*. The messy nature of this treatment is well accepted by patients in return for its rapid and effective results. The main problem is a stubborn stain on clothing, so be careful (ammonia and alcohol are only partially effective in removing stains, but the stains disappear with washing in bleach).

What to do for really resistant and recurrent cases. First make sure that other contributing factors are recognized and if possible eliminated or controlled. This includes diabetes mellitus, the use of antibiotics, oral-genital contact, and immune suppression. Then use continuous therapy for 3–4 weeks. It is not absolutely certain that treatment of a partner is helpful, but there is a high colonization rate with the same species in consorts of women with recurrent infections. For that reason, in extreme cases, both partners should be treated with an oral agent (Ketoconazole 400 mg daily for 14 days) to decrease the candidal reservoir in the gastrointestinal tract and the oral cavity as well as for its systemic action. In addition, the male partner should be given an imidazole cream to use daily during the woman's period of treatment. For the really recalcitrant chronic problem, provide the patient with long-term antifungal suppression, give ketoconazole, half a tablet (100 mg) daily for 6–12 months. (4) But note, liver enzymes must be monitored with long-term ketoconazole therapy. Finally, cryo treatment of the cervix should be given empirical consideration. Routine laundering does not destroy yeast. In recalcitrant cases, it is worth treating underwear, either by boiling, soaking overnight in bleach, or exposure in a high-intensity microwave oven for 5 minutes.

Bacterial Vaginosis

In 1984, a new term was introduced, bacterial vaginosis. This condition is a bacterial vaginitis due to a variety of bacteria, including *Gardnerella vaginalis* (previously called *Haemophilus vaginalis* and *Corynebacterium vaginale*), as well as a newly recognized anaerobic rod named *Mobiluncus*. The prevalence of *G. vaginalis* in symptomatic and asymptomatic women has cast doubt on its etiologic significance as a single agent of infection. Bacterial vaginosis probably represents mixed infections due to an overgrowth of naturally occurring flora, including *G. vaginalis* and *Mobiluncus*, as well as anaerobes of the *Bacteroides* and *Peptococcus* species.

Symptoms. This infection is associated with a characteristic fishy odor due to the presence of amines produced by anaerobic bacteria in an alkaline vagina. Thus this odor may be noticed following intercourse with the introduction of alkaline semen.

Discharge. The discharge is thin, gray and homogeneous (and sometimes frothy).

Diagnosis. The vagina shows little inflammatory response because there is no invasion of the vaginal tissue (thus the term vaginosis rather than vaginitis), and hence, there are no complaints of pruritus or burning. The pH is 4.5 to 6.0. "Clue cells" are vaginal epithelial cells which appear intensely stippled with coccobacilli as the numerous bacteria that are present attach themselves to the surfaces of sloughed epithelial cells. They are no longer considered to be pathognomonic for *G. vaginalis*; however, clue cells are an indicator of pathogenic bacterial vaginosis.

Treatment. The most effective treatment is metronidazole (500 mg bid for 7 days). Intolerance to alcohol while on metronidazole is a well-recognized side effect. The single dose method is definitely less effective. Clindamycin, 300 mg tid for 7 days, is also effective. Oral ampicillin or Keflex can be utilized (500 mg qid for 7 days), but effectiveness is reduced (50–65%). In patients with frequent recurrence, try using the 2% clindamycin cream (available as a preparation for acne) given intravaginally for 7 nights. An old standard, sulfa vaginal creams, is now known to be totally ineffective. (5) Metronidazole treatment of the partner is probably worthwhile with multiple recurrent infections, although studies on the effectiveness of this treatment have not reached consistent conclusions. Women with bacterial vaginosis who undergo hysterectomy are at increased risk for postoperative infection; when present, preoperative treatment is indicated.

Trichomonas Vaginitis

This flagellated protozoa may continue to be a problem for older women in whom the vagina is maintained by hormone replacement therapy. *Trichomonas vaginalis* lives quietly in the paraurethral glands, seeding the vagina and growing optimally in an alkaline pH. (6)

Symptoms. The cardinal symptom is a discharge, and sometimes urinary symptoms are caused by trichomonads. Itching and burning are more characteristic of *Candida*, but can occur with *Trichomonas* infection.

Discharge. The discharge is usually copious, malodorous, white, gray, or greenish. It is usually, but not always, frothy due to the carbon dioxide produced by the organisms.

Diagnosis. The vagina is erythematous. The pH is between 5 and 7. With a pH exceeding 6.0, an infection is almost always due to trichomonads. Those conditions associated with bacterial infections also encourage the growth of trichomonads. The traditional wet mount examination is insensitive, positive only 60% of the time in women with culture-proven infections. New office methods utilizing monoclonal antibodies are superior for accuracy of diagnosis. (7) Until such methods are widely available, there is room for empirical treatment. Indeed, a course of empirical treatment will be more cost effective than repeated efforts at trying to establish a specific diagnosis. It is further worth noting that the identification of trichomonads on Pap smear is not always accurate, and an active infection may not be present.

Treatment. The treatment of choice is metronidazole given either in a short course to both partners (4 tablets, 1000 mg, in the AM, repeated once in the PM) or in a longer course (500 mg bid for 7 days). For recurrent cases resistant to treatment, consider high dose treatment (500 mg qid or 1000 mg bid, plus 500 mg bid given vaginally). The main toxicity risk is peripheral neuropathy. Minor side effects consist of a metallic taste and occasionally vomiting or diarrhea, all of which can be aggravated by alcohol ingestion. For those patients who cannot take metronidazole, topical treatment for 14 days should be prescribed, utilizing Vagisec suppositories or douche.

| Atrophic Vaginitis | A truly atrophic vagina rarely supports infections. Although the usual infections can occur, it is more common that streptococci, gut anaerobes, and coliform bacteria are found in the atrophic, alkaline environment. |

Hormone replacement is the treatment of choice, but a more rapid response can be assured by the temporary addition of vaginal estrogen cream (nightly for 2 weeks). Under the influence of estrogen, the squamous epithelium of the vagina once more becomes many layers thick and the cells rich in glycogen. In the meantime, specific treatment for specific infections can be utilized as noted above.

Older women, beginning estrogen treatment after a lengthy post-menopausal interval, should be cautioned that normal vaginal secretions will return. This "discharge" will be white and opaque, asymptomatic other than wetness, and associated with a normal pH (3.8–4.2). Unnecessary treatment may upset the vaginal ecological balance, yielding a true vaginitis.

Vulvar Disorders

Women should be instructed in vulvar self-examination. This examination should be performed once a month in conjunction with breast self-examination. A hand held mirror is necessary in order to detect moles, warts, ulcers, sores, or changes in pigmentation. The management of vulvar lesions by physicians also requires careful looking, and a readiness to biopsy. Historical information, however, can provide a tip to diagnosis. Even in the absence of an allergic history, attention should be directed to soaps, fabrics, and dyes (e.g. perfumed toilet paper). The patient may not link the vulvar symptoms to other problems such as urinary incontinence or diarrhea.

A magnifying glass (2–4X) is a handy instrument to keep in the examining room. Subtle changes and small lesions need magnification. The colposcope is not useful; it is too focused and time-consuming.

Toluidine blue dye (1% aqueous solution) fixes to the nuclei of cells. Dilute acetic acid (1% aqueous solution applied 3 minutes after the dye) decolorizes any dye not bound to nuclear material. Because there are no surface nuclei on a normal vulva, no blue stain remains on the normal skin surface. The presence of a blue stain indicates the presence of nuclei. This change can be seen in both benign and malignant lesions, and the toluidine blue dye is used to direct a biopsy. While this test is useful, it is not absolute. *Anything that doesn't look right, no matter what the appearance, should be biopsied.*

The vulvar biopsy is best performed with the Keyes dermal punch (also available as the disposable Baker's biopsy punch, Key Pharmaceuticals, Inc, Miami, FL 33169 or the Acu-Punch, Acuderm, Fort Lauderdale, FL 33309) to remove a small core of tissue. The vulva is richly innervated and local infiltration with a small needle and a local anesthetic is necessary. Hemostasis can be achieved with silver nitrate sticks; a suture is rarely required.

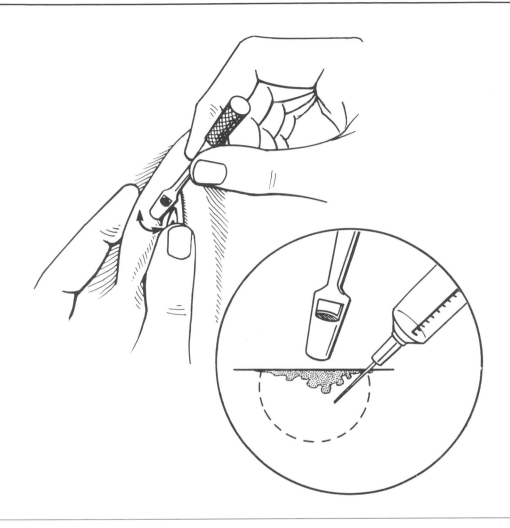

White Lesions

The vulvar dystrophies (white lesions) consist of a spectrum extending from atrophic to hypertrophic lesions, with a common symptom of pruritus. ***These conditions are now classified under the pathologic heading of "nonneoplastic epithelial disorders of skin and mucosa," which replaces the old dystrophy terminology.*** The whiteness is typical of a hyperkeratotic area of the skin which is moist. In addition, these lesions are characterized by loss of skin pigment and decreased vascularity, also contributing to the loss of color. In the past, white lesions of the vulva (leukoplakia is a term no longer used) were erroneously considered to be all premalignant. However, atypia is found in only 5% of nonneoplastic vulvar disorders, and most are mild and respond to medical treatment. *Nevertheless, all white lesions should be biopsied to detect the presence of atypia and for accuracy of diagnosis in order to direct the correct treatment. The dystrophies are best defined by their histology.* A final important clinical note: be sure to examine all vulvar disorders periodically in order to ascertain response to treatment and to detect any unfavorable changes.

231

Lichen Sclerosus

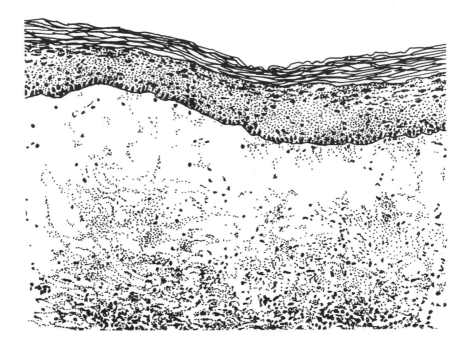

CLASSIFICATION OF VULVAR NONNEOPLASTIC DISORDERS

Lichen Sclerosus:
>   thinning of squamous epithelium,
>   loss of rete pegs,
>   acellular, homogeneous dermis,
>   inflammatory cells deep in dermis,
>   keratin layer thin or normal.

Squamous Cell Hyperplasia:
>   thickening of squamous epithelium,
>   elongated, thickened rete pegs,
>   inflammatory cells throughout dermis,
>   hyperkeratosis.

Mixed Dystrophy:
>   both lichen sclerosus and
>   squamous cell hyperplasia
>   existing on same vulva.

Squamous Cell Hyperplasia

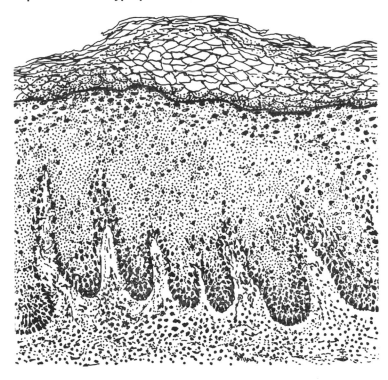

Lichen Sclerosus. The cause of lichen sclerosus is unknown. Older names used to describe this lesion included lichen sclerosus et atrophicus, atrophic leukoplakia, and kraurosis vulvae. This is the most common (70%) of the vulvar disorders. Pruritus is usually present and gets worse with time. The lesion is white and wrinkled like tissue paper, and frequently involves the entire vulva. The labia minora first adhese to the majora then atrophy and disappear. Without regular coitus, the vaginal opening shrinks in size (kraurosis). Treatment consists of the local application of testosterone or progesterone as described below. The recurrence rate (50% after total vulvectomy) argues against surgery, including laser vaporization.

Squamous Cell Hyperplasia (formerly hyperplastic dystrophy). This lesion may occur as a consequence of a chronic irritation or infection. Older names included lichen simplex chronicus, hypertrophic vulvitis, chronic reactive vulvitis, and neurodermatitis. In a significant difference when compared to lichen sclerosus, the labia minora do not disappear and the lesion is usually localized. In large lesions, toluidine blue should be used to direct biopsies in order to assess the presence of atypia. In cases of severe atypia, the invasive potential is about 5%. Atypia requires consultation and individualized surgical management; severe atypia should be treated as carcinoma-in-situ. Lesions with atypia should be considered part of the spectrum of vulvar intraepithelial neoplasms (VIN). In the absence of severe atypia, topical application of corticosteroid preparations is the treatment. Unlike lichen sclerosus, once effectively treated, recurrence is uncommon. But like lichen sclerosus, recurrence does occur after vulvectomy.

233

Lichen Sclerosus With Associated Squamous Cell Hyperplasia (formerly mixed dystrophy). About 15% of white lesions contain mixed dystrophy, which simply means that both lichen sclerosus and squamous cell hyperplasia are present. Only multiple biopsies, preferably with toluidine blue staining, can provide accurate diagnosis. The atypia incidence is slightly higher than in pure squamous cell hyperplasia. Treatment is first directed to the hyperplastic component with 6 weeks of topical corticosteroid, then treatment switches to long-term testosterone or progesterone. One can alternate the corticosteroid and testosterone, but the response is slower.

Topical Treatment
of White Lesions

Topical treatment of vulvar disorders utilizes creams and ointments containing steroids. A cream is a suspension of oil in water; an ointment is a suspension of water in oil. Creams are preferred, being more delicate and gentle to the tissue. However, some drugs can be prepared only as ointments (e.g. testosterone) as they are not absorbed from water-soluble bases.

Crotamiton (Eurax) is a synthetic agent with antipruritic action which is available as a cream and is useful in combination (approximately one-third Eurax) with the steroid preparations to combat itching.

Corticosteroid Preparations. The corticosteroid preparations are applied bid for 1–2 months and are commercially available in the following products, listed in *descending* order of potency:

> Halcinonide (Halog)
> Fluocinonide (Lidex)
> Triamcinolone acetonide (Aristocort, Kenalog, Mycolog)
> Fluocinolone acetonide (Synalar)
> Betamethasone (Diprolene, Diprosone, Valisone)
> Hydrocortisone

Testosterone Ointment. Testosterone is a trophic hormone for the skin, producing a thicker, more oily skin, while estrogen has the opposite effect. Estrogen-containing creams have no impact on the vulvar disorders. Testosterone ointment should be applied bid for 4–6 months. Combine it with Eurax to control itching. Following this initial treatment, long-term maintenance therapy of atrophic lesions is mandatory. Control can be achieved with treatment once or twice a week. Testosterone ointment must be prepared on order by the pharmacist as follows:

> testosterone propionate 2% in white petrolatum
> (30 ml testosterone proprionate in sesame oil, 100 mg/ml, mixed with 120 gm white petrolatum, an 8-week supply).

Progesterone Ointment. One may have to switch to progesterone ointment because of excessive libido and clitoral stimulation with testosterone. The effectiveness of progesterone is probably due to its ability at high concentrations to bind to androgen receptors. The formula is as follows:

> progesterone in oil, 400 mg, mixed in 120 gm hydrophilic ointment or cream (4–6 week supply).

Dark Lesions	A dark lesion is due to localized stimulation in the number of melanocytes or in the production rate of melanin. Lentigo (or melanosis) is a freckle-like concentration of melanocytes and is the most common dark lesion. The remaining dark lesions consist of nevi, reactive hyperpigmentation, carcinomas, and melanoma. ***All dark lesions should be excised regardless of their appearance. Only in this way will atypia and melanomas be detected.*** Incisional biopsy of a melanoma does not affect the prognosis provided correct diagnosis and therapy promptly follow.
Paget's Disease of Skin	Paget's disease is diagnosed from the biopsy specimen by the pathologist. The lesion is marked by nests of large clear cells at the tips of the rete ridges, usually associated with hyperkeratosis. Early lesions look erythematous and velvety. Later, hyperkeratosis gives a mottled appearance. The presence of Paget's disease is a warning signal. About 20–30% of the patients will have a vulvar adenocarcinoma in the underlying apocrine glands. These patients are also at high risk for adenocarcinoma of the breast, colon, cervix, and uterus. Treatment is surgical with wide local excision, often requiring vulvectomy.
Vulvodynia	Vulvodynia, a term coined in 1982, is simply chronic vulvar discomfort. It is manifested by a variety of sensations, including burning, stinging, irritation, or rawness. Grossly abnormal signs are seldom found on examination of the external genitalia. Not surprisingly, many of these patients have been labeled as psychosomatic. Several specific conditions might be considered from an etiologic point of view. (8) Cyclic candidiasis may be present and long-term empirical treatment could be tried. Other possibilities include vulvar vestibulitis or squamous papillomatosis (perhaps a subclinical infection with the human papilloma virus). Consider also overcleaning, which can lead to physical irritation, as well as the use of allergens and irritants.

References

1. **Friedrich EG Jr,** *Vulvar Disease*, 2nd edition, W.B. Saunders Co., Philadelphia, 1983.

2. **Semmens JP, Tsae CC, Semmens EC, Loadhold CB,** Effects of estrogen therapy on vaginal physiology during menopause, Obstet Gynecol 66:15, 1986.

3. **Larsen B, Galask RP,** Vaginal microbial flora composition and influences of host physiology, Ann Intern Med 96:926, 1982.

4. **Sobel JD,** Recurrent vulvovaginal candidiasis: a prospective study of the efficacy of maintenance ketoconazole therapy, New Engl J Med 315:1455, 1986.

5. **Malouf M, Fortier M, Morin G, Dube JL,** Treatment of *Hemophilus vaginalis* vaginitis, Obstet Gynecol 57:711, 1981.

6. **McLellan R, Spence MR, Brockman M, Raffel L, Smith JL,** The clinical diagnosis of trichomoniasis, Obstet Gynecol 60:30, 1982.

7. **Krieger JN, Tam MR, Stevens CE, Nielsen IO, et al,** Diagnosis of trichomoniasis. Comparison of conventional wet mount examination with cytologic studies, cultures, and monoclonal antibody staining of direct specimens, JAMA 259:1223, 1988.

8. **McKay M,** Vulvodynia versus pruritus vulvae, Clin Obstet Gynecol 28:123, 1985.

15   Thyroid and Parathyroid Disorders

Older people develop anatomic and functional changes in the endocrine glands and their target tissues. Recognition and treatment of endocrine disorders in older women require knowledge of these age-related changes, the effects on the clinical expression of endocrine diseases, and the effect of non-endocrine diseases.

Glandular atrophy, fibrosis, and nodule formation in endocrine glands occur commonly with aging. Functional alterations include changes in some hormone levels, basal metabolism, metabolic clearance rates, and target tissue resistance, along with reduced glandular sensitivity to negative feedback. Older women often demonstrate atypical clinical presentations of endocrine disease, and the changes associated with normal aging can impair the recognition of endocrine disorders. For example, fatigue, psychomotor retardation, and constipation may be attributed to normal aging but may actually be manifestations of hypothyroidism or hyperthyroidism. In addition, treatment may require adjustments due to changes in drug metabolism.

THYROID DISEASE

Normal Physiology

Thyroid hormone synthesis depends in large part upon an adequate supply of iodine in the diet. In the small intestine iodine is absorbed as iodide and is transported to the thyroid gland. Plasma iodide enters the thyroid under the influence of thyroid stimulating hormone (TSH), the anterior pituitary thyrotropin hormone. Within the thyroid gland, iodide is oxidized to elemental iodine which is then bound to tyrosine. Monoiodotyrosine and diiodotyrosine combine to form thyroxine (T_4) and triiodothyronine (T_3). These iodinated compounds are part of the thyroglobulin molecule, the colloid which serves as a storage depot for thyroid hormone. TSH induces a proteolytic process which results in the release of iodothyronines into the bloodstream as thyroid hormone. In the blood, thyroid hormone is tightly associated with a group of proteins, chiefly thyroxine binding globulin (TBG).

Although T_4 is secreted at 20 times the rate of T_3, it is T_3 which is responsible for most if not all of the thyroid action in the body. T_3 is 3–4 times more potent than T_4. About one third of the T_4 secreted each day is converted in peripheral tissues, largely liver and kidney, to T_3, and about 40% is converted to the inactive, reverse T_3 (rT_3).

Thyroid hormones regulate TSH by both suppressing thyroid releasing hormone (TRH) secretion and affecting the pituitary sensitivity to TRH (by reducing the number of TRH receptors). While some tissues depend mainly on the blood T_3 for their intracellular T_3, the brain and the pituitary depend on their own intracellular conversion of T_4. The measurement of T_4 and TSH, therefore, provides the most accurate assessment of thyroid function. Drugs taken orally for cholecystograms inhibit the peripheral conversion of T_4 to T_3, and can disrupt normal thyroid levels for up to 30 days.

Functional Changes with Aging

Thyroxine (T_4) metabolism and clearance decrease in older people, and thyroxine secretion decreases in compensation to maintain normal serum thyroxine concentrations. The metabolic rate is determined to a large degree by the relative production of T_3 and rT_3. During periods of stress, when a decrease in metabolic rate would conserve energy, the body produces more rT_3 and less T_3, and metabolism slows. Upon recovery, this process reverses and metabolic rate increases. With aging, conversion of T_4 to T_3 decreases. (1) TSH levels increase in older women, but it is unclear whether this is caused by normal aging or thyroid dysfunction. The TSH response to TRH is normal in older women. (2) TBG concentrations decrease slightly in postmenopausal women, but not enough to alter measurements in serum. However, postmenopausal women receiving oral estrogen replacement usually have increased levels of TBG, which affects the measurement of total T_4.

Thyroid Function Tests

Free Thyroxine (FT_4). Assays are now available to measure free T_4. These are usually displacement assays using an antibody to T_4. The result is not affected by changes in TBG and binding. The free T_4 level has a different range of normal values from laboratory to laboratory.

Total Thyroxine (TT_4). The total thyroxine, both the portion bound to TBG and the free unbound portion, is measured by displacement assays, and in the absence of hormone therapy or other illnesses estimates the thyroxine concentration in the blood. However, the free thyroxine assay is now available and preferred.

Free Thyroxine Index (FTI or T_7). The free thyroxine index is calculated from the TT_4 and the T_3 resin uptake measurements. This test too has been replaced by the free T_4 assay.

Total T_3 and Reverse T_3. Both of these thyronines can be measured by sensitive radioimmunoassays; however, in most clinical circumstances they add little to what is learned by the free T_4 and TSH measurements. The clinical situations where measurement will be useful will be discussed under the specific diseases and indicated on the algorithm.

Thyroid Stimulating Hormone (TSH). TSH can now be measured by highly sensitive assays utilizing monoclonal antibodies. The normal levels vary from laboratory to laboratory. TSH is a very sensitive indicator of thyroid hormone action at the tissue level. In the absence of hypothalamic or pituitary disease, the sensitive TSH assays will provide the best indication of excess or deficient thyroxine.

238

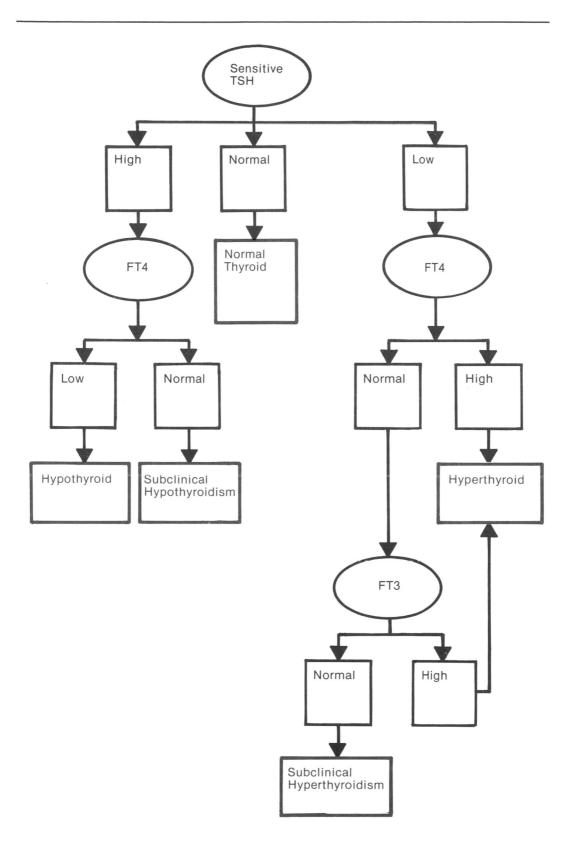

The Laboratory Evaluation. The algorithm represents a cost effective and accurate clinical strategy. (3) For screening purposes, or when there is a relatively low clinical suspicion of thyroid disease, the initial step is to measure the TSH by a sensitive assay. A normal TSH essentially excludes hypothyroidism or hyperthyroidism. A high TSH requires the measurement of free T_4 to confirm the diagnosis of hypothyroidism.

In early hypothyroidism, with undetectable symptoms or signs, a compensated state can be detected by an elevated TSH and normal T_4 (called subclinical hypothyroidism). Many of these patients will eventually become clinically hypothyroid with low T_4 concentrations. A good reason to treat subclinical hypothyroidism is to avoid the appearance of a goiter. Furthermore, some patients in retrospect (after treatment) recognize improved physical and mental well-being. With only very slight elevations of TSH, it is reasonable not to treat, and to check thyroid function every year to detect further deterioration.

If the initial TSH is low, especially less than 0.08 μU/ml, then measurement of a high T_4 will confirm the diagnosis of hyperthyroidism. If the T_4 is normal, the T_3 level is measured, since some patients with hyperthyroidism will have predominantly T_3 toxicosis. If the T_3 is normal, it implies that thyroxine secretin is autonomous from TSH, and this is called subclinical hyperthyroidism. Some of these patients will eventually have increased T_4 or T_3 levels with true hyperthyroidism.

Hyperthyroidism

The prevalence of hyperthyroidism in women older than 60 is between 0.5–1.9%. (4) Twenty percent of hyperthyroid patients are over 60. Twenty-five percent of older women with hyperthyroidism present with an apathetic or atypical syndrome. Symptoms are often concentrated in a single organ system, especially the cardiovascular or central nervous system. Goiter is absent in 40%. Sinus tachycardia occurs in less than half, but atrial fibrillation occurs in 40% and is resistant to cardioversion or spontaneous reversion to sinus rhythm. The ventricular response is usually rapid and resistant to slowing with digoxin. There is often a coexistent disease, such as an infection or coronary heart disease that dominates the clinical picture.

The triad of weight loss, constipation, and loss of appetite, suggesting gastrointestinal malignancy, occurs in about 15% of older patients with hyperthyroidism. Ophthalmopathy is rare in older patients. Hyperthyroidism in older women is sometimes described as "apathetic hyperthyroidism" because the clinical manifestations are different. The clinician should consider the diagnosis in older patients with "failure to thrive," those who are progressively deteriorating for unexplained reasons, and those with heart disease, unexplained weight loss, and mental or psychologic changes.

Hyperthyroidism in Elderly and Young Patients (5)		
Features	Elderly	Young
Tachycardia	50%	100%
Goiter	63%	100%
Nervousness	55%	99%
Hyperhidrosis	38%	91%
Heat intolerance	63%	89%
Palpitation	63%	89%
Fatigue or weakness	52%	88%
Weight loss	75%	85%
Thyroid bruit	27%	77%
Dyspnea	66%	75%
Eye signs	57%	71%
Polyphagia	11%	65%
Diarrhea	12%	23%
Atrial fibrillation	39%	10%
Anorexia	36%	9%
Constipation	26%	4%

Diagnosis

The diagnosis requires laboratory testing. A suppressed TSH with a high T_4 or a high T_3 confirms the diagnosis. Hyperthyroidism caused by high levels of T_3 is more common in older women. Most patients should have a radioactive iodine thyroid uptake and scan after laboratory confirmation of the diagnosis. If the uptake is suppressed, then drug therapy is indicated. The scan will indicate whether the patient has a diffuse toxic goiter, a solitary hot nodule, or a hot nodule in a multinodular gland. Toxic multinodular goiters occur more frequently in the elderly.

Treatment

There are multiple objectives of therapy: control of thyroid hormone effects on peripheral tissues by pharmacologic blockade of beta-adrenergic receptors, inhibition of thyroid gland secretion and release of thyroid hormone, and specific treatment of nonthyroidal systemic illnesses which can exacerbate hyperthyroidism or be adversely affected by hyperthyroidism. Antithyroid drugs are usually administered first to achieve euthyroidism, then definitive therapy is accomplished by radioactive iodine treatment.

Antithyroid Drugs. The drug of choice in most circumstances will be methimazole because it has fewer adverse effects. The drug inhibits organification of iodide and decreases production of T_4 and T_3. The dose is 10–15 mg, q 8 h, orally. The onset of effect takes 2–4 weeks. Remember that the half life of thyroxine is about one week, and the gland usually has large stores of T_4. Maximal effect occurs at 4–8 weeks. The dose can be titrated down once the disease is controlled. The major side effects are rash, gastrointestinal symptoms, and granulocytopenia. Propranolol and other beta blockers are effective in rapidly controlling the effects of thyroid hormone on peripheral tissues. The dose is usually 20–40 mg, q 6 h, orally, and the dose is titrated to maintain a heart rate of about 100 beats/minute. The drug may cause bronchospasm, worsening congestive heart fail-

241

ure, fatigue, and depression. Rarely, inorganic iodine will be needed to block release of hormone from the gland. Lugol's solution, 2 drops in water daily, is sufficient. The onset of effect is 1–2 days, with maximal effect in 3–7 days. There may be an escape from protection in 2–6 weeks, and the drug can cause rash, fever, and parotitis.

After the symptoms are controlled, and the patient is euthyroid, a dose of radioactive iodine can be selected, the thiouracil withheld temporarily, and definitive therapy accomplished. Patients with solitary nodules will be treated in the same fashion. Some patients with hot nodules in multinodular glands will require surgery because of the size of the gland and because the hyperthyroidism tends to recur in new nodules after the ablation of the original hot nodule. This can result in repetitive treatments with substantial doses of radioactive iodine, and surgery may be preferable.

Hypothyroidism

Hypothyroidism increases with aging and is more common in women.(6) Up to 45% of thyroid glands from women over age 60 contain thyroiditis.(7) The incidence of anti-thyroglobulin antibodies is 7.4% in women over age 75 years, while 16.9% of women age 60 and 17.4% of women over age 75 have elevated TSH levels. In women admitted to geriatric wards, 2–4% have clinically apparent hypothyroidism. *Therefore, hypothyroidism is frequent enough to warrant consideration in most older women, justifying screening even in asymptomatic older women. We recommend that older women be screened with the highly sensitive TSH assay at age 45, then every 2 years beginning at age 60, or with the appearance of any symptoms suggesting hypothyroidism.*

Many of the clinical manifestations of hypothyroidism, including constipation, cold intolerance, psychomotor retardation, and decreased exercise intolerance may be erroneously attributed to aging. Patients often appear asymptomatic. Close evaluation can reveal mental slowness, decreased energy, fatigue, poor memory, somnolence, slow speech, a low pitched voice, water retention, periorbital edema, delayed reflexes, or a low body temperature and bradycardia. Hypothyroidism may cause hypertension, cognitive abnormalities, pericardial effusion, asymmetric septal myocardial hypertrophy, myopathy, neuropathy, ataxia, anemia, elevated LDL-cholesterol, or hyponatremia. Serum enzymes may be elevated because of decreased clearance (including creatine phosphokinase [CPK], aspartate aminotransferase [AST,SGOT], alanine aminotransferase [ALT, SGPT], lactic dehydrogenase [LDH], and alkaline phosphatase), triggering a fruitless search for other organ disease.

Diagnosis

With primary thyroid failure, the circulating thyroid hormone levels fall, stimulating the pituitary to increase TSH output. Elevated TSH and low T_4 confirm the diagnosis. Hypothyroidism can occur due to pituitary failure in which case the TSH will be inappropriately low for the T_4. The most common cause will be immune thyroid disease in areas with normal iodine intake. However, making an etiologic diagnosis in older women adds little to the clinical management.

Treatment	Initial therapy is straight forward with synthetic thyroxine, T_4, given daily. Mixtures of T_4 and T_3, such as desiccated thyroid, provide T_3 in excess of normal thyroid secretion. It is better to provide T_4 and allow the peripheral conversion process to provide the T_3. (8) "Natural" thyroid preparations are not better, and in fact are potentially detrimental. Patients taking biological preparations should be switched to synthetic thyroxine. Because of a risk of coronary heart disease in older women, the initial dose should be 25–50 μg per day for about 5 weeks, at which time the dosage is adjusted according to the clinical and biochemical assessment. Usually the dose required will be close to 1.5 μg/lb of body weight, but it may be less in very old women. (9) The average final dose required in the elderly is approximately 70% of that in younger patients. Patients who have been on thyroid hormone for a long time may have their medication discontinued. Recovery of the hypothalamic-pituitary axis usually requires 3–4 weeks, at which time the TSH and free T_4 levels can be measured.
	Evaluation of Therapy. When the patient appears clinically euthyroid, evaluation of TSH levels will provide the most accurate assessment of the adequacy of thyroid hormone replacement. If the sensitive TSH assay is low, then the free T_4 should be measured to help adjust the thyroxine dose. (10)
Osteoporosis and Hyperthyroidism	Because postmenopausal women are at increased risk for osteoporosis, and frequently develop hyperthyroidism or receive levothyroxine treatment for hypothyroidism, the clinician needs to understand how thyroid hormone affects bones. (11) Thyroid hormone excess alters bone integrity via direct effects on bone and gut absorption, and indirectly through the effects of vitamin D, calcitonin, and parathyroid hormone.
	Thyroid hormone increases bone mineral resorption. In addition, total and ionized calcium increase in hyperthyroid women, leading to increases in serum phosphorous, alkaline phosphatase, and bone Gla protein (osteocalcin), a marker of bone turnover. Parathyroid hormone decreases in response to the increased serum calcium, and this results in decreased hydroxylation of vitamin D. Intestinal calcium and phosphate absorption decrease, while urinary hydroxyproline and calcium excretion increase. The net effect is increased bone resorption and a subsequent decrease in bone density—osteoporosis. (12)
	These effects become more clinically important in prolonged exposure to excessive thyroid hormone. This has raised concern that mild chronic excess thyroid hormone replacement, especially in postmenopausal women, might increase the risk of osteoporosis, and indeed, this subsequently was documented. (13,14) Bone density has even been found to be reduced (9%) in premenopausal women receiving enough thyroxine to suppress TSH for 10 years or more. (15) In another study finding lower bone densities in women being treated with levothyroxine, the hormone levels indicated that many were being overtreated for their hypothyroidism. (16) This can likely be prevented by using TSH measurements to ensure that levothyroxine doses are "physiologic." Some patients who require TSH

243

suppressive doses of thyroxine, such as patients with nodules, goiters, and cancer, must be considered at increased risk of osteoporosis. The use of hormone replacement and exercise programs must be seriously considered for these patients. Thus, hyperthyroidism must be added to the risk factors for osteoporosis. (Chapter 17)

Thyroid Nodules

The major concern with thyroid nodules is the potential for thyroid cancer. Carcinoma of the thyroid is nearly 3 times more common in women than in men. The incidence rises steadily from age 56. Mortality from thyroid cancer occurs predominantly in the middle-aged and the elderly. There are 4 major types of primary thyroid carcinoma: papillary, follicular, anaplastic, and medullary. Solitary nodules are common in women, and in nodules that are "cold" (those which do not take up radioactive iodine or pertechnetate on thyroid scan), 12% prove to be malignant. This also means that the majority are benign. Surgical excision of nodules can result in vocal cord paralysis, hypoparathyroidism, and other complications. Therefore, the goal is to select patients for curative surgery who have the greatest likelihood of having cancer in the nodule.

Epidemiologic and Clinical Data

The major risk factors for thyroid cancer are family history of this disease and a history of irradiation to head or neck. In those who have received thyroid irradiation, about one-third will have thyroid abnormalities, and about one-third of those with abnormalities will have thyroid cancer (about 10% overall). The carcinogenic risk has been estimated to be 1% per 100 rads in twenty years. A rapidly growing nodule, a hard nodule, the presence of palpable regional lymph nodes, or vocal cord paralysis greatly increase the chance of thyroid cancer.

Thyroid nodules in multinodular thyroid glands not previously exposed to thyroid irradiation have no greater risk of thyroid carcinoma than normal glands. Therefore, predominant thyroid nodules in multinodular glands should be followed, and if a nodule grows, then biopsy or surgery should be considered.

Diagnostic Strategy

Detection of a thyroid nodule is followed by clinical characterization of the nodule, examination of the lymph nodes, and inquiry regarding rapid growth, family history, and history of thyroid irradiation. In the presence of any of these findings, surgery is recommended for excision of the nodule. If none of these is present, proceed directly to fine needle aspiration biopsy or thyroid scan. If the scan is chosen, hot nodules are evaluated independently. Cold nodules should be fine needle aspirated for histological evaluation. If the patient prefers, one can treat with suppressive doses of levothyroxine and evaluate over time. Unfortunately, many of these thyroid nodules do not regress with thyroid treatment, but it is very reassuring if they do. Growth with thyroid suppression is an indication for fine needle aspiration biopsy. Thyroid ultrasound can be utilized to more accurately establish size for comparison over time.

If the fine needle aspiration biopsy reveals suspicious cells, a subtotal thyroidectomy should be performed for diagnosis and treatment. If the aspiration biopsy is benign some would repeat the biopsy in one year to avoid false negatives. Most would provide euthyroid hormone suppressive therapy and follow for growth of the nodule. (17,18) Growth indicates the need for biopsy or surgery. In some cases,

244

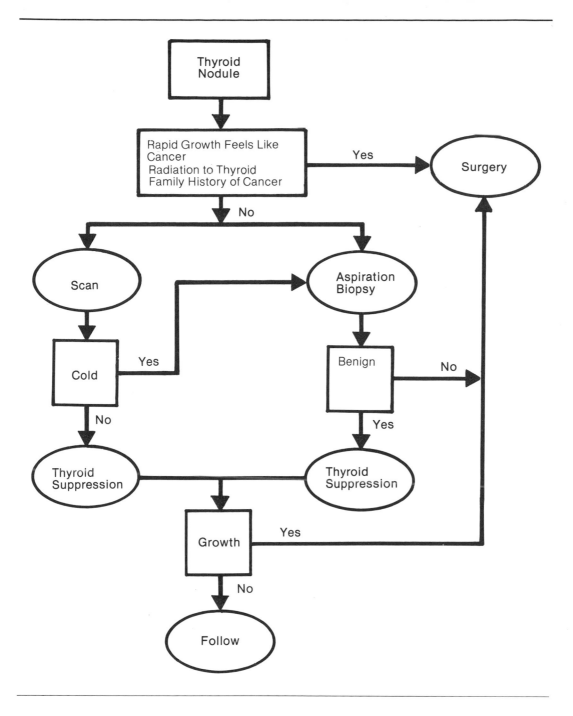

especially in older women, nodules can be followed with no therapy and little risk. One of the reasons many are treated with levothyroxine is because of the known growth promoting effects of TSH in carcinoma of the thyroid, and the hope that TSH suppression will inhibit the growth of early carcinoma.

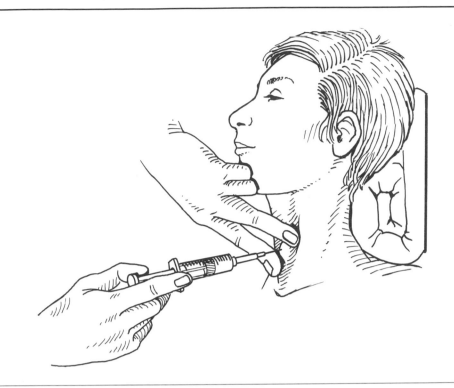

Fine Needle Aspiration. The method for fine needle aspiration biopsy requires no anesthetic. Using sterile technique and a 23 gauge needle on a 10 ml syringe, fix the nodule with two fingers of one hand and enter the nodule and aspirate with the syringe while making several passes through a vertical distance of about 2 mm in the nodule. Stop applying suction when biopsy material becomes visible in the hub of the needle. The contents of the needle should be expelled onto a slide and fixed for pathology. Gentle pressure is applied over the nodule for 10 minutes. Occasionally, a patent will have some bleeding into the nodule or surrounding tissues, but it is usually self-limiting.

Hyperparathyroidism The feedback loop between serum ionized calcium and parathyroid hormone (PTH) secretion remains normal with increasing age. In women, the marked decrease in estrogen at the time of menopause is associated with a small increase in serum calcium. Serum PTH levels increase with age, thought to be due to the reduction in renal function with aging. Older women with inadequate sun exposure or vitamin D intake have decreased 25-hydroxyvitamin D and 1,25-dihydroxyvitamin D levels with lower ionized serum calcium concentrations, resulting in increased PTH levels.

Today, the frequent use of screening chemistry panels in well outpatients identifies a large population of women with asymptomatic hypercalcemia. When malignancy or other disorders cause hypercalcemia, they are usually clinically obvious. Therefore, the older woman who has no clinical, radiological, or biochemical evidence of malignancy, thyrotoxicosis, sarcoidosis, or thiazide treatment will nearly always be suffering from hyperparathyroidism.

The prevalence of hyperparathyroidism is estimated at 1.5% of the elderly. Fifty percent of all patients with this condition are asymptomatic women older than 50, and 35% are older than 65. The incidence in women is twice that in men and increases with age. For about 5 years after recognition, this hyperparathyroidism is clinically inactive in 80% of patients, but thereafter results in increasing complications of parathyroid hyperfunction. (19,20)

Symptoms

Less than half of patients actually have any symptoms or complains. However, asymptomatic osteoporosis may be quite frequent. The symptoms that can be associated with hyperparathyroidism include bone pain, joint pain, polydipsia, polyuria, constipation, pruritus, and muscular weakness. Peptic ulcer disease and renal stones are less common today. Dementia and depression can be aggravated by hyperparathyroidism.

Diagnosis

Hyperparathyroidism is by far the most common cause of hypercalcemia in ambulatory women. The increased serum calcium should be confirmed with repetitive testing, and for accuracy, the level of ionized calcium should be measured. Clinical evidence of a malignancy should be pursued, including unexplained weight loss, breast examination and mammography, chest x-ray, urine for hematuria, and pelvic examination with Pap smear. Further evaluation should include evaluation of thiazide use, clues for sarcoidosis and myeloma, use of vitamin D or milk or alkali, complete blood count, chemistry panel, and thyroid function tests. The demonstration of an elevated midportion or whole molecule serum PTH by radioimmunoassay confirms the diagnosis. Calcium excretion (in a 24 hour urine collection) is measured to evaluate for the familial hypocalciuric hypercalcemia. Localization procedures have been disappointing and therefore are of little value except in patients who have previously had surgery.

Treatment

The definitive treatment is removal of the parathyroid adenoma or hyperplastic glands by an experienced surgeon performing an exploratory operation with full identification of all parathyroid glands. The cure rate is 95%. Surgery is ordinarily recommended for all healthy individuals with a life expectancy of greater than 5 years and for all symptomatic individuals without a surgical contradiction. However, asymptomatic old women with mild increases in serum calcium and no bone disease may be followed with no therapy. Since estrogen replacement therapy will decrease serum calcium and decrease bone resorption through a multitude of actions (including a decrease in the calcium set point for parathyroid response), it is strongly recommended. (21,22) If the serum calcium increases and averages over 11.5 mg/dl or if the bone density decreases with observation, then surgery is recommended. In general, the clinician should have a low threshold for recommending surgery if there is an experienced surgeon available since the results of surgery are so good and the risks minimal. If the serum PTH is low or normal with hypercalcemia, consultation with an endocrinologist is in order.

References

1. **Harman SM, et al,** Pituitary-thyroid hormone economy in healthy aging men: Basal indices of thyroid function and thyrotropin responses to constant infusions of thyrotropin releasing hormone, J Clin Endocrinol Metab 58:320, 1984.

2. **Melmed S, Hershman J,** The thyroid and aging, in Korenman SG, editor, *Endocrine Aspects of Aging,* Elsevier Science Publishing, New York, 1982, pp 33–53.

3. **Caldwell G, Gow SM, Sweeting VM, Kellett HA, Beckett GJ, Seth J, Toft AD,** A new strategy for thyroid function testing, Lancet i:1117, 1985.

4. **Davis PJ, Davis FB,** Hyperthyroidism in patients over the age of 60 years, Medicine 53:161, 1974.

5. **Davis PJ, Davis FB,** Endocrine diseases, in Rossman I, editor, *Clinical Geriatrics,* J.B. Lippincott, Co., Philadelphia, 1986, p 425.

6. **Robuschi G, Safran M, Braverman LE, Gnudi A, Roti E,** Hypothyroidism in the elderly, Endocrine Rev 8:142, 1987.

7. **Felicetta JV,** Thyroid changes with aging: Significance and managment, Geriatrics 42:86, 1987.

8. **Cooper DS,** Thyroid hormone treatment: New insights into an old therapy, JAMA 261:2694, 1989.

9. **Rosenbaum RL, Barzel US,** Levothyroxine replacement dose for primary hypothyroidism decreases with age, Ann Intern Med 96:53, 1982.

10. **Watts NB,** Use of a sensitive thyrotropin assay for monitoring treatment with levothyroxine, Arch Intern Med 149:309, 1989.

11. **Cooper DS,** Thyroid hormone and the skeleton, JAMA 259:3175, 1988.

12. **Wartofsky L,** Osteoporosis: A growing concern for the thyroidologist, Thyroid Today 11:1, 1988

13. **Barsony J, Lakatos P, Foldes J, Feher T,** Effect of vitamin D_3, loading and thyroid hormone replacement therapy on the decreased serum 25-hydroxyvitamin D level in patients with hypothyroidism, Acta Endocrinol 113:329, 1986.

14. **Ettinger B, Wingerd J,** Thyroid supplements: Effect on bone mass, West J Med 136:473, 1982.

15. **Ross DS, Neer RM, Ridgway EC, Daniels GH,** Subclinical hyperthyroidism and reduced bone density as a possible result of prolonged suppression of the pituitary-thyroid axis with L-thyroxine, Am J Med 82:1167, 1987.

16. **Paul TL, Kerrigan J, Kelly AM, et al,** Longterm L-thyroxine therapy is associated with decreased hip bone density in premenopausal women, JAMA 259:3137, 1988.

17. **VanHerle AJ,** The thyroid nodule, Ann Intern Med 96:221, 1982.

18. **Hamberger B, Gharib H, Melton LJ, Goellner JR, Zinsmeister AR,** Fine-needle aspiration biopsy of thyroid nodules, Am J Med 73:381, 1982.

19. **Christensson T, Hellstrom K, Wengle B, Aloveryd AS, Wikland B,** Prevalence of hypercalcemia in a health screening in Stockholm, Acta Med Scand 300:131, 1976.

248

20. **Scholz DA, Purnell DC,** Asymptomatic primary hyperparathyroidism: 10-year prospective study, Mayo Clin Proc 56:473, 1981.

21. **Selby PL, Peacock M,** Ethinyl estradiol and norethindrone in the treatment of primary hyperparathyrodism in postmenopasual women, New Engl J Med 314:1481, 1986.

22. **Boucher A, D'Amour P, Hamel L, Fugere P, Gascon-Barre M, Lepage R, Ste-Marie LG,** Estrogen replacement decreases the set point of parathyroid hormone stimulation by calcium in normal postmenopausal women, J Clin Endocrinol Metab 68:831, 1989.

16   Diabetes Mellitus

Diabetes mellitus is a chronic metabolic syndrome of glucose intolerance which generally involves absolute or relative insulin availability, or insulin resistance, or both. The hallmark of the disease is hyperglycemia, but the abnormalities in metabolism of carbohydrates, lipids, and proteins lead to the development of chronic microvascular complications

Diabetes mellitus is exceedingly common, with a prevalence of 8.9% in women older than 65. (1) Approximately 20% of those above 80 years old have diabetes mellitus. (2) It is estimated that two-thirds of all diabetic patients hospitalized are over 65 years of age. (3) Diabetes mellitus, therefore, represents one of the major chronic disorders in older women.

The two major risk factors for diabetes mellitus are obesity and age. More women are overweight than men, which probably accounts for the increased prevalence of diabetes in women as they age. The other significant risk factor for diabetes is a family history, indicating a genetic predisposition.

Classification of Diabetes

Type I diabetes is defined as a patient who has insulin-dependent diabetes. The word "dependent" is the key. These patients cannot survive without exogenous insulin. This is the type of diabetes which commonly occurs in young onset diabetics who are prone to ketosis. Physiologically this form of diabetes is characterized by insulin deficiency.

Type II diabetes is non-insulin dependent diabetes. These patients may take insulin but do not require insulin for survival. This type of diabetes is characterized by insulin resistance. Type II diabetes is much more common in older patients and will be the most frequent form of diabetes in older women.

Prognosis

About 20–25% of Type II diabetics who are older will die within 8 years of treatment. (4) A great majority die from cardiovascular disease. However, Type II diabetics develop all of the microvascular complications of diabetes if they survive long enough. Smoking and hypertension have marked adverse effects on the prognosis of older diabetics. The prospect for the development of retinopathy is related to the one hour plasma glucose after a glucose challenge. There is a slight increase in the risk of retinopathy with modest increases in plasma glucose, but a dramatic increase occurs with levels above 200 mg/dl (which approximates fasting levels of 140 mg/dl). This

251

finding has led to new diagnostic criteria and treatment goals which are based upon an understanding of the threshold level at which complications are likely to develop. (5) It is worth noting that there is no statistically significant increase in mortality due to diabetes when the diagnosis is made beyond the age of 75. (6)

Pathophysiology of Type II Diabetes

Under normal circumstances, plasma glucose levels are maintained within a narrow range of approximately 70–100 mg/dl between meals. During this phase, plasma glucose levels are maintained by hepatic glucose production, and plasma insulin levels are relatively low. On ingestion of carbohydrates and proteins, insulin is secreted, hepatic glucose production ceases, and the liver becomes a glucose-storing organ as peripheral tissues take up glucose in response to the increasing insulin.

Type II diabetes mellitus is characterized by the following abnormalities:

1. Insulin resistance.

2. Alterations in insulin action with decreased receptor numbers and post-receptor abnormalities.

3. Increased hepatic glucose production.

4. Insulin secretion may be high, normal, or low depending upon the time of measurement in the clinical course.

These alterations result in fasting plasma glucose levels which are fairly constant, but which are regulated around a higher basal setpoint than in normal individuals. The hyperglycemia re-establishes nearly normal basal insulin secretion, hepatic glucose output, and peripheral glucose uptake. However, this effect occurs at the expense of an elevated fasting plasma glucose level and significant postprandial hyperglycemia.

Complications

Atherosclerosis. Type II diabetics have 2 to 3 times more complications due to atherosclerosis, including coronary heart disease, cerebrovascular disease, and peripheral vascular disease, but these complications do not appear to be related to duration or severity of the diabetes. Family history, smoking, hypertension, lipid disorders, and obesity remain as important risk factors. Coronary artery disease occurs prematurely and is more severe in diabetics than in nondiabetics. (7,8) Diabetics have a different form of coronary artery disease in that it is more diffuse with more frequent myocardial infarctions. Myocardial infarctions have been said to be more commonly painless than in nondiabetics. Short-term mortality from coronary heart disease is not higher, but the prognosis over 1–5 years is much worse. Peripheral vascular disease contributes to marked disability in diabetics with claudication, foot ulcers, ischemia, and amputations. It is unclear whether these complications can be prevented by improved glucose control in older patients.

Retinopathy. Diabetic retinopathy in older Type II patients is somewhat different with more macular edema and other complications rather than the proliferative form commonly seen in the Type I diabetic. The role of Photocoagulation in the treatment of macular changes is not yet well established; however, it may be possible to prevent loss of vision through improved glucose control and early photocoagulation treatment to prevent vitreous hemorrhages, retinal retraction, and increased ocular pressure. There is an association between systolic blood pressure and retinal changes, and therefore treatment of hypertension is important.

Cataracts. Cataracts occur more frequently in diabetics under the age of 70. Those patients with significant impairment beyond a 20/40 to 20/60 level due to cataracts are surgical candidates if diabetic retinopathy is not so severe that it will preclude improvement of vision after extraction of the cataracts.

Nephropathy. End stage renal disease occurs in 5–20% of Type II diabetics. (1) Proteinuria is thought to be the first manifestation of diabetic nephropathy. Other forms of renal disease, however, occur commonly in the elderly and must be considered in the differential diagnosis of any renal dysfunction in older women. It has been proposed that control of hypertension and the use of moderate to low protein diets may prevent the progression of renal dysfunction in Type II diabetics. It is definitely advantageous to institute strict glucose control before the occurrence of microalbuminuria. End stage renal disease must be handled on an individual basis. The choices (hemodialysis, peritoneal dialysis, and renal transplantation) must be based upon personal preference, the availability of resources, and the needs of the family.

Neuropathy. Neuropathy may affect the peripheral nerves, isolated cranial or spinal nerves, or the central nervous system. The most common neuropathy is the typical stocking glove bilateral peripheral sensory and motor neuropathy with pain, paresthesias, loss of reflexes, and decreased vibratory and other sensory sensation. Once the neuropathy is established there are a number of treatment modalities, but none is well established. Autonomic neuropathy is an important complication and often results in iatrogenic orthostatic hypotension, disturbed gastrointestinal motility, and gastroparesis.

Lipid Disorders. An elevated LDL-cholesterol, elevated triglycerides, and decreased HDL-cholesterol in diabetics add to the risk for coronary heart disease. These abnormal lipid changes occur more frequently in poorly controlled diabetics. Only after improved glucose control has been achieved should other treatments for the lipid changes be considered.

Smoking. There is no question that smoking accelerates the complications of diabetes mellitus. Smoking cessation should be mandated for all older women who have diabetes.

Infections. Malignant otitis externa is a dramatic complication specific to elderly diabetics with a mortality rate of more than 50%. This condition is easily recognized, presenting with pain and purulent discharge from the ear, tenderness and swelling of the surrounding tissues, and polyps on the floor of the external auditory canal. Facial paralysis can occur early in the course of illness. The treatment of choice combines carbenicillin or ticarcillin with tobramycin or gentamicin, and surgical debridement.

Mastoiditis occurs with aerobic bacteria such as staphylococcus or pseudomonas acting in synergism with anaerobic organisms such as bacteroides. This is a life threatening condition seen in elderly diabetics. Diabetes further increases the increased prevalence of cholecystitis in older women.

Clinical Symptoms

Patients commonly present with mild to moderate acute symptoms of weight loss, fatigue, weakness, polyuria, polydipsia, and or polyphagia. The latter three symptoms often occur in association with an acute infection. The infections are usually minor, such as candidal vulvovaginitis, an infected tooth, or a viral or bacterial respiratory infection. An uncommon, but important, presentation in older women is hyperglycemic, hyperosmolar coma which is marked by seizures or focal neurologic signs, and marked hyperglycemia. This presentation is often due to an infection combined with decreased renal function and an inability to consume sufficient water. Rarely an older patient will present with ketoacidosis, usually associated with a severe illness.

Diagnostic Criteria

There are 3 possible ways to establish the diagnosis of type II diabetes in older patients: (5)

1. Fasting plasma glucose of 140 mg/dl or greater, on at least 2 occasions in the nonstressed state.

2. Sustained hyperglycemia after an oral glucose tolerance test, with plasma glucose at least 200 mg/dl at two hours and one other time point within the two hours.

3. Manifestation of classic symptoms of diabetes mellitus with unequivocal elevation of plasma glucose greater than 200 mg/dl.

Impaired glucose tolerance requires all 3 of the following:

1. Fasting plasma glucose between 115 and 140 mg/dl.

2. During an oral glucose tolerance test, one value greater than or equal to 200 mg/dl between the baseline and two hours.

3. During an oral glucose tolerance test, plasma glucose between 140–200 mg/dl at two hours.

After excluding those older patients who have diabetes mellitus by the above criteria, another 10–30% have abnormalities in carbohydrate tolerance. (9) These abnormalities represent a change per decade after age 40 of the following: a small increase in the fasting plasma glucose ranging from 1–2 mg/dl and a moderate increase of 8–20 mg/dl in the 1–2 hour postprandial glucose. In addition, older patients with these mild abnormalities have increased levels of glycosylated hemoglobin A_{1c}. (10) Individuals with these mild abnormalities in glucose tolerance have a significant increase in coronary artery disease. (11) Furthermore, there is evidence that the progression to diabetes can be delayed or prevented by treatment with diet and weight reduction.

| Treatment | The principal goal of treatment of Type II diabetes is to relieve symptoms; however, most clinicians believe (although clinical trial evidence is lacking) that reduction of the plasma glucose level to less than 140 mg/dl fasting and 200 mg/dl postprandial will either slow or decrease the onset and progression of the vascular complications. |

Definition of Control

	Fasting	Postprandial	Hemoglobin A_{1c}
Excellent Control:	<115 mg/dl	<140 mg/dl	Normal
Good Control:	115–140	<200	Elevated 100–130%
Poor Control:	>140	>200	Elevated >130%

The goal for most diabetics would be to try to achieve good control and only to accept poor control under circumstances of poor compliance, where there is a risk of hypoglycemia, when patients are very old, or when better control cannot be achieved despite a therapeutic trial. Eventually all Type II diabetics and those with some impairment of glucose tolerance should be treated with diet and exercise. Oral agents or insulin should be prescribed in most symptomatic patients (usually with fasting levels greater than 140 mg/dl and postprandial levels greater than 200 mg/dl).

Diet. Dietary treatment aims at both weight reduction and limitation of refined carbohydrates. (12)

Complex carbohydrates —55%
Saturated fats   —10%
Unsaturated fats   —10%
Monosaturated fats   —10%
Protein   —15%

In most Type II diabetics, 3 meals a day without snacks is reasonable. Some patients who are taking insulin will require snacks to avoid periods of hypoglycemia. If the patient is obese, a decrease in total calories is necessary to achieve weight reduction.

Exercise increases insulin sensitivity and is an important component of treatment. If the response to diet and exercise is inadequate, then oral agents should be considered.

Oral Agents. In the presence of high glucose levels, oral agents acutely increase the endogenous insulin secretion. (13) They also have a chronic effect by reducing hepatic glucose production. Oral agents potentiate insulin action by increasing insulin receptors or post receptor responsiveness. More than 85% of patients will respond to oral agents. Failure due to a lack of compliance or a change in the diabetic state occurs at a rate of about 3% per year. About 3–5% of patients have side effects, including gastrointestinal effects, liver function abnormalities, rashes, and hypoglycemia. The drugs should not be prescribed for patients who will not eat 3 meals a day.

255

There are a number of medications from which to choose. The first generation sulfonylureas include tolbutamide, chlorpropamide, acetohexamide, and tolazamide. In our view, the second generation sulfonylureas are superior for most older women because they have fewer drug interactions with commonly prescribed drugs. In addition, they have less active or inactive metabolites. These drugs are very potent in lowering blood glucose and should be prescribed to elderly patients at the lowest possible daily dose.

Second Generation Sulfonylureas	
Glyburide	2.5–15 mg/day
Glipizide	2.5–40 mg/day

Insulin Therapy. Patients who fail diet and exercise, those who fail oral agents, and those who have a preference for insulin can usually take a single dose of intermediate acting human insulin such as NPH or Lente once a day.

A reasonable starting dose of human insulin is 0.5–0.7 unit of intermediate acting insulin per kg per day. If short acting insulin is required because of inadequate control, premixed insulin preparations with a 70:30 combination of intermediate:regular insulin are easier for older patients to administer correct doses. Many obese older individuals have insulin resistance and their programs may require split doses of intermediate and regular insulin. With split insulin regimens, two-thirds of the insulin is given in the morning before breakfast and the remainder before supper.

Monitoring. Home monitoring of finger stick blood glucose can be accomplished with automatic finger sticking devices and glucose oxidase impregnated strips or digital glucose meters. In clinical studies, these devices have been shown to be very accurate, comparable to laboratory measurements. Compliance is sometimes a problem, however, and the self reports from patients may not be real. Compliance in older women is influenced by dexterity and visual acuity. Changes in color perception may account for some errors if a metered device is not being used. Periodic measurements (every 2–3 months) of hemoglobin A_{1c} and fasting and postprandial glucose are important to assess the accuracy of the patient's method. In addition, elderly diabetics should have medic alert bracelets or some other information device.

Foot Care

Diabetics must be taught and practice good foot care. Elderly diabetics who have additional problems of decreased sensation, foot deformities, peripheral vascular disease, and visual changes must be especially careful with foot care. The physician must inspect the feet at each office visit, and patients must inspect their feet daily. Diabetics are taught to palpate the foot for pressure points, warm spots, and to detect breaks and lesions in the skin. It is recommended that diabetics wear well-fitted leather shoes; walking barefoot should be avoided. Once a foot ulcer occurs in a diabetic it is slow healing. Penetrating ulcers must be aggressively treated with hospitalization and intravenous antibiotics.

References

1. **Lipson LG,** Diabetes in the elderly: Diagnosis, pathogenesis, and therapy, Am J Med 80 (Suppl 5A):10, 1986.

2. **Bennett PH,** Diabetes in the elderly: Diagnosis and epidemiology, Geriatrics 39:37, 1984.

3. **Harrower ADB,** Prevalence of elderly patients in a hospital diabetic population, Br J Clin Pract 34:131, 1980.

4. **Schor S,** A statistician looks at the mortality results, JAMA 217:1671, 1971.

5. **National Diabetes Data Group,** Classification and diagnosis of diabetes mellitus and other categories of glucose intolerance, Diabetes 28:1039, 1979.

6. **Fitzgerald MG,** Diabetes, in Brocklehurst JC, editor, *Textbook of Geriatric Medicine and Gerontology*, Churchill-Livingstone, Edinburgh, 1973, pp 458–575.

7. **Kannel WB,** Lipids and diabetes in coronary heart disease, Am Heart J 110:1100, 1985.

8. **Minaker KL,** Aging in diabetes mellitus is a risk factor for vascular disease, Am J Med 82 (Suppl 113):47, 1987.

9. **Bennett PH,** Report of the working group on epidemiology, National Commission of Diabetes, U.S. Dept Health, Education and Welfare, Pub. No. (NIH) 76-10211, 1976, pp 65–133.

10. **Arnetz BB, Kallner A, Theorell T,** The influence of age on hemoglobin A_{1c} (HBA$_{1c}$), J Gerontol 37:648, 1982.

11. **Jarrett RJ, McCartney P, Keen H,** The Bedford Survey: 10-Year mortality rates in newly diagnosed diabetics, borderline diabetics, and normal glycemic controls, and risk indices for coronary artery disease in borderline diabetics, Diabetologica 22:79, 1983.

12. **American Diabetes Association,** Nutritional recommendations and principles for individuals with diabetes mellitus: 1986, Diabetes Care 10:126, 1987.

17   Joint and Bone Problems

"Rheumatism" is derived from the Greek word meant to indicate that mucus was an evil humor which flowed from the brain to joints and provided pain. Today, rheumatic disease includes any condition which causes pain and stiffness in some portion of the musculoskeletal system. Approximately 50% of people age 65 or older have arthritis or rheumatism. X-ray evidence of osteoarthritis of the extremities can be found in approximately 85% of people 75–80 years old. Musculoskeletal symptoms are the foremost daily problem for older people, being twice as frequent as any other symptoms. (1)

Knobby fingers and stiffness and creaking of the knees are consequences of aging, but these are conditions which can be ameliorated by the physician. In this chapter, we will consider inflammatory and noninflammatory joint problems, arteritis, postmenopausal bone loss, and Paget's disease of bone.

INFLAMMATORY JOINT PROBLEMS

Rheumatoid Arthritis

Rheumatoid arthritis can begin at any age, even in the very old. Many older patients will enter old age with rheumatoid arthritis which has run its course, leaving damaged joints, but this is now more accurately labeled as osteoarthritis. There is evidence that estrogen replacement before the onset of joint disease is associated with protection against rheumatoid arthritis. (2) Experimental studies of synovial cells in culture have identified the presence of large amounts of both estrogen and progesterone receptors. (3) This represents another argument for estrogen treatment of postmenopausal women since rheumatoid arthritis is chronic, relapsing, and potentially disabling.

Pathophysiology.   Rheumatoid arthritis is a systemic inflammatory disease of unknown etiology. It is widely believed that an immunological mechanism is involved in the pathogenesis. (4) Type II collagen is a major constituent of joint cartilage and may act as an autoantigen stimulating the autoimmune reaction which then presents as rheumatoid arthritis. Antibodies to type II collagen are found in patients with rheumatoid arthritis, but not in patients with osteoarthritis. (5) Of the autoimmune diseases, only rheumatoid arthritis is common in older people.

Signs and Symptoms. The presentation in older patients is usually the same as in younger people, characterized by symmetrical synovitis of the distal joints, wrists, fingers, and toes. In older patients with pre-existing osteoarthritis, the diagnosis can be easily missed or delayed. With rheumatoid arthritis, morning stiffness usually lasts more than 30 minutes, and grip strength decreases. The signs of articular inflammation are swelling, pain, and warmth. The first joints to be involved are the small joints of the hands and feet. The pattern in the hands is characteristic, involving the proximal interphalangeal (PIP) joints, and sparing the distal interphalangeal (DIP) joints. Systemic manifestations may include fever and weight loss.

Diagnostic Tests. The diagnosis is based upon the clinical manifestations. An elevated erythrocyte sedimentation rate is often accompanied by anemia, but the rheumatoid factor may be negative. The rheumatoid factor is composed of antibodies specific to portions of immunoglobulin G and derived from B-lymphocytes which migrate into the inflamed joints. It is not unique to rheumatoid arthritis. In general, 70–80% of patients with rheumatoid arthritis are positive for the rheumatoid factor. The anemia is a recalcitrant normochromic or hypochromic, normocytic anemia. The lupus erythematous factor and antinuclear antibodies are positive in 10–15% of patients.

Management. All treatment is symptomatic; the course of the disease is unaltered. Aspirin in full doses (3–6 gr/day) is the cornerstone of therapy. Many older women do not eat 3 times per day. A regular eating pattern is important in reducing aspirin toxicity. Tinnitus is a dependable sign of salicylate toxicity in younger adults, but may not be reliable in older people. Buffered aspirin does not but enteric-coated aspirin does reduce the incidence of gastric side effects. One can measure salicylate levels to assess the therapeutic concentration (10–20 ng/dl) and to avoid toxicity.

The efficacy of the nonsteroidal anti-inflammatory drugs (NSAIDs) is not better than aspirin at full doses. In appropriate studies, no significant difference in efficacy exists among the various types of NSAIDs; however, indomethacin is not recommended for use in the elderly because of its potential for serious toxicity. The response to specific NSAIDs appears to be varied and each agent should be tried to identify the most satisfactory for a given patient. The risk of renal toxicity is greatest in the elderly, especially in users of diuretics and those with compromised renal or cardiac function. Serum creatinine must be monitored. Mental side effects occur in the elderly, including confusion, memory loss, depression, and even paranoid behavior. Hepatic injury can occur, and therefore, annual monitoring of liver function tests is recommended.

The incidence of gastrointestinal side effects with NSAIDs ranges from 8 to 34%, but in older patients it is 31–38%. (6) Combining the NSAID with a synthetic E prostaglandin significantly lowers the incidence. (6) This combination can allow some patients to avoid the NSAID-induced ulcers. The side effect problem with NSAIDs should not be underrated. It has been argued that this is the most severe and frequent drug side effect in the United States, occurring most often in older patients and accounting for a significant number of hospitalizations and deaths. (7) To minimize gastrointestinal side effects, NSAIDs should be taken with food.

Because older people are more susceptible to the side effects of aspirin and the NSAIDs, low doses of corticosteroids (5.0 mg prednisone daily) may be preferred.

Because patients with rheumatoid arthritis are subject to disability, reduced ambulation, and steroid use, they are prone to develop osteoporosis. Hormone replacement therapy is highly recommended for these patients to avoid an increased risk of fractures.

Nonpharmacologic measures include rest, splinting, and appropriate exercise. All patients with active disease should be referred to a therapist for a good exercise program (for muscle strengthening and to maintain range of motion). Patients refractory to conventional therapy should be referred to a rheumatologist.

Felty's Syndrome.   Chronic rheumatoid arthritis associated with splenomegaly, leukopenia, and pigmented skin spots on the lower extremities.

Sjögren's Syndrome.   Chronic inflammation of the exocrine glands, thus decreased lacrimal and salivary gland secretion leading to the complaints of the sicca (dry) syndrome: dry mouth (xerostomia) and dry eyes (keratoconjunctivitis sicca). These complaints associated with rheumatoid arthritis are more common in older women. Enlargement of the parotid glands and the submaxillary glands is common but not always present.

Polymyalgia Rheumatica

This rheumatic disease is found mainly in white older women.

Pathophysiology.   Polymyalgia rheumatica is thought to be due to a synovitis, and it is often difficult to distinguish from rheumatoid arthritis. (8) The onset is usually insidious, but occasionally it is so abrupt that it occurs overnight.

Signs and Symptoms.   The aching and stiffness of polymyalgia rheumatica are centered at the pelvis and shoulders and neck. Characteristically patients report difficulty in getting out of bed in the morning. The pain may be widespread, but it is usually symmetrical and confined to the shoulders and hips. Morning stiffness is very prolonged, and movement causes pain. Fever and malaise are common.

Diagnostic Tests.   The only abnormal laboratory test is a very high erythrocyte sedimentation rate. A sedimentation rate greater than 50 mm/hr is almost diagnostic of polymyalgia rheumatica and giant cell arteritis. (9) X-rays show only the characteristic findings of osteoarthritis usually seen at the age of the patient. The rheumatoid factor and antinuclear antibodies are negative.

Management.   Whether the problem is truly polymyalgia rheumatica or whether it is rheumatoid arthritis is not crucial since the treatment is the same. The symptomatic response to moderate doses of corticosteroids (10–20 mg prednisone daily) is dramatic. This rapid response (often within one day) can be considered diagnostic. Patients can be maintained on low doses of corticosteroids (5.0–7.5 mg prednisone daily). Although some patients will have a limited course, long-term treatment for several years will be required for a large number. (10)

Giant Cell Arteritis

Giant cell arteritis is found often in patients with polymyalgia rheumatica, and these two conditions may actually represent the same disease. (11) Any patient with polymyalgia rheumatica who fails to respond to treatment should undergo temporal artery biopsy.

Pathophysiology. Giant cell arteritis is a pathologic diagnosis, necrotizing granulomatous arteritis, of a disease of unknown etiology. Any of the medium or larger arteries may be involved. The most serious consequence is sudden and irreversible blindness due to ischemic optic neuritis.

Signs and Symptoms. Headache and the symptoms of polymyalgia rheumatica are the most common presenting complaints. A pathognomonic complaint is pain with chewing. The patient may present with a fever of unknown origin. The involved arteries are often palpably enlarged and tender.

Diagnostic Tests. In the presence of a very elevated sedimentation rate (greater than 40 mm/hr), temporal artery biopsy should be considered. The biopsy is almost always positive in the presence of signs of cranial nerve involvement (headache, diplopia, jaw claudication, blurred vision), but can also be positive when the artery is clinically normal in the presence of systemic symptoms. The anemia of chronic inflammation is commonly encountered. Sometimes liver function tests are abnormal (and return to normal with treatment).

Management. Higher doses of corticosteroids are necessary, starting with 60 mg prednisone daily, which is maintained for one month. The dose is then gradually reduced according to symptoms and sedimentation rate. The patient eventually can be maintained on a low dose (5.0–7.5 mg prednisone daily) which is in fact necessary to avoid the risks of blindness and a dissecting aortic aneurysm. These diseases are self-limiting and treatment is usually necessary no longer than 2 years. Because the arteries are involved in a patchy fashion, a biopsy may be falsely negative. When the clinical story is strong, empirical treatment is indicated.

A diagnosis of polymyalgia rheumatica and/or giant cell arteritis should be considered in any elderly patient who has the following:

1. Unexplained aching and stiffness.

2. Acute onset of headaches.

3. Visual disturbances.

4. Fever of unknown etiology.

5. Unexplained anemia.

Gout

The term gout is derived from the 13th century, from a Latin word meaning drop, reflecting the notion that a poison was being introduced drop by drop into the joints. Gout is a metabolic disease, a derangement of purine metabolism, characterized by an elevated serum uric acid concentration (greater than 7.0 mg/dl), acute arthritis, tophi (deposits of monosodium urate), renal disease, and urolithiasis. The arthritis is the consequence of an inflammatory response to the presence of uric acid crystals in the synovial fluid. Chronic gouty arthritis takes years to develop and represents a response to tophi, collections of sodium urate crystals surrounded by inflammation. This is less common today with the use of prophylactic treatment.

Pathophysiology.   Women become hyperuricemic only after menopause, and therefore clinical gout does not appear until ages 60–70. (12) (The influence of estrogen replacement on this condition has not been studied.) The strong association between gout and osteoarthritis in the elderly suggests that damaged cartilage is more prone to allow crystal deposition. In the elderly, gout is commonly due to hyperuricemia secondary to the long-term use of diuretics. The exact mechanism for the well-known association of an acute attack with illness (medical or surgical) or stress remains unknown.

Signs and Symptoms.   The acute inflammation can occur in the great toe, knee, wrist, ankle, or elbow. The typical attack is abrupt in onset (often at night) with rapid progression to maximal symptoms within a few hours. The attack lasts from a few days to a few weeks. Fever is often present. Only after many years do patients develop a chronic problem involving multiple joints. The previous period of hyperuricemia may have been asymptomatic, therefore any elderly patient with an inflammatory arthritis may have gout, and the possibility of gout should always be considered in patients with osteoarthritis who present with an inflamed joint.

Diagnostic Tests.   Uric acid levels are too variable and inconsistent to aid in the diagnosis of gout. If synovial fluid is available, the diagnosis of gout can be established by demonstrating the presence of sodium urate crystals in the fluid. Aspiration of the involved joint (arthrocentesis) is highly recommended. Acute attacks are usually accompanied by leukocytosis and an elevated sedimentation rate.

Synovial Fluid Analysis

Inflammatory Disease	Non-Inflammatory Disease
WBC > 3000	WBC < 1000

Urate crystals
  —needle shaped, yellow, with
    negative birefringence	

Calcium pyrophosphate crystals
  —rodlike, bluish, with positive
    birefringence	

Management.   In the elderly, the NSAIDs are a better choice of treatment than colchicine (because of its gastrointestinal side effects). The response to treatment is very prompt. If diuretics cannot be discontinued, prophylaxis against gouty arthritis can be achieved with 0.6 mg bid colchicine, or simply treating the acute episodes with the anti-inflammatory drugs. Probenecid (500 mg daily or bid) and sulfinpyrazone are the most commonly used uricosuric drugs, blocking tubular reabsorption of uric acid. Because of the risk of precipitating stones, they are not the drugs of first choice. If attacks are frequent or there is joint destruction, the drug of choice for hyperuricemic treatment is allopurinol, which inhibits xanthine oxidase and blocks the formation of uric acid. The drug is given once daily (300 mg) along with large volumes of fluids and colchicine (0.6 mg daily) as prophylaxis for the hyperuricemia during the first 3–6 months. Patients with renal impairment are at risk of serious toxicity with allopurinol. Prednisone (40–60 mg per day) will promptly treat an acute episode in those patients intolerant of other drugs.

What To Do With Asymptomatic Hyperuricemia?   Uric acid is the end product of purine metabolism and must be excreted by the kidneys. Therefore either overproduction or underexcretion can cause hyperuricemia. Common causes to keep in mind are thiazide diuretics, prostaglandin synthesis inhibitors, and excessive alcohol intake. Although the risk of gout is increased with asymptomatic hyperuricemia, the cost of prophylaxis far exceeds the cost of waiting for and treating acute attacks. The risk of renal impairment or renal stones due to the hyperuricemia is not significant and also does not warrant prophylactic treatment. Asymptomatic hyperuricemia may last a lifetime without consequences.

CPPD Disease

Pseudogout, more common in the elderly than gout, is due to calcium pyrophosphate deposition rather than urate crystals. (13) Accordingly, this disorder is now named calcium pyrophosphate dihydrate (CPPD) deposition disease. This metabolic problem can be a subtle disorder presenting as an acute problem or as a chronic arthropathy. The acute inflammation usually involves only one joint, most often in the knee rather than the big toe, and also in the wrist, shoulder, and ankle joints. Synovial fluid examination under polarized light microscopy will reveal the calcium pyrophosphate crystals. Corticosteroids can be injected into the knee joint or a short course of the NSAIDs can be used. Often no treatment is necessary, as the acute attack resolves spontaneously. This condition has a characteristic x-ray appearance—chondrocalcinosis (calcification in cartilage). This characteristic x-ray calcification is due to the same calcium pyrophosphate crystals found in the synovial fluid. CPPD disease is often associated with hyperparathyroidism and hemochromatosis in elderly patients. Asymptomatic chondrocalcinosis does not require treatment. Chronic arthropathy with CPPD disease is more severe than osteoarthritis, and because it is inflammatory, it may be difficult to distinguish this disease from rheumatoid arthritis. Of course the demonstration of the characteristic crystals in the synovial fluid will establish the diagnosis. Treatment of the chronic disease is the same as for rheumatoid arthritis.

Inflammatory Joint Disease	Non-Inflammatory Joint Disease
PIPS, MCPs, and carpals	DIPs
Morning stiffness longer than 30 minutes	Pain with activity, relieved by rest
Systemic symptoms	No systemic symptoms
Anemia	Normal CBC
ESR > 40 mm/hr	ESR < 30 mm/hr
Rheumatoid factor and/or ANA may be positive	Rheumatoid factor and/or ANA usually negative

NONINFLAMMATORY JOINT PROBLEMS

Osteoarthritis

The term osteoarthritis is a misnomer. This is not an inflammatory condition. This is a chronic, non-inflammatory deterioration and abrasion of articular cartilage, although cartilage particles can cause inflammation of the synovium. Osteoarthritis of the hands is more common in women. Pain in the early years gives way to the knobby appearance as the main problem, as well as some loss of dexterity. Because the first carpometacarpal joint is involved, the use of the thumb may become impaired. Almost half of people in the 7th, 8th, and 9th decades of life have osteoarthritis of the knee. (14) But not all old people get osteoarthritis, and the severity does not increase with age, being about the same when people in their 60s are compared to people in their 80s and 90s. (14)

Pathophysiology. The deterioration of the articular cartilage usually but not always occurs without the synovial inflammation characteristic of rheumatoid arthritis. The loss of cartilage and the formation of new cartilage and bone (osteophytes) are the characteristic features of osteoarthritis. (15) It is still a mystery why some individuals and some joints are subjected to an accelerated deterioration of cartilage. In only a minority of patients can it be attributed to previous trauma or inflammation. Indeed, in studies of runners ages 50–72, there is no difference in osteoarthritis, bone density is greater, and musculoskeletal disability develops with increasing age at a slower rate in the runners. (16,17)

Signs and Symptoms. *Osteoarthritis involves the distal interphalangeal joints and spares the metacarpophalangeal joints and wrists, the exact opposite of the distribution seen with rheumatoid arthritis.* Other factors which distinguish rheumatoid arthritis from osteoarthritis include loss of grip strength, the elevated sedimentation rate, and the character of the discomfort with rheumatoid arthritis. With osteoarthritis, the pain is deep and aching in the involved joints. It is increased with weight-bearing activity and relieved by rest. Morning stiffness usually lasts 5–15 minutes, and unlike rheumatoid arthritis, no longer than 30 minutes. The joint problem remains localized, usually in the hands, hips, knees, feet, or the cervical and lumbar vertebrae. Osteoarthritis is rarely seen in the metacarpophalangeal joints, wrists, elbows, shoulders, and ankles. The small paired osteophytes at the distal interphalangeal joints are known as *Heberden's nodes*. Similar osteophyte formation affecting the prox-

265

imal interphalangeal joints is known as *Bouchard's nodes*. Women have more multiple joint involvement than men, and higher prevalence and severity of osteoarthritis of the hands, knees, ankles, and feet. A partial explanation for the greater frequency in weight-bearing joints in women is an association with obesity which probably increases the mechanical stress across a joint. (18)

Both the severity of the disease and psychological variables play a role in the degree of functional impairment and pain in the elderly. (19) This underscores the need to provide support for coping and management of depression and anxiety.

Diagnostic Tests. The diagnosis can be confirmed only by x-ray findings. The degeneration of the articular cartilage is accompanied by bone and cartilage overgrowth which gives the characteristic x-ray picture: narrowing of joint spaces, eburnation (subchondral bony sclerosis), and spur (osteophyte) formation. There are no diagnostic blood tests. It is important to keep in mind that an elevated erythrocyte sedimentation rate is not associated with osteoarthritis.

Management. There is no treatment available that can prevent or reverse osteoarthritis. Patients should limit their activity according to their symptoms, but an ordinary level of daily activity does not accelerate progression of the problem. Absolute rest is not recommended; muscle atrophy and osteoporosis will be accelerated. The degree of inflammation involved is minimal, and therefore there is no place for aggressive anti-inflammatory therapy with corticosteroids. Aspirin and the NSAIDs should be used only sporadically in analgesic doses to relieve symptoms, not daily unless necessary to allow exercise and mobility. Acetaminophen is a better choice to avoid the gastric problems associated with the prostaglandin inhibitors. In patients with severe symptoms and disability, response may require 3–4 weeks of treatment, and once relief is obtained, treatment should not be interrupted. Alternate joint rest with exercise. Swimming is an especially good exercise, and referral to a physical therapist is worthwhile.

There are 3 points which are important for patients to know:

1. This is a limited condition, not a generalized disease.

2. The aches and pains get better with time.

3. Hand function will be maintained.

Certain features are associated with the other specific sites of involvement:

The Hip. The chief symptom with hip involvement is pain with walking. The pain may extend to the groin, along the inner thigh to the knee. The diagnosis is made by internally rotating the hip and reproducing the pain. Of course, the diagnosis must be confirmed by x-ray. With progression, total hip arthroplasty is the choice yielding excellent results with resumption of daily activities.

266

The Knee. This site of osteoarthritis is associated with an effusion. Synovial fluid analysis may be necessary to rule out gout, CPPD disease, and rheumatoid arthritis. Treatment is symptomatic until total knee arthroplasty.

The Spine. Osteoarthritis of the spine is found to some degree in everyone over age 65. The most common locations are C4-C6 and L3-S1, but many people with abnormal x-rays are asymptomatic. Progression may lead to spinal stenosis, a narrowing of the spinal canal which produces pain in the thighs.

BONE PROBLEMS

Normal Calcium Metabolism

Bone is a very active organ. A continuous process, called bone remodeling, involves constant resorption (osteoclastic activity) and bone formation (osteoblastic activity). The amount of bone at any point of time reflects the balance of these forces, either of which is influenced by a multitude of stimulating and inhibiting agents. A decrease in calcium intake or absorption lowers the serum level of ionized calcium. This stimulates parathyroid hormone secretion to mobilize calcium from bone by direct stimulation of osteoclastic activity. Increased PTH also stimulates the production of 1,25-dihydroxyvitamin D to increase intestinal calcium absorption. Calcium increases and PTH levels return to normal. A deficiency in estrogen is associated with a greater responsiveness of bone to PTH. Thus for any given level of PTH there is more calcium removed from bone, raising serum calcium which in turn lowers PTH and decreases 1,25-dihydroxyvitamin D and intestinal absorption of calcium.

Postmenopausal Bone Loss

Osteoporosis, the most prevalent bone problem in the elderly, is decreased bone mass with a normal ratio of mineral to matrix, leading to an increase in fractures. Osteomalacia is deficient mineralization with a decreased ratio of mineral to matrix. Osteitis fibrosa is the resorption of bone and replacement by fibrous tissue, mediated by an increase in parathyroid hormone.

Postmenopausal bone loss is a heterogeneous mixture of all of the above conditions. Osteomalacia and osteitis fibrosa are more likely to occur in patients with renal failure, malabsorption, or on anticonvulsants. Thus the diagnosis of osteoporosis requires the demonstration of normal blood chemistry values.

SPECIFIC CAUSES OF BONE DISEASE IN ELDERLY WOMEN

Drugs: Heparin, anticonvulsants, alcohol.

Chronic Disease: Renal and liver.

Endocrine Diseases: Excess glucocorticoids, hyperthyroidism, estrogen deficiency, hyperparathyroidism.

Nutritional: Calcium, phosphorous, vitamin D deficiencies.

The prevention of osteoporosis in aging women now constitutes a major public health problem and one of our greatest health expenses. By virtue of the large number of women living a significant postmenopausal time span, a major reduction in the clinical manifestations of osteoporosis will have a very large impact on our health care system and our patients in terms of quality of life, mortality, and money saved.

An aggressive approach is necessary for two reasons. First, therapy is more effective the closer it is initiated to menopause, and second, once significant amounts of bone have been lost, complete retrieval can never be achieved.

Pathophysiology. There are two types of bone, cortical and trabecular. Cortical bone is the compact outer layer of bones. Trabecular bone refers to the interior meshwork (trabeculae) of bones. Long bones are at least 90% cortical, whereas the spinal vertebrae are mostly trabecular bone. Trabecular bone is more sensitive to changes in estrogen, and therefore the loss of estrogen affects trabecular bone more quickly than cortical bone. While trabecular bone loss begins earlier and occurs faster (accounting for vertebral and wrist fractures), the fact that 40% of white women have sustained hip fractures by age 80–90 indicates the significance and degree of postmenopausal cortical bone loss.

Loss of estrogen is a major factor affecting the risk of osteoporosis for postmenopausal women; 75% or more of the bone loss which occurs in women during the first 20 years after menopause is attributable to estrogen deficiency rather than to aging itself. (20,21) Vertebral bone is especially vulnerable, beginning to decline as early as 20 years of age. (22) Vertebral bone mass can be found to be significantly decreased in perimenopausal and early postmenopausal women who have rising FSH and decreasing estrogen levels, while bone loss from the radius is not found until at least a year out from the menopause. (23) This early loss of axial skeleton bone suggests that the hypoestrogenic postmenopausal state is not the only cause of vertebral osteoporosis. (24) A study of the premenopausal daughters of women with osteoporosis revealed a reduction in bone mass, suggesting either a genetic influence or the sharing of a lifestyle which produces a relatively low peak bone mass. (25) One obvious suspect is a decline in dietary intake of calcium in the premenopausal years; nevertheless, menopause and the loss of estrogen remain as the major contributors to bone loss. The risk of fracture, therefore, depends upon 2 factors: the bone mass achieved at maturity and the subsequent rate of bone loss. The bone density which is the threshold for vertebral fractures is only slightly below the lower limit of normal for premenopausal women. (26)

There is an epidemic of fractures in older people in the parts of the world with a high standard of living. (27) The incidence in Oslo, Norway, was 5 times greater in 1982 than in 1950. (28) This increase is greater than can be explained by the increasing number of elderly people. A favored explanation is the change in dietary practices in affluent societies, notably the elimination of dairy products early in life. Other possibilities include decreasing parity and the loss of a protective effect from the high steroid levels of pregnancy, and an earlier and greater loss of bone because of the impact of smoking.

Signs and Symptoms. The osteoporotic disabilities sustained by the castrate or postmenopausal woman include back pain, decreased height and mobility, and fractures of the vertebral body, humerus, upper femur, distal forearm, and ribs. Back pain is a major clinical symptom of vertebral compression fractures. The pain with a fracture is acute, then it subsides over 2–3 months but lingers as chronic low back pain due to increasing lumbar lordosis. The pain will subside within 6 months unless multiple fractures produce a picture of constant pain.

Loss of mineral content of bone happens in all aging individuals; however, white and oriental women start losing bone earlier and at a more rapid rate than black women; thus, not only a sexual but also a racial difference exists. Epidemiologic studies have revealed the following: (29)

1. *Spinal (vertebral) compression fractures:* Symptomatic spinal osteoporosis, causing pain, loss of height, postural deformities (the kyphotic dowager's hump) with consequent pulmonary, gastrointestinal, and bladder dysfunction, is 5 times more common in white women than men. Approximately 50% of women over 65 years of age have spinal compression fractures. Each complete compression fracture causes the loss of approximately 1 cm in height. The average non-treated postmenopausal white woman can expect to shrink 2.5 inches. The most common sites for vertebral fractures are the 12th thoracic and the first 3 lumbar vertebrae. These physical changes also have a negative impact on body image and self esteem.

2. *Colles' fractures:* There is a 10-fold increase in distal forearm fractures in white women as they progress from age 35 to 60 years. A white woman has approximately a 15% lifetime risk of a forearm fracture. Colles' fractures are the most common fractures among white women until age 75, when hip fractures become more common.

3. *Head of femur fractures:* The incidence of hip fractures also increases with age in white women, rising from 0.3/1000 to 20/1000 from 45 to 85 years. Eighty percent of all hip fractures are associated with osteoporosis. White women have about a 15% lifetime risk of having a hip fracture. This fracture carries a heavy risk of morbidity and mortality. Between 15–20% of patients with hip fracture die due to the fracture or its complications (surgical, embolic, cardiopulmonary) within 3 months, and Beals found that only half of hip fracture victims in Portland, Oregon, survived for 1 year. (30) In addition, the survivors are frequently severely disabled and may become permanent invalids.

Diagnostic Tests. It is not cost effective to attempt to select a high risk group (e.g. bone density measurements to select those at high risk for osteoporosis). (31) Such efforts are useful when an individual woman requires the information in order to make an informed decision regarding hormone replacement. Because smokers have lower estrogen levels on estrogen therapy, it might be worthwhile to document the impact of treatment on bone density in order to consider whether dosage is adequate. The method of choice, in terms of accuracy and sensitivity, is either dual-photon absorptiometry or a quantitative CT scan of the metabolically active trabecular bone in the spine. There is an increased risk of fracture when the bone density is less than 1 gm of mineral/cm^2 by dual photon absorptiometry or below 110 mg/cm^3 by CT scan. A new technique, dual energy x-ray absorptiometry, also called quantitative digital radiography, appears to be superior in terms of resolution and time. (32) Look for this method to become the method of choice.

Patients with apparent osteoporosis should be screened for other conditions which can lead to osteoporosis:

1. Serum parathyroid hormone, calcium, phosphorus, and alkaline phosphatase—for primary hyperparathyroidism.

2. Renal function tests—for secondary hyperparathyroidism with chronic renal failure.

3. Blood count and smear, and sedimentation rate—for multiple myeloma, leukemia, or lymphoma.

4. Thyroid function tests—for thyrotoxicosis.

5. Careful history and, when indicated, appropriate laboratory studies to rule out hypercortisolism.

The presence of osteomalacia, to be suspected in all elderly patients with osteoporosis, can be detected by measuring the serum calcium, phosphorus, alkaline phosphatase, and 1,25-dihydroxyvitamin D levels. These values are all normal in patients with osteoporosis but not osteomalacia.

Management. Unquestionably, exercise and diet have a beneficial effect on bone integrity. In a prospective, population-based study in southern California, calcium intake was low in both men and women with subsequent hip fractures. (33) Those who had the highest calcium intake had a 60% reduction in the risk of hip fracture compared to those with the lowest intake. This protection persisted even after adjustment for smoking, alcohol intake, exercise, and obesity.

Equally impressive is the accumulating evidence that an appropriate estrogen replacement program can have a major impact on the risk of fractures. One can expect a 50 to 60% decrease in fractures of the arm and hip (34–36), and when estrogen is supplemented with calcium, an 80% reduction in vertebral compression fractures can be observed. (37) It should be noted that the addition of vitamin D or its active metabolite has no impact on the fracture rate, and some women develop hypercalcemia with a risk of renal stone formation. (37,38)

Fluoride treatment stimulates osteoblasts leading to new bone formation. The resulting bone is less responsive to resorption. The addition of fluoride does offer some benefit; however, a high rate of side effects (40%) has been encountered, including joint and tendon inflammation, anemia, and gastrointestinal disturbances. A new slow release form that bypasses the stomach may prove to be effective with an acceptable level of side effects. (39) In the meantime, the optimal regimen is a combination of sex steroids and calcium.

An analysis of aging women's calcium needs indicated a greater requirement than previously appreciated. (40) In order to remain in zero calcium balance, women on estrogen replacement require a total

270

of 1,000 mg elemental calcium per day. Since the average woman receives only 500 mg of calcium in her diet, the minimal daily supplement equals an additional 500 mg. Women not on estrogen replacement require a daily supplement of at least 1,000 mg. Unfortunately in the absence of estrogen, there is significant impairment of calcium absorption. Even with the commonly used therapeutic doses of calcium, nearly 40% of postmenopausal women will have inefficient absorption. (41) Therefore estrogen improves calcium absorption and makes it possible to utilize supplemental calcium in effective doses (500 mg daily) without the side effects associated with higher doses (constipation and flatulence) which diminish compliance.

There are dozens of calcium supplements on the market. Most contain one of three calcium compounds: calcium carbonate, calcium lactate, or calcium gluconate. Calcium carbonate tablets are the cheapest and contain the most elemental calcium (40%). Calcium lactate tablets contain 13% calcium, and calcium gluconate only 9%. The calcium carbonate antacids are excellent, inexpensive sources. One should be aware that aluminum-containing antacids such as Maalox, Mylanta, Gelusil, and Riopan can inhibit gastrointestinal absorption of calcium. Bone meal and dolomite as sources of calcium should be avoided because they can be contaminated with lead.

Despite the important role for calcium, older women cannot totally substitute for the effectiveness of estrogen by compensatory increases in calcium supplementation. In the absence of estrogen, calcium, even in supplemental doses of 2000 mg/day, has only a little impact on trabecular bone and a minor impact on compact bone. (42,43) Furthermore, studies have been unable to detect any impact of dietary calcium intake (high or low) on the bone density of women in the early postmenopausal period. (44) Thus only a minimal level of calcium supplementation is necessary with hormonal replacement, and high calcium intake neither replaces hormone therapy nor adds to its impact.

This makes one think that the action of estrogen, besides its effect on calcium absorption, must include a direct protective mechanism on the bone. Bone resorption is regulated by osteoclasts, whereas osteoblasts form bone. Estrogen receptors have now been identified in osteoblast-like cells, and in addition, it has been demonstrated that this receptor is functional in that it induces the production of mRNA proteins as well as an increase in progesterone receptors. (45,46) The presence of estrogen receptors in osteoblasts strongly indicates that estrogen directly stimulates bone formation, and it is not surprising, therefore, that appropriate estrogen/progestin treatment can be associated with an increase in bone density.

Because progestational agents are anti-estrogenic, it is not illogical to question whether the addition of a progestin to an estrogen program counters the beneficial impact of estrogen on the bone. Fortunately progestational agents independently, in a manner similar to estrogen, reduce bone resorption, and when added to estrogen, no loss of protection against osteoporosis occurs. (47–50)

The positive impact of hormone replacement therapy on bone has been demonstrated to take place even in women over age 65. (48,51) This is a strong argument in favor of treating very old women who have never been on estrogen. Estrogen use between the ages of 65 and 74 has been documented to protect against hip fractures. (36)

The precise mechanism of action for sex steroid protection of bones remains unknown. It is apparent that the beneficial impact is achieved without significant changes in the blood levels of the various calcium regulating hormones. In addition, data do not support a role for calcitonin in postmenopausal osteoporosis. (52) Increased efficiency of calcium absorption and a still to be determined role for the estrogen receptors in the osteoblasts are likely important factors. Local mechanisms within the bone involve a variety of agents, including prostaglandins, interleukins, and growth factors. (53) The answer may be at this molecular level.

The protection of estrogen is maintained only while women are maintained on the replacement hormone. In the 3 to 5 year period following loss of estrogen, whether after menopause or after cessation of estrogen therapy, there is an accelerated loss of bone. (54,55) While this was not confirmed in one study (56), a careful analysis points out that bone mineral must be measured in the same exact sites because of differences in composition. When this is done an effect of estrogen is seen only in current users, and prior users have a prevalence rate of vertebral osteoporosis similar to women who have never taken estrogen. (57) For the greatest impact on fractures, it is vital that estrogen-progestin replacement be initiated as close to the menopause as possible, and it must be maintained long-term, if not life long.

Cigarette smoking is associated with an earlier menopause and an increased risk of osteoporosis. Because estrogen blood levels are lower in smokers who are on estrogen when compared to nonsmokers, it is concluded that smoking increases liver metabolism of estrogen. (58) Others have documented that smoking induces 2-hydroxylation of estradiol; the metabolic products, 2-hydroxyestrogens, have minimal estrogenic activity and are cleared rapidly from the circulation. (59) In addition, constituents of cigarette smoke inhibit granulosa cell aromatase, providing a further explanation for an earlier menopause in smokers. (60) Lower blood levels of estrogen in smokers have been correlated with a reduced bone density, and therefore, estrogen replacement does not totally counteract the predisposition toward osteoporosis in smokers.

Patients who already have clinically significant osteoporosis should be treated more vigorously. In addition to hormone replacement, treatment should include the active metabolite of vitamin D and either fluoride or calcitonin or both, depending upon the severity of the condition. Calcitonin inhibits osteoclast activity, and when compared to estrogen in postmenopausal women, it is just as effective in reducing vertebral bone loss. (61) Calcitonin is administered subcutaneously, 50–100 units every 1 to 3 days. The dose of sodium fluoride is 40–60 mg/day, and that of vitamin D 800–1000 IU/day. These treatments should be accompanied by adequate calcium supplementation.

Finally, we would be remiss if we did not promote the benefits of exercise. Physical activity (weight-bearing), as little as 30 minutes a day, 3 times a week, will increase the bone mineral content of bone in older women. (62,63) The exercise need not be extreme.

Walking 1.5 miles and ordinary calisthenics will suffice. The impact of exercise on vertebral trabecular bone is significantly less, however, and women require the full combination of hormone replacement, calcium supplementation, and exercise in order to fully minimize the risk of vertebral compression fractures.

Paget's Disease of Bone

Paget's disease of bone, also called osteitis deformans, is a chronic condition now believed to be a slow virus infection of the skeleton. There is increased bone resorption with haphazard formation of relatively weak and immature bone so that the bones are thickened, but weakened and distorted. Rare before 40, the incidence increases steadily to almost 10% in the 9th decade. The disease occurs more commonly in women, but equally in all races. Sarcoma develops in less than 1% of the patients.

The diagnosis is usually made on x-rays obtained because of an elevated serum alkaline phosphatase. Bone pain and fractures are a late presentation. Paget's affects the pelvis, femurs, and tibiae most frequently, followed by the skull and lumbar vertebrae. Bone remodeling can cause enlargement of the skull or bowing of bones such as the femur. Cranial nerves may be compressed because of bone overgrowth resulting in corresponding signs and symptoms (as well as spinal compression syndromes). The increase in bone blood flow can be so marked that high cardiac output failure may ensue.

Indications for treatment include pain, bending and deformities, fractures, and nerve damage (especially hearing loss), but severe symptoms occur in a minority of patients. Symptoms are usually treated with aspirin or NSAIDs, but severe disease requires more vigorous therapy. Calcitonin and diphosphates (sodium editronate) are the drugs of choice. Diphosphates bind to hydroapatite crystals and inhibit bone turnover. An intravenous form of bisphosphonate is available with long-term action, an especially good option for elderly patients in whom compliance is a problem. (64) Calcitonin as a nasal spray has been utilized, but antibodies form, reducing its effectiveness. (65) Mithramycin is very potent with acute renal, hepatic, and hematological toxicity; it is reserved for last resort treatment. Hearing loss can be halted and reversed with treatment. (66)

Patients with Paget's disease of bone often present with symptoms of degenerative joint disease. The arthritis in these patients does not respond to calcitonin, and standard arthritis treatment is necessary.

References

1. **Verbrugge LM,** From sneezes to adieux: Stages of health for American men and women, Soc Sci Med 22:1195, 1986.

2. **Vandenbroucke JP, Witteman JCM, Valkenburg HA, Boersma JW, Cats A, Festen JJM, Hartman AP, Huber-Bruning O, Rasker JJ, Weber J,** Non-contraceptive hormones and rheumatoid arthritis in perimenopausal and postmenopausal women, JAMA 255:1299, 1986.

3. **Ghosh SN, Seshadri R,** Expression of tumor cell properties in synovial cells in culture, Acta Cytol 31:77, 1987.

4. **Decker JL, Malone DG, Haraoui B, Wahl SM, Schrieber L, Klippel JH, Steinberg AD, Wilder RL,** Rheumatoid arthritis; evolving concepts of pathogenesis and treatment, Ann Intern Med 101:810, 1984.

5. **Choi EKK, Gatenby PA, McGill NW, Bateman JF, Cole WG, York RJ,** Autoantibodies to type II collagen: Occurrence in rheumatoid arthritis, other arthritides, autoimmune connective tissue diseases, and chronic inflammatory syndromes, Ann Rheum Dis 47:313, 1988.

6. **Graham DY, Agrawal NM, Roth SH,** Prevention of NSAID-induced gastric ulcer with misoprostol: Multicentre, double-blind, placebo-controlled trial, Lancet ii:1277, 1988.

7. **Fries JF, Miller SR, Spitz PW, Williams CA, et al,** Toward an epidemiology of gastropathy associated with nonsteroidal antiinflammatory drug use, Gastroenterology 96 (Suppl):647, 1989.

8. **Healey LA,** Late-onset rheumaoid arthritis vs polymyalgia rheumatica: Making the diagnosis, Geriatrics 43:65,69,1988.

9. **Sox HC, Liang MW,** The erythrocyte sedimentation rate, Ann Intern Med 104:515, 1986.

10. **Ayoub WT, Franklin CM, Torretti D,** Polymyalgia rheumatica. Duration of therapy and long-term outcome, Am J Med 79:309, 1985.

11. **Healey LA,** The spectrum of polymyalgia rheumatica, Clin Geriatr Med 4:323, 1988.

12. **Campbell SM,** Gout: How presentation, diagnosis, and treatment differ in the elderly, Geriatrics 43:71, 1988.

13. **Bonafede RP,** Evaluating CPPD crystal deposition, an important disease of aging, Geriatrics 43:59, 1988.

14. **Forman MD, Malamet R, Kaplan D,** A survey of osteoarthritis of the knee in the elderly, J Rheumatol 10:282, 1983.

15. **Hamerman D,** The biology of osteoarthritis, New Engl J Med 320:1322, 1989.

16. **Lane NE, Bloch DA, Jones HH, Marshall WH Jr, Wood PD, Fries JF,** Long-distance running, bone density, and osteoarthritis, JAMA 255:1147, 1986.

17. **Lane NE, Bloch DA, Wood PD, Fries JF,** Aging, long-distance running, and the development of musculoskeletal disability, Am J Med 82:772, 1987.

18. **Davis MA, Ettinger WH, Neuhaus JM, Hauck WW,** Sex differences in osteoarthritis of the knee, Am J Epidemiol 127:1019, 1988.

19. **Summers MN, Haley WE, Reveille JD, Alarcon GS,** Radiographic assessment and psychologic variables as predictors of pain and functional impairment in osteoarthritis of the knee or hip, Arthritis Rheumatism 31:204, 1988.

20. **Richelson LS, Wahner HW, Melton LJ III, Riggs BL,** Relative contributions of aging and estrogen deficiency to postmenopausal bone loss, New Engl J Med 311:1273, 1984.

21. **Nilas L, Christiansen C,** Bone mass and its relationship to age and the menopause, J Clin Endocrinol Metab 65:697, 1987.

22. **Avioli LV,** Calcium and osteoporosis, Annu Rev Nutr 4:471, 1984.

23. **Johnston CC Jr, Hui SL, Witt RM, Appledorn R, Baker RS, Longcope C,** Early menopausal changes in bone mass and sex steroids, J Clin Endocrinol Metab 61:905, 1985.

24. **Riggs BL, Wahner HW, Melton LJ III, Richelson LS, Judd HL, Offord KP,** Rates of bone loss in the appendicular and axial skeletons of women, J Clin Invest 77:1487, 1986.

25. **Seeman E, Hopper JL, Bach LA, Cooper ME, Parkinson E, McKay J, Jerums G,** Reduced bone mass in daughters of women with osteoporosis, New Engl J Med 320:554, 1989.

26. **Riggs BL, Wahner HW, Dunn WL, Mazess RB, Offord KP, Melton LJ III,** Differential changes in bone mineral density of the appendicular and axial skeleton with aging: Relationship to spinal osteoporosis, J Clin Invest 67:328, 1981.

27. **Lindsay R, Herrington BS,** Estrogens and osteoporosis, Seminars Reprod Endocrinol 1:55, 1983.

28. **Falch JA, Ilebekk A, Slungaard U,** Epidemiology of hip fractures in Norway, Acta Orthoped Scand 56:12, 1985.

29. **Cummings SR, Kelsey JL, Nevitt MC, O'Dowd KJ,** Epidemiology of osteoporosis and osteoporotic fractures, Epidemiol Rev 7:178, 1985.

30. **Beals RK,** Survival following hip fracture: Long term follow-up of 607 patients, J Chronic Dis 25:235, 1972.

31. **Hall FM, Davis MA, Baran DT,** Bone mineral screening for osteoporosis, New Engl J Med 316:212, 1987.

32. **Wahner HW, Dunn WL, Brown ML, et al,** Comparison of dual-energy x-ray absorptiometry for bone mineral measurements of the lumbar spine, Mayo Clin Proc 63:1075, 1988.

33. **Holbrook TL, Barrett-Connor E, Wingard DL,** Dietary calcium and risk of hip fracture: 14-year prospective population study, Lancet ii:1046, 1988.

34. **Weiss NC, Ure CL, Ballard JH, Williams AR, Daling JR,** Estimated incidence of fractures of the lower forearm and hip in postmenopausal women, New Engl J Med 303:1195, 1980.

35. **Ettinger B, Genant HK, Cann CE,** Long-term estrogen replacement therapy prevents bone loss and fractures, Ann Intern Med 102:319, 1985.

36. **Kiel DP, Felson DT, Anderson JJ, Wilson PWF, Moskowitz MA,** Hip fracture and the use of estrogens in postmenopausal women: The Framingham Study, New Engl J Med 317:1169, 1987.

37. **Riggs BL, Seeman E, Hodgson SF, Taves DR, O'Fallon WM,** Effect of the fluoride/calcium regimen on vertebral fracture occurrence in postmenopausal osteoporosis, New Engl J Med 306:446, 1982.

38. **Jensen GF, Christiansen C, Transbol I,** Treatment of postmenopausal osteoporosis. A controlled therapeutic trial comparing oestrogen/gestagen, 1,25-dihydroxy-vitamin D3, and calcium, Clin Endocrinol 16:515, 1982.

39. **Pak CYC, Sakhaee K, Zerwekh JE, Parcel C, Peterson R, Johnson K,** Safe and effective treatment of osteoporosis with intermittent slow release sodium fluoride: Augmentation of vertebral bone mass and inhibition of fractures, J Clin Endocrinol Metab 68:150, 1989.

40. **Heaney RP, Recker RR, Saville PD,** Menopausal changes in calcium balance performance, Lab Clin Med 92:953, 1978.

41. **Heaney RP, Recker RR,** Distribution of calcium absorption in middle-aged women, Am J Clin Nutrition 43:299, 1986.

42. **Riis B, Thomsen K, Christiansen C,** Does calcium supplementation prevent postmenopausal bone loss? New Engl J Med 316:173, 1987.

43. **Ettinger B, Genant HK, Cann CE,** Postmenopausal bone loss is prevented by treatment with low-dosage estrogen with calcium, Ann Int Med 106:40, 1987.

44. **Stevenson JC, Whitehead MI, Padwick M, Endacott JA, Sutton C, Banks LM, Freemantle C, Spinks TJ, Hesp R,** Dietary intake of calcium and postmenopausal bone loss, Brit Med J 297:15, 1988.

45. **Komm BSD, Terpening CM, Benz DJ, Graeme KA, Gallegos A, Korc M, Greene GL, O'Malley BW, Haussler MR,** Estrogen binding, receptor mRNA, and biologic response in osteoblast-like osteosarcoma cells, Science 241:81, 1988.

46. **Eriksen EF, Colvard DS, Berg NJ, Graham ML, Mann KG, Spelsberg TC, Riggs BL,** Evidence of estrogen receptors in normal human osteoblast-like cells, Science 241:84, 1988.

47. **Abdalla HI, Hart DM, Lindsay R, Leggate I, Hooke A,** Prevention of bone mineral loss in postmenopausal women by norethisterone, Obstet Gynecol 66:789, 1985.

48. **Selby PL, Peacock M, Barkworth SA, Brown WB, Taylor GA,** Early effects of ethinyl oestradiol and norethisterone treatment in postmenopausal women on bone resorption and calcium regulating hormones, Clin Sci 69:265, 1985.

49. **Christiansen C, Nilas L, Riis BJ, Rodbro P, Deftos L,** Uncoupling of bone formation and resorption by combined oestrogen and progestagen therapy in postmenopausal osteoporosis, Lancet ii:800, 1985.

50. **Munk-Jensen N, Nielsen SP, Obel EB, Eriksen PB,** Reversal of postmenopausal vertebral bone loss by oestrogen and progestogen: A double blind placebo controlled study, Brit Med J 296:1150, 1988.

51. **Quigley MET, Martin PL, Burnier AM, Brooks P,** Estrogen therapy arrests bone loss in elderly women, Am J Obstet Gynecol 156:1516, 1987.

52. **Tiegs RD, Body JJ, Wahner HW, Barta J, Riggs BL, Heath H,** Calcitonin secretion in postmenopausal osteoporosis, New Engl J Med 312:1097, 1985.

53. **Raisz LG,** Local and systemic factors in the pathogenesis of osteoporosis, New Engl J Med 318:818, 1988.

54. **Lindsay R, MacLean A, Kraszewski A, Clark AC, Garwood J,** Bone response to termination of estrogen treatment, Lancet i:1325, 1978.

55. **Horsman A, Nordin BEC, Crilly RG,** Effect on bone of withdrawal of estrogen therapy, Lancet ii:33, 1979.

56. **Christiansen C, Christiansen MS, Transbol IB,** Bone mass in postmenopausal women after withdrawal of oestrogen/gestagen replacement therapy, Lancet i:459, 1981.

57. **Wasnich R, Yano K, Vogel J,** Postmenopausal bone loss at multiple skeletal sites: Relationship to estrogen use, J Chronic Dis 36:781, 1983.

58. **Jensen J, Christiansen C, Rodbro P,** Cigarette smoking, serum estrogens, and bone loss during hormone replacement therapy early after menopause, New Engl J Med 313:973, 1985.

59. **Michnovicz JJ, Hershcopf RJ, Naganuma H, Bradlow HL, Fishman J,** Increased 2-hydroxylation of estradiol as a possible mechanism for the anti-estrogenic effect of cigarette smoking, New Engl J Med 315:1305, 1986.

60. **Barbieri RL, McShane PM, Ryan KJ,** Constituents of cigarette smoke inhibit human granulosa cell aromatase, Fertil Steril 46:232, 1986.

61. **MacIntyre I, Stevenson JC, Whitehead MI, Wimalawansa SJ, et al,** Calcitonin for prevention of postmenopausal bone loss, Lancet i:900, 1988.

62. **Chow RK, Harrison JE, Brown CF, Hajek V,** Physical fitness effect on bone mass in postmenopausal women, Arch Phys Med Rehabil 67:231, 1986.

63. **Dalsky GP, Stocke KS, Ehsani AA, Slatopolsky E, Lee WC, Birge SJ Jr,** Weight-bearing exercise training and lumbar bone mineral content in postmenopausal women, Ann Intern Med 108:824, 1988.

64. **Thiebaud D, Jaeger P, Gobelet C, Jacquet AF, Burckhardt P,** A single infusion of the bisphosphonate AHPrBP (APD) as treatment of Paget's disease of bone, Am J Med 85:207, 1988.

65. **Levy F, Muff R, Dotti-Sigrist S, Dambacher MA, Fischer JA,** Formation of neutralizing antibodies during intranasal synthetic salmon calcitonin treatment of Paget's disease, J Clin Endocrinol Metab 67:541, 1988.

66. **Lando M, Hoover LA, Finerman G,** Stabilization of hearing loss in Paget's disease with calcitonin and etidronate, Arch Otolaryngol Head Neck Surg 114:891, 1988.

67. **Winfield J, Stamp TCB,** Bone and joint symptoms in Paget's disease, Ann Rheum Dis 43:769, 1984.

277

18 Common Infectious Problems

Infectious diseases are responsible for 30% of all mortality in older people. (1) Aging is associated with a greater susceptibility to infections, probably due to a decline of host defense mechanisms. An altered pharmacology of antibiotics in older people affects treatment choices and outcomes. Although the signs and symptoms of infection in older people are essentially the same as in younger people, it is the impression of clinicians that many infections in the elderly present in a vague way. Mild general symptoms such as confusion, weakness, loss of appetite, decline in performance, or a lessened interest in an individual's social and physical environment may indicate the presence of infection. ***When an older person is sick and there is no apparent etiology, always consider infection.***

Aging and Infection

Diagnosis.   Infection in the elderly is often a problem of recognition. As a general rule, infection in elderly people who are physiologically young will present in the usual, typical fashion. But aged patients with reduced reserves who are under stress because of the presence of an infection frequently present with common geriatric problems which reflect relative functional impairment of other systems: confusion or delirium, falling or postural instability, immobility, urinary incontinence, fecal incontinence.

Older patients are often unable to date the onset of an illness. Any change in well-being requires careful assessment, but infection may be totally silent because of the attenuation of symptoms and signs due to aging. Temperature response is lower, often normal, and sometimes hypothermic. (2) Afebrile bacteremia is not rare in geriatric patients. The most common association is with an alteration in mental status or unexplained leukocytosis. (3) The leukocyte response to infection is usually similar in old and young patients; however, older people often respond to acute bacterial infection with a significant lymphopenia, the severity of which has prognostic value. (4) With an unclear history, the lack of fever, and a pre-existing cardiac or respiratory problem, an older patient with an infection is likely to be misdiagnosed.

279

ASSESSMENT FOR THE PRESENCE OF INFECTION

History: Acute symptoms, chills, weakness, malaise, minor changes in daily function.

Examination: Fever or hypothermia, hyperventilation, tachycardia.

Laboratory: CBC with differential, ESR, chest x-ray, urinalysis, cultures.

Treatment. In older people who are physiologically young, it is not critical whether an antimicrobial compound is bactericidal or bacteriostatic. In an older individual who is immunologically less competent and who has an underlying illness which interferes with the response to infection, it is important to choose agents which are bactericidal.

BACTERICIDAL ANTIMICROBIAL AGENTS

Penicillin and its homologues
Cephalosporins
Aminoglycosides
Vancomycin
Metronidazole
Fluoroquinolones

The initial dose of antibiotics is not altered by age, but maintenance doses are usually less. Also keep in mind that antibiotics may interfere with other medications and with certain laboratory tests. Some important pharmacologic principles are as follows:

1. A decline in gastric acidity with aging leads to greater absorption and a need for lesser doses.

2. Blood levels are affected by renal function, therefore both serum drug levels and renal function should be monitored.

3. Patients with congestive heart failure may require higher doses because of a greater volume of distribution.

4. Dehydrated patients require lower doses.

5. Diseases affected by electrolyte concentrations and diseases that limit electrolyte excretion can be influenced by the sodium content of antibiotics.

6. Renal excretion of antibiotics can enhance urinary potassium and hydrogen ion losses, leading to hypokalemic alkalosis.

7. The elderly have an increased frequency of adverse reactions.

Urinary Tract
Infections

The most common bacterial infection in the elderly is that of the urinary tract. It is the most common source of bacteremia in older people. Although infection is usually associated with the familiar symptoms of dysuria and frequency, atypical presentations are common in the elderly. Therefore, the urine should be examined and cultured in all elderly people with fever, new onset of incontinence, or renal impairment.

Clinical studies have generally supported empiric treatment for acute, uncomplicated urinary tract infections in women. From a cost effective point of view, it is acceptable to omit a culture in this circumstance. However, with repeated episodes, it becomes important to culture the urine prior to a course of antibiotics. The drugs of choice are trimethoprim, trimethoprim/sulfamethoxazole, nitrofurantoin, or sulfa. Ampicillin is not recommended for first-line therapy. Treatment regimens for cystitis range from single dose to 10 days. For upper tract infections, longer courses are indicated.

It is important to identify patients with recurrent infections because of the significant risk of renal impairment. Urinary tract infections usually are secondary to stepwise colonization of the vaginal introitus and urethral mucosa by uropathogenic organisms from the rectal flora. Bacterial adherence to epithelial receptors is an important part of the mechanism. Although not documented, it is likely that estrogen replacement therapy will reduce the frequency of urine infections in the postmenopausal years because of its support of a normal vaginal flora.

Women with recurrent infections should have urologic evaluation, including urography and cystoscopy, to identify correctable causes for reinfection, e.g. a urethral diverticulum. The urethral diverticulum is probably an acquired problem following trauma, catheterization, labor and delivery, or infections. The classic symptoms are dysuria, post voiding dribbling, and a purulent exudate expressible from the urethra. Surgical repair is necessary.

In women with repeated infections, a midstream clean catch specimen which yields a positive result should be confirmed by a urine sample obtained by catheterization. (Single catheterization for diagnostic purposes should be followed by single dose prophylaxis of an antimicrobial agent). The traditional requirement for a colony count of 100,000 or more per ml is no longer acceptable. Lower counts (as low as 100/ml) can be associated with significant infections.

Recurrent reinfection without an identifiable cause should be given a course of low-dose prophylaxis (maintained for at least 6 months). (5) An agent must be used that has no risk of causing resistance in the fecal flora.

Agents for Low-Dose Prophylaxis

1. Nitrofurantoin 100 mg qhs.

2. Cephalexin 250 mg qhs.

3. Trimethoprim-sulfamethoxazole (Bactrim, Cotrim, Septra) 40–200 mg qhs or trimethoprim 50 mg qhs.

4. Cinoxacin 250–500 mg qhs.

For difficult, recalcitrant cases, the patient can be educated to utilize self-start therapy. Treatment follows the demonstration of infection with one of the home testing kits. A 3 day full dose, empirical broad spectrum antimicrobial agent is used. Full dose nitrofurantoin, cinoxacin, or norfloxacin are recommended. Ampicillin, tetracycline, sulfisoxazole, and cephalexin all should be avoided because of the propensity for resistant bacteria. Bacteriuria persistent 10 days after treatment requires follow-up evaluation. The fluoroquinolones are bactericidal broad spectrum drugs, well tolerated by elderly people. (6) Norfloxacin is especially effective for the treatment of urinary tract infections due to resistant organisms.

Asymptomatic Bacteriuria. Asymptomatic bacteriuria (a colony count greater than 100,000/ml in an asymptomatic patient) is more common in older women. A lack of estrogen lowers the vaginal pH, promoting colonization of the vagina by uropathogens. Pelvic floor relaxation can lead to urinary tract obstruction and incomplete voiding. It is not cost-effective to routinely culture all older women. However, if asymptomatic bacteriuria is identified, single-dose antibiotic therapy is worthwhile: 3 tablets of double-strength trimethoprim sulfamethoxazole (Bactrim DS, Septra DS) or 3 gm of amoxicillin. If asymptomatic bacteriuria persists, repeated treatment is not indicated.

Pneumonia

Most cases of pneumonia occur in the elderly and are associated with a significant mortality rate. Approximately two-thirds of the cases are bacterial, usually streptococcus. But Gram-negative pneumonia is more common in the elderly than in younger people. Bacterial pneumonia is usually due to aspiration of oral fluids, therefore the organism which causes pneumonia is related to the bacterial colonization of the oropharynx. Oropharyngeal colonization with Gram-negative bacteria is more common in elderly patients, and especially more common in the institutionalized elderly. Because of the frequency of Gram-negative infections, it is appropriate to treat initially with a broad spectrum antibiotic until cultures demonstrate the presence of streptococcus, *Haemophilus influenzae*, or pneumococcus.

Older people with pneumonia may not present with the typical cough, sputum, and rales. Therefore older, febrile patients usually require a chest x-ray. Despite this proviso, most older patients with pneumonia *will* have a cough with sputum production, hyperventilation, and fever. X-ray patterns are somewhat different in the elderly with pneumonia. Lobar consolidation is not common, infiltrates are less extensive, and resolution is slower.

Influenza	Most patients who die of influenza are elderly. The flu usually presents as a mild pneumonic illness which becomes complicated by a bacterial superinfection. Vaccination has been documented to significantly reduce hospitalizations and deaths in the elderly population during epidemics. (7) While the illness may not be prevented, the vaccine is effective in reducing complications and mortality. In susceptible populations, amantadine can be used for effective prophylaxis and therapy against influenza A. The dose is 100 mg bid until age 65, after which the dose is reduced to 100 mg daily. (8) When used for treatment, it should be started within the first 48 hours of the illness.

Tuberculosis	The largest group of patients with active tuberculosis in the U.S. is the elderly. (9) Most cases of tuberculosis are due to activation of an infection acquired earlier in life. This occurs in the elderly as defense mechanisms wane with aging. Thus it is not surprising that reactivation of dormant disease occurs when an elderly person's immune system is compromised by a significant illness or malnutrition. The majority of undiagnosed and fatal cases of miliary tuberculosis occur in patients over age 60. Also now more common in older people are genitourinary tuberculosis and tuberculosis meningitis.

Tuberculosis in the elderly can present in many and often atypical manifestations. Tuberculosis should always be considered in an elderly patient with any of the following:

1. Puzzling pleuropulmonary symptoms.

2. Unexplained fever.

3. Anorexia.

4. Weight loss.

5. Change of behavior, mental state.

6. Impaired organ function.

7. Unexplained physical findings.

8. Unexplained laboratory abnormalities.

Several precautions are in order with PPD skin testing in the elderly. A boosted response occurs more often in the elderly, and a false positive may appear up to a year after the initial negative skin test. Thus nonreactors should be retested one week after the initial negative test to document this effect. The skin test is often negative in older people with severe pulmonary tuberculosis and with active miliary tuberculosis.

Treatment of tuberculosis in the elderly consists of isoniazid and rifampin in the usual recommended doses, with monthly assessment of SGOT levels. Peripheral neuropathy (which is potentially incapacitating in an older person) can be prevented with a daily 50 mg dose of pyridoxine.

Dermatologic Infections	The two main dermatologic problems which increase with advancing age are infected skin ulcers and herpes zoster.

Herpes Zoster. It is likely that acute episodes of herpes zoster in older life are due to reactivation of previous varicella-zoster viral infections. (10) Why the latent virus lying dormant in ganglia becomes activated is unknown, although the increase in frequency with aging is thought to reflect the decrease in immunocompetency.

In about 20% of patients, the eruption involves the trigeminal nerve. In the remaining patients, the rash usually occurs on the neck, trunk, or abdomen. Bladder and anal involvement occur, but complete recovery of function is the rule. The acute phase lasts 10–14 days.

Contrary to younger people, the older patient with herpes zoster is prone to develop a neuralgia that persists for over a year. Although controversial, the overall course can probably be shortened and neuralgia prevented with acyclovir.

Infected Skin Ulcers. The elderly are prone to decubitus ulcers and skin ulcers of the lower extremities due to vascular insufficiency. Infections are usually due to staphylococci, streptococci, and aerobic Gram-negative bacilli, but the presence of gas and/or a putrid odor suggests infection with anaerobes. Surgical debridement is an important component of treatment, combined with parenteral antibiotics if systemic signs of infection are present. Enzymatic debriding can be utilized between the periodic surgical debridements. Patients with skin infections should receive a booster of tetanus toxoid.

Otitis	External otitis due to pseudomonas is seen principally in older people who are diabetic. The infection frequently spreads to adjacent soft tissue and the skull. Pain and discharge are the most common complaints. At least a 3 week course of an aminoglycoside along with an anti-pseudomonal penicillin should be administered. Aminoglycoside blood levels and the serum potassium must be monitored. Treatment must be aggressive and prompt to avoid spread of the infection.

Immunizations	Only about 22% of people 65 years of age and older receive influenza vaccine annually and only 10% have ever received the pneumococcal vaccine. (11) These low percentages indicate the need for physicians to become more aggressive in promoting the availability, efficacy, and safety of immunization.

Influenza Immunization. Influenza viruses belong to the myxovirus group. There are 3 major immunologically distinct groups: influenza A, B, and C. A and B are encountered most frequently, and the A group contains major subgroups. Type B occurs principally in young people, while type A occurs in the older population. Therefore it is not surprising that excess mortality is associated with type A outbreaks.

Every 10–15 years a major antigenic variant appears, resulting in a significant epidemic. This variation is a critical problem in the use of influenza vaccines. Specific strains of influenza viruses are identified regularly throughout the world, and each February a decision is made regarding which strains to include in the vaccine which is then administered annually.

284

It is argued that the vaccine effectively reduces complications and mortality and should be administered to all people 65 years old and older. (8,12,13) Elderly people considered to be at high risk for influenza include adults with chronic cardiovascular or pulmonary disorders, and older people who are living in chronic care facilities. Healthy people over 65 years of age are considered to be a moderate risk. The Australians have contended that vaccinating healthy people aged 45–64 is even more cost-effective than vaccinating the high risk groups. (14)

We recommend that influenza vaccine be administered annually (best in the Fall) to all women, beginning at age 65. Reaction to the vaccination includes redness and swelling at the site as well as fever. People who have anaphylactic hypersensitivity to eggs should not receive the influenza vaccine.

Pneumococcal Immunization. Pneumococcal polysaccharide vaccine should be offered to all people at age 65. Even though data on its efficacy for the elderly are not available, this recommendation is made because of its safety, inexpensive cost, and the increased incidence of pneumonia with advancing age. Certainly patients with chronic illnesses are appropriate candidates for this vaccine. This vaccine is effective against about two-thirds of the bacterial pneumococcal infections encountered in the U.S. Only a single immunization is necessary, and it can be given simultaneously with the influenza vaccine.

Diphtheria and Tetanus Immunization. The highest number of unprotected people are those over 60. (15) Tetanus-diphtheria toxoids must be administered to older people with the same frequency as recommended for younger adults (every 10 years). This should not be neglected, since the elderly represent the greatest risk for these diseases.

References

1. **Mostow SR,** Infectious diseases in the aged, in Schrier RW, editor, *Clinical Internal Medicine in the Aged*, W.B. Saunders Co., Philadelphia, 1982, pp 256–273.

2. **Finkelstein MS, Petkun WM, Freedman ML, Antopol SC,** Pneumococcal bacteremia in adults: Age-dependent differences in presentation and outcome, J Am Geriatrics Soc 31:19, 1983.

3. **Gleckman R, Hibert D,** Afebrile bacteremia: A phenomenon in geriatric patients, JAMA 248:1478, 1982.

4. **Proust J, Roxenzweig P, Debouzy C, Moulias R,** Lymphopenia induced by acute bacterial infections in the elderly: A sign of age-related immune dysfunction of major prognostic significance, Gerontology 31:178, 1985.

5. **Schaeffer AJ,** Recurrent urinary tract infections in women, Postgrad Med 81:51, 1987.

6. **Gantz NM,** Quinolones: Their uses in geriatric infections, Geriatrics 43:41, 1988.

7. **Barker WH, Mullooly JP,** Influenza vaccination of elderly persons: Reduction in pneumonia and influenza hospitalizations and deaths, JAMA 244:2547, 1980.

8. **Arden NH, Patriarca PA, Fasano MB, Lui K-J, Harmon MW, Kendal AP, Rimland D,** The roles of vaccination and amantadine prophylaxis in controlling an outbreak of influenza A (H3N2) in a nursing home, Arch Intern Med 148:865, 1988.

9. **Nagami PH, Yoshikawa TT,** Tuberculosis in the geriatric patient, J Am Geriatrics Soc 31:356, 1983.

10. **Ragozzino MW, Melton LJ III, Kurland LT, et al,** Population-based study of herpes zoster and its sequelae, Medicine 61:310, 1982.

11. **Williams WW, Hickson MA, Kane MA, Kendal AP, Spika JS, Hinman AR,** Immunization policies and vaccine coverage among adults: The risk for missed opportunities, Ann Intern Med 108:616, 1988.

12. **Thompson MP,** Is routine influenza immunization indicated for people over 65 years of age? An affirmative view, J Fam Pract 26:211, 1988.

13. **Gross PA, Quinnan GV, Rodstein M, LaMontagne JR, et al,** Association of influenza immunization with reduction in mortality in an elderly population. A prospective study, Arch Intern Med 148:562, 1988.

14. **Evans DB, Hensley MJ, O'Connor SJ,** Influenza vaccination in Australia: A review of the economic evidence for policy recommendatins, Med J Aust 149:540, 1988.

15. **Kjeldsen K, Simonsen O, Heron I,** Immunity against diphtheria and tetanus in the age group 30–70 years, Scand J Infect Dis 20:177, 1988.

19   Chronic Pain and Hypochondriasis

Pain is the most common reason patients see a physician. The most common types of pain are headaches, abdominal pain, and low back pain. (1,2) Chronic low back pain is the most common reason for time lost from work and accounts for 20 million visits to physicians each year. (2–4) Most often pain is adaptive and essential for the health and well-being of an individual. It frequently provides the first clue that an important disease is present. Clinically, we use pain characteristics to enable us to diagnose a treatable condition promptly when the chance of cure is best. However, chronic pain can become maladaptive and a challenge to manage.

Pain Perception

Two types of peripheral nerve fibers transmit pain signals: large, myelinated A fibers which rapidly conduct impulses associated with sharp pain sensation, and small, unmyelinated C fibers which slowly transmit impulses associated with dull pain. (5) Type A nerve fibers are involved with acute traumatic pain and are responsible for spinal reflex withdrawal from the source of pain. Type C fibers are more involved with chronic pain states.

Acute and chronic pain differ neuroanatomically in the pain pathways involved. Pain sensation signals travel to the dorsal root zone of the spinal cord and then divide into ascending and descending branches of Lissauer's tract, the posterolateral fasciculus of the spinal cord. After synapsing with posterior horn neurons, nerve fibers cross anterior to the spinal cord's central canal in the anterior white commissure. They then proceed rostrally in the lateral spinothalamic tract, carrying information to the limbic system, several thalamic nuclei, and the hypothalamus. Fibers from the thalamus transmit information to the secondary somatic sensory area of the cerebrum, and some fibers go from the ventral posterolateral nucleus of the thalamus to the hypothalamus and to the primary somatic sensory area.

There are two basic types of pain, fast pain and slow pain. Fast pain is characterized as sharp or pricking and is associated more with acute pain with little emotional counterpart. Fast pain pathways are somatotypically organized, and the pain is typically very localized. Slow pain pathways are not so systematically organized. The pain is difficult to precisely localize or characterize and close integration with emotional factors is typical. Descending neural pathways modify

287

pain perception at various levels. Conscious perception of pain occurs when impulses reach the thalamus, and the pain can be localized and its intensity perceived when the impulses reach the parietal cortex. Memory and cortical association also play a role in modifying the reaction to pain.

Normal healthy people perceive pain at about the same threshold for pain stimuli, but the threshold may be substantially decreased by behavioral modification, analgesics, placebos, or euphoric mental states. (6) The central nervous system is capable of utilizing endogenous opiates (endorphins) to produce analgesia, which is the probable explanation for the variability in analgesic requirements in patients. Naloxone (an endorphin antagonist) can reverse placebo-induced analgesic effects or analgesia induced by acupuncture, suggesting that these techniques operate through endogenous opiates.

The psychologic state of the patient can affect pain perception and tolerance. Patients with depression, anxiety, and panic disorders can be exquisitely sensitive to pain. Schizophrenics can suffer significant trauma and yet experience little or no pain. The neurotransmitter imbalances in these clinical states and their effects on pain modification are complex and poorly understood.

Most clinicians have heard of the "gate control theory of pain" in which cells in the spinal cord synapse on pain pathway neurons to open or close a "gate" through which pain stimuli must travel to reach a higher level. These transmitting neurons reportedly alter the number of pain stimuli reaching higher levels and are modulated by other inhibitory and facilatory neurons from peripheral nerves and the brain. (7) It is hypothesized that white noise used by dentists and transcutaneous nerve stimulators work through these mechanisms to change pain threshold and perception.

Pain perception can also be affected by the psychological meaning the pain has for the patient. About 80% of civilians with gunshot wounds and major trauma request analgesics compared to one-third of soldiers with similar wounds suffered in battle. The soldiers with wounds were probably happy to be alive and leaving the battlefield, whereas there is no perceived benefit from trauma or wounds in civilians. (8)

COMMON PAIN DISORDERS (9)

Headache disorders: Tension
Vascular
Psychogenic

Abdominal disorders: Irritable bowel syndrome
Peptic ulcer disease

Musculoskeletal disorders: Low back pain
Arthritis

Psychiatric disorders: Depression
Hypochondriasis
Anxiety, panic disorders
Conversion symptoms
Compensation neurosis
Malingering
Delusions

Ischemic disorders: Angina pectoris
Peripheral vascular disease

Neoplastic disorders

Neurologic disorders: Post-traumatic neuritis
Neuromas
Coccydynia
Scar pain
Neuralgia

Others: Temporomandibular joint syndrome
Gout
Chronic pancreatitis

Diagnosis

The clinical assessment of chronic pain should focus on the following key items:

1. The precise location and referral, if any, of the pain.

2. The quality and severity.

3. The duration and course of the pain.

4. Fluctuating quality of the pain.

5. Intensity and variation of the pain.

6. Precipitating, alleviating, or aggravating factors.

7. Associated signs and symptoms.

The diagnostic approach and treatment of acute pain syndromes are usually straightforward, but patients with chronic pain present a different challenge to the clinician. Chronic pain patients tend to be complex and difficult to diagnose. The clinician becomes frustrated

289

when unable to make a specific diagnosis and treatment interventions fail to help. It is understandable why clinicians develop an aversive response to many chronic pain patients. The clinician is often tempted to "turf" the patient to other specialists or refer to the patient as a "crock." The physician may conclude that the patient's pain must be psychogenic and tell the patient "it's all in your head, and you need to see a psychiatrist." However, with appropriate strategies, many of these patients can be managed successfully enough to enable them to return to normal function and cease being a "pain in the physician's neck."

Many patients presenting with pain have no identifiable organic cause for their pain. (10) Some seek medical evaluation so early in their illness that the problem cannot be diagnosed, but they are motivated to seek a physician because they are obsessed about physical disability, deformity, cancer, or death. Chronic pain patients frequently suffer from hypochondriasis, anxiety, depression, or another psychiatric disorder which increases their preoccupation and decreases their tolerance for pain. (11)

In patients without serious psychiatric illness, and those with less severe pain and disability of relatively short duration, reassurance and education may resolve the pain syndrome. Follow-up care is important, and physician availability should be emphasized for worsening of symptoms.

Pain and its severity and chronicity may be influenced by sociocultural factors. Some cultures, social groups, religions, and families value pain and suffering differently. Some cultures are noted for their stoicism, and others have a low threshold with exaggerated responses to pain. For most patients with chronic pain, there is a reason the patient has adopted the identified symptoms. Chronic pain is frequently associated with secondary gain, but the gain comes in differing forms and is sometimes unusual. The patient may get attention from the family, while some families may avoid the patient altogether. The pain or illness may serve an individual or social purpose, to prevent divorce or to keep from working. Some expect compensation for their pain and disability.

Chronic pain or illness may be welcomed by some individuals. The pain and illness may provide them with justification and rationalization for personal failures or decisions with bad outcomes.

Chronic pain patients often abuse alcohol, over-the-counter medications, prescribed medications, and illicit drugs. The patient is usually reluctant to reveal these abuses, providing a challenge to the physician who needs to seek such behavior in the evaluation of chronic pain.

It is most important to carefully consider organic etiologies such as migraine headaches, arthritis, or intervertebral disc disease. However, one must be prudent with diagnostic testing, utilizing tests critically to prevent unnecessary expense, iatrogenic disease, unrealistic expectations, and misdiagnoses. Even in those patients with organic causes for pain, the therapy is often not specific but empiric.

Psychiatric Disorders	A careful psychiatric examination is important in the evaluation of chronic pain patients. If a patient is not responding well to management, a psychiatric consultation should be obtained, not with the goal of convincing the patient that the pain is psychologic, but to identify important and often treatable psychiatric disorders.

Depression. Chronic pain frequently causes depression, and depression increases the risk of developing chronic pain. (12) In some patients, the chronic pain may be the major manifestation of the depression with few psychologic or somatic symptoms. In others, the pain is associated with the classical symptoms of depression. The symptoms of depression are often atypical in the elderly, and chronic pain should alert the physician to the possibility of depression.

If depression is associated with chronic pain, the depression should be treated aggressively. We recommend treatment with imipramine titrated to 150 mg/day or another tricyclic antidepressant for at least 4–6 weeks. Physicians are often reluctant to increase the antidepressant dosage to an effective level in old women or in debilitated patients. If the patient has no side effects at a particular dose and has not improved sufficiently, a serum drug level can be measured to determine compliance and to decide about increasing the dose to achieve more therapeutic levels. Many chronic pain patients can be treated empirically with tricyclic agents even when the manifestations of depression are debatable. Tricyclic antidepressants are quite safe in most patients, and the dysfunction of the pain and depression are much greater than the risks of the medication. The major side effects are dry mouth, constipation, difficulty emptying the bladder, increased heart rate, and orthostatic hypotension.

Depressed patients who have delusions associated with the chronic pain, such as bizarre thoughts about organ decay or bizarre explanations for the cause of the pain, require psychiatric care as part of their management.

Munchausen Syndrome. Munchausen syndrome should be considered in patients with chronic pain syndromes, especially if the patient has had extraordinary diagnostic or exploratory procedures or traveled to famous doctors or medical centers in search of a diagnosis. Most have a phobia about psychiatrists and will become agitated and angry if psychiatric consultation is proposed. On the other hand, most chronic pain patients will consider psychiatric evaluation if the physician does not imply that the patient is crazy, or the pain is imaginary, or attempt to transfer responsibility to the psychiatrist. Munchausen syndrome is an important diagnosis to make since serious disability and even mortality can occur because of over testing and over treatment.

Grieving. Grieving may result in the development of pain symptoms. The pain may be perceived in the anatomic area involved in the cause of death in a loved one, such as abdominal pain in gastrointestinal cancer. These patients deserve attention because patients with broken hearts are at increased risk of morbidity and mortality during the acute grieving period. (13)

291

Narcissism. Borderline and narcissistic personalities are predisposed to develop chronic pain. The patients often describe feeling empty, hollow, and chronically bored. They prefer to feel pain or to inflict pain on themselves to demonstrate to themselves that they are people, alive with feelings. (9) The narcissistic patient is so involved with appearance and functional perfection that minimal pain will motivate the patient to seek a physician.

Alexithymia. Alexithymia is the inability to verbalize and discuss emotional states. About one-third of chronic pain patients have alexithymia. It is more common in older patients and probably explains older patients who use somatic complaints to express emotional distress. (14) Hypochondriacs frequently have alexithymic features. When the patient has clear cut psychosocial stresses sufficient to result in emotional reactions and illness, but does not recognize the obvious relationship with his or her somatic manifestations, it is probable that the patient does not percieve and correctly interpret emotional factors and stress in life. Since these patients have little ability to express emotions verbally, they are not ordinarily good candidates for psychotherapy. (3,15)

Somatoform Disorders. In hypochondriasis emotional distress is expressed in the form of a somatic complaint. These patients tend to be anxious and frightened that they have a serious illness, and the chief complaint is often a fear of multiple illnesses. Patients with somatization disorder have similar physical complaints, but not the fear and desperation of the hypochondriac. Both groups of patients with pain as their major symptom are sometimes referred to as ''pain prone.'' The need for pain is due to an underlying psychodynamic reason. A variant group is characterized by sadomasochistic behavior, behavior which produces pleasure by suffering.

Management

A careful history, examination, and appropriate laboratory tests demonstrate that the physician takes the complaints seriously with recognition of their importance. In the absence of organic disease, it is still important to maintain close follow-up. Many patients will not respond to simple reassurance—patients should not be told or given the impression that there is nothing wrong. Quite the contrary, the patient needs to perceive that the physician believes the pain is real even if there is uncertainty regarding the cause. Optimism should be demonstrated that treatment will be provided and pain can be managed, but it is best not to imply that the pain can be eradicated. It is important to discuss the interaction between chronic pain and depression and how each affects the other. This allows the introduction of emotions as a contributor to pain without saying the pain is psychologic in origin.

It is definitely counterproductive to struggle with patients, trying to convince them they are not sick. The pain is a symptom of a need, a way of expressing emotional distress. Confrontation should be avoided in preference for a caring and supporting role. This should help to prevent doctor shopping, multiple testing, multiple referrals, and the risks of medication abuse. Be slow to introduce therapy if the patient is involved in litigation, divorce, or a disability claim.

The management plan should include rewards for being more functional, taking less medication, complaining less rather than acting ill and unable to function. Positive feedback from the family and physician should be provided for healthy behavior and minimal feedback for complaints of illness or pain. The physician must recognize his or her power and importance as a therapeutic modality, which may be more important than technology or pharmacology. The doctor-patient relationship becomes a major force in managing the patient with chronic pain. With some older women, the physician is their only resource. Rather than ask, "Can I talk with you for 30 minutes every 4 weeks, I'm lonely," patients present with chronic pain hoping the physician will recognize their emotional needs. On the other hand, with chronic pain patients, it is important to set limits on time, drug use, and other aspects of care through either a verbal or written contract.

The clinician must be sensitive to what is not being said as much as to what is being said. Be attentive to nonverbal clues of emotional reactions. The ideal relationship involves free communication between patient and physician. When things are not going well, the physician must assess the relationship to diagnose what is wrong and effectively manage the interaction.

Analgesics

Most experts recommend classifying pain as "malignant" (due to cancer or other serious organic pathology) or "benign" prior to choosing pharmacologic treatment. (5,16) Patients with malignant pain should be treated aggressively with narcotic analgesics, nerve blocks, and neuroablative procedures to control pain. Physicians are often reluctant to prescribe adequate doses of narcotics. In cases of malignant pain, one should not worry extensively about addiction or withdrawal, and worry more about whether the pain has been relieved.

USEFUL GUIDELINES FOR THE USE OF NARCOTICS

1. Know the pharmacology of the drug.

2. Choose the route of administration to meet the patient's needs.

3. Administer on a regular schedule.

4. Use combinations to reduce side effects.

5. Avoid combinations that increase sedation.

6. Anticipate side effects (sedation, respiratory depression, nausea and vomiting, constipation).

7. Watch for development of tolerance.

8. Prevent acute withdrawal.

9. Anticipate complications (overdose, seizures).

Nonnarcotic Analgesics.   Aspirin is the most efficacious oral analgesic and should be considered the "gold standard" of nonnarcotic analgesics. Aspirin has been demonstrated to be as effective as codeine in relieving cancer pain. (9) Acetaminophen has equal efficacy with aspirin and can be easily substituted. Several nonsteroidal anti-inflammatory drugs are available as analgesics, but none is more effective than aspirin or acetaminophen.

Analgesics for Mild to Moderate Pain

	Equivalent Doses	Duration
Aspirin	650 mg	4–6 hr
Acetaminophen	650 mg	4–6 hr
Propoxyphene	65 mg	4–6 hr
Codeine	32 mg	4–6 hr
Meperidine	50 mg	4–6 hr
Pentazocine	30 mg	4–6 hr

It is preferable to prescribe analgesics at appropriate scheduled intervals rather than "prn." The latter approach requires the patient to develop the pain to get the "reward." The patient should not have to increase suffering in order to get attention or treatment.

Opiates are frequently combined with other analgesics or other medications to enhance analgesic activity, to reduce opiate dosage, or to counteract side effects. For example, combination of opiates with minor tranquilizers will potentiate the analgesic effect of the opiate, allowing a lesser dosage with less adverse effects.

"Benign" pain should generally be treated with nonnarcotic analgesics, appropriate psychotropic agents (including antidepressants and stimulants), and with psychotherapy and behavioral modification.

Cognitive-Behavioral Treatment.   Most physicians can manage the skills of cognitive-behavioral treatment. (17)

1. Reconceptualize the problem from overwhelming to manageable.

2. Convince the patients that skills necessary for responding to problems more adaptively will be included in treatment.

3. Change patients' views of themselves from passive, reactive, and helpless to active, resourceful, and competent.

4. Help patients to learn how to monitor thoughts, feelings, and behavior; and how to interrupt automatic, maladaptive patterns.

5. Teach patients how to employ and execute behavioral changes required for adaptive responses to problems.

6. Encourage patients to recognize their own efforts in sucessful control of pain.

7. Anticipate and discuss problems.

294

Identifying the problem of pain comes first, then building a commitment to adopt a new management plan with contracts; teaching self-awareness by keeping a diary of pain frequency, severity, associations, drug use, and functional disabilities; and developing an action plan. Evaluate the success in controlling (not necessarily curing) the pain, then maintain the improvement through regularly scheduled follow-up visits.

Hypochondriasis

Ill health and impairment in activities of daily living are the most important sources of stress and strain in older people. Although women are more likely to live alone and be subject to strains on life, they have larger social networks, more social contacts, and greater support. Therefore, older women are no more likely than men to demonstrate psychosomatic or emotional symptoms of distress. (18)

The clinician often has an inaccurate picture; the majority of the elderly are doing very well. Most elderly people describe themselves as being in good health and do not need help with their care. In a study from Connecticut, the combined rate of severe cognitive impairment and psychiatric disorders in the elderly was 10.8%, a rate lower than that in people under age 65.

But most of us have played sick at one time or another to escape a difficult situation, and it is not surprising that older people would use this same technique. However, it usually lasts longer and can become on-going. Clinical experience and research have argued that hypochondriasis in the elderly is significantly correlated with underlying depression. Some would argue that hypochondriasis is more a function of the underlying personality, and less a direct function of stressful life events. (20)

Symptom formation in hypochondriasis is largely unconscious. There are four standard diagnostic criteria: (21)

1. Unrealistic interpretation of physical signs or sensations as abnormal, leading to a fear or belief of having a disease.

2. Failure of medical evaluation to support any diagnosis of any physical disease to account for the signs or symptoms.

3. Impairment of functioning (social, occupational, or recreational).

4. Other specific psychiatric disorders are not present.

True hypochondriasis can lead to unnecessary procedures and surgery; but unfortunately, the failure to find anything does not solve the problem, but reinforces the hypochondriasis and makes treatment even more difficult. The most effective therapeutic approach is to identify the factors in the patient's social environment that are providing stress, and then to help the patient to deal with the stress. Examine the patient's personal relationships and seek out possible life situations that provide reasons for hypochondriasis. For example, look for threatening psychological problems, hostile or vengeful feelings toward others, or failures to meet personal or social expectations.

295

References

1. **Hackett TP,** The pain patient, evaluation and treatment, in Hackett TP, Cassem NH, editors, *Massachusetts General Hospital Handbook of General Hospital Psychiatry*, C.V. Mosby, St. Louis, 1978, p 41.

2. **Thompson TL II,** Chronic pain, in Kaplan HI, Sadock BJ, editors, *Comprehensive Textbook of Psychiatry*, Williams & Wilkins, Baltimorre, 1985, p 1212.

3. **Thompson TL II, Steele BF,** The psychological aspects of pain, in Simons RC, editor, *Understanding Human Behavior in Health and Illness*, Williams & Wilkins, Baltimore, 1985, p 60.

4. **Long DM,** The evaluation and treatment of low back pain, in Hendler NH, Long DM, Wise TN, editors, *Diagnosis and Treatment of Chronic Pain*, John Wright, Littleton, Mass., 1982, p 31.

5. **Luce JM, Thompson TL II, Getto CJ, et al,** New concepts of chronic pain and their implications, Hosp Pract 14:113, 1979.

6. **Strain JJ,** The problem in pain, in Strain JJ, editor, *Psychological Care of the Medically Ill*, Appleton-Century-Crofts, New York, 1975, p 93.

7. **Melzack R,** *The Puzzle of Pain*, Basic Books, New York, 1973.

8. **Beecher HK,** Relationship of significance of wound to pain experience, JAMA 161:1609, 1956.

9. **Thompson TL II, Byyny RL,** Pain problems in primary care medical practice, in Tollison DC, editor, *Handbook of Chronic Pain Managment*, Williams & Wilkins, Baltimore, 1989, pp 532–549.

10. **Devine R, Merskey H,** The description of the pain in psychiatric and general medical patients, J Psychosom Res 9:311, 1965.

11. **Rhine MW, Thompson TL II,** Hypochondriasis, in Simons RC, editor, *Understanding Human Behavior in Health and Illness*, Williams & Wilkins, Baltimore, 1985. p 73.

12. **Mersky H, Boyd D,** Emotional adjustment and chronic pain, Pain 5:173, 1978.

13. **Parkes CM, Benjamin B, Fitzgerald RG,** Broken heart: A statistical study of increased mortality among widowers, Br Med J 1:740, 1969.

14. **Postone N,** Alexithymia in chronic pain patients, Gen Hosp Psychiatry 8:163, 1986.

15. **Lipsitt DR,** Medical and psychological characteristics of "crocks," Int J Psychiatr Med 1:15, 1970.

16. **Reuler JB, Girard DE, Nardone DA,** The chronic pain syndrome, misconceptons and management, Ann Intern Med 93:588, 1980.

17. **Turk DC, Rudy TE,** A cognitive-behavioral perspective on chronic pain: Beyond the scalpel and syringe, in Tollison DC, editor, *Handbook of Chronic Pain Managment*, Williams & Wilkins, Baltimore, 1989, pp 222–236.

18. **Arling F,** Strain, social support, and distress in old age, J Gerontol 42:107, 1987.

19. **Weissman MM, Myers JK, Tischler GL, Holzer CE III, Leaf PJ, Orvaschel H, Brody JA,** Psychiatric disorders (DSM-III) and cognitive impairment among the elderly in a U.S. urban community, Acta Psychiatr Scand 71:366, 1985.

20. **Brink TL, Janakes C, Martinez N,** Geriatric hypochondriasis: Situational factors, J Am Geriatrics Soc 29:37, 1981.

21. **Busse EW,** Hypochondriasis in the elderly, AFP 25:199, 1982.

20

Depression and Dementia

Depression is as treatable or more treatable than many medical conditions. Prognosis in most cases is excellent. Older women often avoid a psychiatrist and attribute somatic complaints to an organic illness, resulting in the seeking of care from a family physician, internist, or gynecologist. Physicians interacting with older women need to be skilled in the recognition, diagnosis, and treatment of common psychiatric problems in this group of patients, but more than that, physicians need to be sensitive to the everyday emotional needs of older women.

Life Adjustments

As people get older, they master tasks less easily, occasionally giving the erroneous impression that there is a medical impairment or psychological problem. Perceptual problems, especially impairment of eyesight and hearing, can lead to confusion, and even result in paranoia in older women. Elderly women frequently fear losing control and becoming dependent upon others. Learning to accept appropriate assistance from others without losing self pride represents a major developmental task for older people. A major consideration is the financial situation of our patients. Many older people have difficulty affording adequate housing and food, let alone other items which we now regard as necessities, like eyeglasses, hearing aids, telephones, and even television.

In the U.S., older women frequently find themselves geographically separated from their families. Nevertheless families continue to provide most of the support for older people, and consultation with family members regarding medical decisions and plans is always important.

In helping older women, physicians should recognize their need for human closeness, warmth, sexuality, independence, social support, and respect. These are almost universal, and deserve the interest and attention of physicians.

Psychiatric disorders become more prevalent with each decade of life. (1) Approximately 15% of the elderly need treatment for some type of mental disorder. Approximately 14% of people over age 65 have a significant functional disorder such as hypochondriasis, reactive depression, paranoia, or neurosis. As much as 5% of those over 65 and 25% of those over age 80 have a severe dementia.

However, as these figures indicate, most older people are very contented with their lives, and tolerate losses relatively well, because they are expected.

Depression

Depression is common (about 10% incidence) and often very serious in older women. (2) Only 1–2% have a major depression, and about 2% have dysthymic or neurotic depression. Indeed, major depression is less prevalent among older individuals than in younger people. (3) However, depression accounts for 25% of suicides. (4) Risk factors for suicide include physical illness, divorce, living alone, social isolation, bereavement, use of alcohol, and dementia. Poor nutrition and noncompliance with medication may be a form of passive suicide and motivation must be considered when these situations are encountered. If a patient is suicidal, an appointment with a physician may be made with the hope that the physician will discover their suicidal thoughts. Obviously, many patients cannot offer these depressed thoughts spontaneously. Older patients should be routinely asked about depression, and whether life is worth living. The features in the following table are useful for the clinician to differentiate between depression and dementia.

Differential Diagnosis of Depression and Dementia (5)

	Depression	Dementia
Initial presentation:	Complaints of memory loss and other deficits	Denial and concealment of deficits
Recent memory:	Normal, although concentration may be necessary	Impaired with intact remote memory
Intellect:	Normal, although patient may have to be motivated	Deterioration in higher, abstract thinking
Judgment:	Poor judgment, can't do things right	Bad decisions because of focus on irrelevant
Diurnal variation:	Worse in morning	Worse in evening and night
Affect:	Sad, hopeless, helpless	Labile and inappropriate
Out of touch with life:	Not present	Present
Delusions, psychotic symptoms:	Delusions of death common	Varied in content
Response:	Better with antidepressants, worse with tranquilizers	Better with low doses of major tranquilizers, worse with minor tranquilizers, antidepressants

Older people suffering from depression often have predominantly somatic and vegetative symptoms, such as loss of appetite, loss of weight, decreased energy, decreased motivation, and sleep disturbance. They are usually not guilt-ridden and self-accusatory as is the case with younger depressed people. A slowing of perceptual or psychomotor functioning may be falsely attributed to "senility" when an underlying depression is actually the responsible factor. Depression may be responsible for cognitive dysfunction and memory complaints, and this can present in a state labeled as pseudodementia (a depression that presents as cognitive impairment). However, pseudodementia is rare in older life.

There is a physiologic basis for the greater susceptibility to depression among older people. For example, changes occur with aging in neurotransmitter concentrations. Monoamine oxidase levels increase and norepinephrine levels steadily decrease with age. Laboratory assessment is indicated to rule out other illnesses, anemia, and hypothyroidism.

Many medications commonly produce depression. As many as 15% of patients taking reserpine for hypertension will develop dose-related depression. Propranolol and methyldopa are associated with depression in 20% of patients. Depression may be associated with organic dementia (Alzheimer's disease), and treatment of the depression improves mood and function but the cognitive dysfunction persists.

There are more and more reasons for reactive depression as we get older. Losses of loved ones and losses of functional abilities accumulate with age. Grief reactions due to the inevitable death of spouses, friends, colleagues, and sometimes children may be almost continuous in the elderly. The grief process is not always benign and self-limited. The clinician's responsibility is to be attentive to the higher likelihood that older patients will be depressed and their manifestations of depression may be different than in younger people. Recognition should lead to treatment.

Treatment of Depression. A physician should constantly demonstrate respect for older patients. The laying on of hands in response to physical complaints provides a sense of physical closeness and contact. Sitting near the patient or placing a hand on the shoulder, or holding a hand, especially if the patient is frightened, is reassuring. The secret in caring for patients is in "caring" for the patient.

The best therapy for a patient who is grieving over a loss is to discuss the loss, with an effort to uncover any previous hidden emotions such as anger at a spouse for dying and leaving the patient alone, or guilt. A grieving process also occurs for physical and mental functions which have been lost. These too need to be discussed at length, on repetitive occasions, in order to resolve the grief.

A physician should be supportive with a focus on helping the patient enjoy the here and now. It is a common mistake to attempt to cure all of the patient's complaints. It is often more important to help a patient adjust to problems. A sympathetic ear and reassurance that a condition is not life threatening are frequently the best therapy. One should be careful to remove any reversible causes (especially drugs, both prescriptive and over the counter). Self-help books can be recommended. Especially good are: *Control Your Depression*, by Lewinsohn et al, *The Self-Talk Solution*, by Helmstetter, and *Feeling Good*, by Burns. (6–8)

Melancholic depression usually responds to antidepressant medication and is characterized by the following:

—Decreased interest in activities and former pleasures.
—Lack of reaction to pleasurable stimuli.
—Early morning awakening.
—Diurnal mood variation (worse in morning).
—Weight loss.

Antidepressive Medication. Tricyclic or tetracyclic antidepressants are especially useful in managing depression in older patients. (9) These drugs have a very long half-life in the elderly, and therefore, 3–5 weeks are usually required for stable drug levels to be reached. A small trial dose should initially be given to test sensitivity, then the dosage should be increased slowly. A therapeutic level can be achieved with a dose of 25–75 mg per day of imipramine or doxepin, but some older patients may require larger doses.

Amitriptyline (Elavil) causes the most sedative and anticholinergic effects of any drugs in this class. It is not the drug of choice for older patients. Doxepin (Sinequan, Adapin) may also cause excessive sedation. Nortriptyline (Pamelor), imipramine (Tofranil), or desipramine (Norpramin, Pertofrane) are better choices for initial therapy. Desipramine has the fewest anticholinergic properties. Nortriptyline has the added advantage of a "therapeutic window" (about 75 mg daily) which is effective in a large majority of patients. Low doses should be prescribed initially (10–25 mg at night) and then increased by 10–25 mg per day every 3–5 days until one develops side effects. A usual maintenance dose is 25 mg bid or 50 mg qhs. The most common side effect is postural hypotension. If the drug does not lead to symptomatic improvement or if side effects persist after several weeks at a therapeutic dose, another drug should be tried. If simple counseling and the use of antidepressant drugs do not resolve the depression, the patient should be referred to a psychiatrist.

It is important to continually assess compliance. Noncompliance is a symptom of depression and dementia. Furthermore, one should be sure that the patient can repeat therapeutic instructions, otherwise someone else should take over the administration of critical medications.

Sedatives and Hypnotics. The chronic use of sedative-hypnotics should be discouraged, especially in the elderly. A change in sleep patterns may be normal. It is not necessary to medicate the elderly into the sleep patterns of a younger person. Excessive use of sedative medication can actually cause delirium or dementia, or worsen depression. The long acting sleep medications should definitely be avoided (such as Valium). If there is a need to treat a sleep or anxiety disorder, temazepam (Restoril) or oxazepam (Serax) is preferable. These drugs have a shorter half-life and do not produce as much sedation during the day. Chloral hydrate can also be used. Other benzodiazepines and barbiturates should be avoided.

Estrogen for Depression. There is no doubt that the immediate postmenopausal period is associated with a sleep disorder, probably secondary to hot flushes and adrenergic activation due to estrogen deficiency. This sleep disorder can be disruptive or subtle (although asleep, the quality of sleep is less, leaving a woman less well-rested to face the next day). Fatigue and decreased productivity can contribute to depression, and therefore, restoration of good sleep with estrogen treatment can have an impact on depression. However, there is little evidence that estrogen is directly an antidepressant. In older women, years beyond the menopause, a sleep disorder is unlikely to be related to estrogen deficiency, and an impact on depression by estrogen treatment is not to be expected.

Normal Aging of the Nervous System.   Approximately 5–10% of brain weight is lost by 80–90 years of age, although this is not universal. (10) This is probably the reason why subdural hematomas occur more frequently in the elderly, since there is more room for brain movement.

CT scanning has disclosed that there is a small but gradual increase in ventricular size through the first 6 decades of life, followed by a dramatic increase to the 8th and 9th decades. There are no good standards, however, to diagnose cerebral atrophy and to correlate brain size with function, except in extreme cases where cerebral atrophy can be determined with accuracy. Aging of the brain is a later process. At age 60, the middle cerebral artery looks like the radial artery at age 40 and the coronary artery at age 20–30.

By 80–90 years of age, approximately 45% of the neurons are lost in the superior frontal and temporal gyri and in the frontal pole and area striata. By the 9th decade, 85% of the Betz cells in each hemisphere disappear. Even those neurons which remain may not be functionally normal. There is an increased lumpiness of proximal dendrites, progressive loss of horizontal dendrites and spines, and eventual loss of the apical shafts in the frontal and superior temporal cortex, the adjacent entorhinal cortex, and the dentate nucleus. These may be the most important losses, since these areas are involved in modulating cortical activity.

The neurologic examination of the older individual commonly demonstrates irregular pupils with a sluggish light reflex for accommodation. Cogwheel tracking movements of the eyes and irregular pursuit eye movements can be detected. There is muscle wasting in the hands and feet in the absence of local joint and bone disease. Tremor is not common in a normal elderly individual; however, it occurs occasionally in the head, face, hands, and voice, but rarely in the legs. The tremor is usually intermittent and exaggerated by movement and motion. There is no known pathology associated with this tremor.

Many older individuals assume an attitude of mild general flexion and develop some rigidity and slowness of movement. This is not Parkinsonism. However, many elements of Parkinson's are present in older people. Small steps contribute to unsteadiness of gait. Reflexes diminish, and superficial reflexes disappear. The plantar response can be difficult to elicit. There is a decreased threshold for light touch and pain. Vibration sense decreases and special senses dull. Older people do less well on performance tests compared to verbal tests. Most of the difficulty with impairment of acquisition, retention, and retrieval of information falls into an area best called benign forgetfulness, quite different from dementia.

Dementia or senility is a progressive loss of intellectual capacity with gradual regression of physical and mental ability to a point of near or absolute helplessness. (11) What is due to disease and what is due to normal aging after 70 years of life has been a problem for generations of physicians.

All dementia illnesses interfere with the degree of memory and cognitive functioning. At times a person may be so depressed that this is recognized as pseudodementia. It is important to differentiate true dementia from depression. While some depression is common early in the course of progressive dementia, it usually is not severe. As dementia worsens, depression lightens as insight decreases. Patients with Alzheimer's disease rarely commit suicide. Reliance on past history, psychometric testing, a trial of antidepressant medication, and the course of the illness will all be necessary. There are physicians who believe that depression in older individuals can cause an organic dementia, which is alleviated as the depression lifts.

Alzheimer's Disease. Alzheimer's disease predominates in women. Although the disease is usually sporadic, it can be transmitted as an autosomal dominant. The risk for acquisition of the disease if present in a first degree relative has been estimated to vary from 10% to 30%. (10) The clinical features of Alzheimer's disease are as follows: (10)

1. Slow progression of memory impairment, mainly for recent memory, although later, remote memory also becomes impaired.

2. Language disturbances range from halting speech and perseveration through dysosmia, paraphasia, dysphasia, and aphasia. Patients usually retain the ability to articulate.

3. Patients have difficulty with comprehension.

4. Abstract abilities fail quite early.

5. Visual-spatial difficulties commonly involve right-left disorientation.

6. Constructional disturbance or apraxia is noted, involving fragmentation, rotation, and perseveration of diagram copying, inability to dress properly, and occasionally inability to sit properly.

7. Agitation and restlessness or hypokinesia and mild depression appear; moods may be labile.

8. Delusion and paranoia are occasionally noted.

9. Patients may harm themselves or others because of a loss of social control.

10. Late in the disease, the use of body parts, such as the limbs, may become difficult.

11. Any of the above signs and symptoms may predominate, and not all symptoms occur in single individuals.

12. Patients often manifest general good health and alertness, particularly early in the disease.

The neurological examination of an Alzheimer patient may include difficulty with eye-hand coordination, paratonia, a flexed posture in advanced cases, slowness of movement, presence of sucking and snout reflexes, and an exaggerated jaw jerk. In early cases, no neurologic abnormalities may be present except those relating to mentation. A variety of simple bedside mental status tests have been developed, investigating orientation, recent and remote memory, and arithmetic ability (forward and backward counting, serial 7's, proverb interpretation). It is useful to have the patient memorize 3 items (e.g. a street address, automobile type and year, and an object) to be repeated 5 minutes later. In addition, formal testing is used for diagnosis and for following patients.

Vascular Dementia. Vascular dementia, usually referred to as multi-infarct dementia, accounts for 20–25% of dementia. (10) This diagnosis can often be made on CT scan, whereas the Alzheimer's brain looks normal on CT scanning. The key to diagnosis, however, is the history. An abrupt event or a series of events (strokes) can often be designated, with a maximal neurologic defect at onset followed by some improvement. Focal neurologic signs are usually present in contrast to patients with Alzheimer's disease.

Other Causes of Dementia. Alcohol, drugs, and other toxins can result in dementia. Nutritional, endocrine, and metabolic abnormalities cause only 1–2% of dementia. Tumors and other space occupying lesions occasionally cause dementia, but usually have other manifestations.

Treatment of Dementia. Patients must be taught to utilize methods to substitute for lost functions. For example, the use of lists and other reminders can assist patients with memory impairments. Correctable conditions should be addressed, such as poor vision or hearing, poor nutrition, and any other medical or physical limitations. As disease progresses, the use of day hospitals and outpatient facilities is recommended for mental stimulation in the form of art and music therapy.

It is important to make as little environmental change as possible to avoid any increase in confusion. Clinicians performing surgery must be constantly alert and aware of dementia related to environmental change. This is one of the major causes for iatrogenic disease in the elderly who are hospitalized. All efforts should be made to maximize stimuli for patients both at home and in the hospital. The use of television, newspaper, and other daily information to keep the patient oriented and intact with the here and now are critical.

Drug therapy is disappointing. Hydergine is believed by some to improve alertness and decrease confusion, but the results have not been dramatic.

Conclusions

Depression and dementia are common disorders in the elderly and require prompt recognition and management, the earlier the better. Hospitalization can be a precipitating event, and this important psychosocial and neurological disorder should always be considered in the care of hospitalized patients.

References

1. **Butler RN,** The geriatric patient, in Usdin G, Lewis JM, editors, *Psychiatry in General Medical Practice*, McGraw-Hill, New York, 1979.

2. **Blazer D,** Depression in the elderly, New Engl J Med 320:164, 1989.

3. **Blazer D, Hughes DC, George LK,** The epidemiology of depression in an elderly community population, Gerontologist 27:281, 1987.

4. **Resnik HL, Cantor JM,** Suicide and aging, J Am Geriatr Soc 18:152, 1970.

5. **Thompson TL,** Psychosocial and psychiatric problems of the aged, in Schrier RW, editor, *Clinical Internal Medicine in the Aged*, W.B. Saunders Co., Philadelphia, 1982, pp 29–40.

6. **Lewinsohn PM, Munoz RF, Youngren MA, et al,** *Control Your Depression*, Prentice-Hall, Englewood Cliffs, New Jersey, 1979.

7. **Helmstetter S,** *The Self-Talk Solution*, William Morrow, New York, 1987.

8. **Burns D,** *Feeling Good: The New Mood Therapy*, William Morrow, New York, 1980.

9. **Thompson TL, Moran MG, Nies AG,** Psychotropic drug use in the elderly, New Engl J Med 308:134,194, 1983.

10. **Schneck SA,** Aging of the nervous system and dementia, in Schrier RW, editor, *Clinical Internal Medicine in the Aged*, W.B. Saunders Co., Philadelphia, 1982, pp 41–50.

11. **Cummings TL, Benson DF,** *Dementia: A Clinical Approach*, Butterworths, Boston, 1983, pp 1–14.

Index

Page numbers in *italics* denote figures; those followed by "t" denote tables.

effect on sexual functioning, 117
evaluation of, 206
signs and symptoms of, 206
vaginal pessaries for, 207–211, *208–211*
Pentazocine, 294t
Peptic ulcer, 198
  diagnosis of, 198
  prophylaxis for, 198
  signs and symptoms of, 198
  treatment of, 198
Peptococcus, 228
Periodontal disease, 26
Peripheral nervous system, effects of aging on, 23
Peripheral vascular disease, 183
  diabetes mellitus and, 252
  diagnosis of, 183
  prevalence of, 183
  treatment of, 183
Pertofrane. *See* Desipramine
Pessaries. *See* Vaginal pessaries
Phenoxybenzamine, for overflow incontinence, 220t
Phenylpropanolamine, for stress incontinence, 220t
Phobias, 53
Phospholipids, 60
Physical activity, 43–46, *44–45*
  coronary heart disease and, 43
  effect on HDL-cholesterol, 84
  hypercholesterolemia and, 73
  maintenance of function and, 52
  obesity and, 125–126, 130
  osteoporosis and, 82, 272–273
  recommendations for, 44–45
  threshold for training effect, 44
Physical examinations, recommendations for, 31–32, 38
Pneumonia, 191, 282
  causative organisms of, 191, 282
  diagnosis of, 191, 282
  immunization against, 50, 285
  signs and symptoms of, 191
  treatment of, 191
Polymyalgia rheumatica, 261
  diagnostic tests for, 261
  giant cell arteritis and, 262
  management of, 261
  pathophysiology of, 261
  signs and symptoms of, 261
Polyps, colonic, 199
Population distribution
  determinants of age structure, 6
  men vs. women, 4t-5t, 4–5, *5–6*
  postmenopausal women, 75
  U.S., 2, *2–3*
  world-wide, 4
Poverty, effect on health status, 30
PPD test, 191, 283
Prazosin, for overflow incontinence, 220t
Prednisone, for gout, 264
Pregnancy, protective effect against breast cancer, 134
Presbycusis, 24
Presbyesophagus, 196
Preventive medicine, 29–55. *See also* Health promotion
  for accidents/injuries, 50
  for alcoholism, 52
  behavioral strategies in, 54–55
  for cancer, 47–50
  for cardiovascular disease, 39–42

considerations in, 34–36
  acceptance of death, 36
  diagnosis in elderly, 35
  health care team, 36
  individualized therapy, 35
  patients at risk of losing independence, 35
  patient's preferences, 35
  physician's attitude, 34
  recognition of screening/intervention opportunities, 35, 36t
  test differences in aged, 35
  variations in therapeutic response in aged, 35
  for diabetes mellitus, 51
  encouraging physical activity, 43–46, *44–45*
  general principles of, 32–33
  for hypothyroidism, 51
  for iatrogenic disease, 51
  for infectious disease, 29
  levels of, 33
  for obesity, 46–47
  recommendations for, 36–37
  screening measures for, 33–34
  for women ages 40–59, 53
  for women ages 60–74, 31–32
  for women ages 75t, 32
Prinzmetal's angina, 176
Pro-Banthine. *See* Propantheline
Probenecid, for gout, 263
Progesterone ointment, for vulvar white lesions, 234
Progesterone receptor assay, 144
Progestins, for dysfunctional uterine bleeding, 89
Propantheline, for urge incontinence, 218, 220t
Propoxyphene, 294t
Propranolol
  for hypertension, 169t
  for hyperthyroidism, 241
Prostate surgery, sexuality and, 115
Protriptyline, for sleep apnea, 193
Pseudodementia, 300, 303
Pseudogout, 264
Pseudohypertension, 162
Psychiatric disorders. *See also* specific disorders
  alexithymia, 292
  chronic pain and, 291–292
  dementia, 303–305
  depression, 291, 300–302
  hypochondriasis, 295
  life adjustments and, 299
  Munchausen syndrome, 291
  narcissism, 292
  prevalence of, 299
  somatoform disorders, 292
Pulmonary problems, 188–193. *See also* specific disorders
  bronchial asthma, 190–191
  chronic bronchitis, 188–189
  chronic obstructive pulmonary disease, 189–190
  clinical manifestations of, 188
  interstitial lung diseases, 192
  lung cancer, 192
  pneumonia, 191
  sleep apnea, 192–193
  tuberculosis, 191
Pulmonary system, aging of, 25–26, 187–188

Q-Tip test, *214,* 215

Ranitidine
  for peptic ulcer, 198

316

This volume may circulate for 2 weeks.

Renewals may be made in person or by phone: X6-6050; from outside dial 746-6050. No VMX renewals please. Fines are charged for overdue items. Please renew promptly. Thank you.

Date Due	Date Returned
MAR. 20 1991	
MAY 1 1991	MAY 9 1991
NOV 04 1999	

Preventive Screening For Well Women

AGE	40	41	42	43	44	45	46	47	48	49	50	51	52
Interval history and physical examination:	✓	✓	✓	✓	✓	✓	✓	✓	✓	✓	✓	✓	✓
Smoking	At every visit												
Alcohol and drug use	At every visit												
Weight and height	At every visit												
Blood pressure	At every visit												
Breast examination	✓	✓	✓	✓	✓	✓	✓	✓	✓	✓	✓	✓	✓
Pelvic examination	✓	✓	✓	✓	✓	✓	✓	✓	✓	✓	✓	✓	✓
Rectal examination/ occult blood	✓	✓	✓	✓	✓	✓	✓	✓	✓	✓	✓	✓	✓
Pap smear	✓	✓	✓	✓	✓	✓	✓	✓	✓	✓	✓	✓	✓
Hearing assessment	✓										✓		
Visual assessment	✓										✓		
Immunizations:													
Tetanus-diphtheria booster	✓										✓		
Influenza immunization													
Pneumovax													
Laboratory work:													
Total cholesterol	✓					✓					✓		
STD screen	High risk only												
Tuberculosis screen	High risk only												
Hematocrit or hemoglobin	✓										✓		
Thyroid assessment (TSH)						✓							
Special items:													
Proctosigmoidoscopy											✓		
Mammography Baseline at 35	✓		✓		✓		✓		✓		✓	✓	✓
Regular counseling:	Nutrition, smoking, exercise, breast and skin self examinations,												

Based on references 4–11, Chapter 3.